# South Asian Perspectives in Mental Health and Psychology

**Series Editors**

S. M. Yasir Arafat, Bangladesh Specialized Hospital, Dhaka, Bangladesh

Sujita Kumar Kar, Department of Psychiatry, King George's Medical University, Lucknow, Uttar Pradesh, India

This series of books is an endeavor to gather and present a comprehensive understanding of the various aspects of mental health that are relevant to people living in South Asia. The books aim to provide in-depth guidance and practical solutions to the mental health challenges that are unique to these areas. The content covers a wide range of topics, including but not limited to, climate change and its impact, prison mental health, perinatal mental health, social psychiatry, mental health and disorder among the elderly population, psychiatry education and training, suicide, SDGs and mental health, trauma, addiction, and social isolation. The books also emphasize the importance of early intervention and provide resources for seeking help. The ultimate goal of this series is to empower individuals and communities to take proactive steps toward enhancing their mental wellbeing. The proposed books will fill the existing unmet need in the region with huge populations in low and middle-income country (LMIC) settings.

South Asia, home to about 2 billion people, is a region of diverse cultures, languages, and religions. It caters to about 25% of the global population. This densely populated region faces a myriad of challenges, both natural and man-made. The frequent occurrence of natural disasters, such as earthquakes, floods, and landslides, threaten the lives and livelihoods of millions of people. War, terrorism, and political instability have caused significant disruptions to the region's socio-political fabric. Poverty, migration, and tropical infectious diseases remain major challenges that hinder progress towards sustainable development. Climate change exacerbates these challenges, causing widespread environmental degradation, food insecurity, and water scarcity. Despite these obstacles, South Asian people have shown remarkable resilience and strength in the face of adversity.

Mental health issues in the South Asian region significantly contribute to the global burden of mental illnesses. However, the region faces plenty of challenges such as high stigma, low mental health literacy, poor budgetary allocation, high out-of-pocket expense for mental health services, lack of adequate infrastructure, and limited human resources are significant barriers in mental healthcare. The majority of research on mental health issues is produced by the western countries which may not fit all in the South Asian culture, albeit evidence is needed to test. There is a paucity of research and evidence-based strategies that are region-specific. This series of books is an attempt to compile the important dimensions of mental health that will benefit the regional people.

S. M. Yasir Arafat · Amit Singh · Sujita Kumar Kar
Editors

# Social Psychiatry in South Asia

Springer

*Editors*
S. M. Yasir Arafat
Bangladesh Specialized Hospital
Dhaka, Bangladesh

Amit Singh
Department of Psychiatry
King George's Medical University
Lucknow, Uttar Pradesh, India

Sujita Kumar Kar
Department of Psychiatry
King George's Medical University
Lucknow, Uttar Pradesh, India

ISSN 3059-3646 ISSN 3059-3522 (electronic)
South Asian Perspectives in Mental Health and Psychology
ISBN 978-981-96-8077-1 ISBN 978-981-96-8078-8 (eBook)
https://doi.org/10.1007/978-981-96-8078-8



This Springer imprint is published by the registered company Springer Nature Singapore Pte Ltd.
The registered company address is: 152 Beach Road, #21-01/04 Gateway East, Singapore 189721, Singapore

*N N Wig*

# Foreword by Dinesh Bhugra, CBE

For a considerable period, there has been a clear recognition and an acknowledgement that psychiatric disorders are influenced by underlying bio-psychosocial models which help in our understanding of both aetiology and therapeutic interventions in order to manage these illnesses. In many parts of the world in the past few decades there has been an increasing awareness of the role social determinants play in the health of population, communities and individuals. Understanding such core factors in aetiology of psychiatric disorders and how these can influence individual, community, national and international levels but are also in turn influenced at these levels, can be incredibly helpful not only in public health but also interventions at individual levels as well as helping develop and deliver policy objectives. With advances in technical investigations in the past thirty years or so, increased attention is being paid to the role these investigations play in our understanding of psychiatric disorders at various levels.

The role of social determinants in having a major impact on causation of various psychiatric disorders cannot be underestimated. On the other hand, recent interest in supra-national factors such as conflicts, wars, disasters, climate change, famines, pandemics which have been identified as influencing social determinants directly and indirectly means that we need to look at aetiological and therapeutic factors in different ways. These causes can lead to internal and cross-border migration which brings certain challenges with it. In addition, commercial, cultural, economic, geographical and political factors appear to have a major impact on causation and perpetuation of various mental illnesses both through impacting upon physical health but also direct and indirect effect on mental health and wellbeing. For example, research has shown that social factors such as attachment patterns in childhood affect brain development and structures which in turn influence brain functioning thereby modulating a child's development and into young age and adulthood and thus make them prone to psychiatric disorders. It is clear from both clinical practice and research that social factors are clearly important facets in aetiology, patient engagement and clinical outcomes which are very often ignored. Social factors are also likely to be affected by cultural expectations and similar factors. Cultures influence expectations people have of medication along with ethnic differences in pharmacokinetic and pharmacodynamics are not taken into account in research or clinical practice. Recent suggestions that we need to move to a socio-bio-psycho-cultural-spiritual with more emphasis on social factors deserve serious attention by clinicians, researchers and policymakers. Another complicating factor has been inexorable rise of global health and global mental health which has often been accused of Western imperialism in telling low- and middle-income countries what to do and how to do it. It is important to recognize cultural relativism which can play a major role in understanding social causation of mental illnesses.

It is refreshing to see this volume bringing together perspectives in clinical experience and research findings from Southeast Asia which houses a significant proportion of world's populations across different cultures and settings. Another striking finding from this part of the world is that many of these cultures are in transition moving from agrarian to industrial societies which makes research fascinating. Furthermore, wealth disparity, rapid urbanization and industrialization are significant factors which highlight urgent need for recognition of these ongoing changes and their potential impact on population, community and individual levels.

In this volume, editors have brought together an impressive array of clinical academics and others to share their ideas and experiences. It is to their credit that they are sharing these so that the academic world can learn from some innovative ideas. Congratulations to the contributors for their significant input.

Dinesh Bhugra, CBE
MA, M.Sc., M.B.B.S, D.Sc.(Hon), Ph.D., F.R.C.P, FRCPE, FRCPsych, FFPHM, F.R.C.Psych(Hon), F.H.K.C.Psych(Hon), FACPsych(Hon), FAMS(Singapore), FKCL, M.Phil., LMSSA, FAcadME, FRSA, DIFAPA
Professor Emeritus, Mental Health & Cultural Diversity, IoPPN
Kings College, London, UK
President, Royal College of Psychiatrists (2008–2011)
President, World Psychiatric Association (2014–2017)
President, British Medical Association (2018–2019)
Editor, International Journal of Social Psychiatry (2000–2024)

# Foreword by Afzal Javed

I am pleased that Dr. S. M. Yasir Arafat and his colleagues have edited this important book on Social Psychiatry in South Asia.

Developments in psychiatry and mental health are gaining more visibility across the globe as rapid changes in policies are shaping the services and practices in most countries. South Asia, home to about 2 billion people, is a region of diverse cultures, languages and religions. Developments in mental healthcare and delivery in South Asian Region are of greater significance and like many other fields in psychiatry; social psychiatry is also assuming a major importance at different levels of care. Social psychiatry is a discipline that focuses on the social dimension of mental health, mental illness and mental healthcare. As relevant social and cultural factors play an important role in the future developments, understanding and acknowledgement of psycho-social perspectives of mental illnesses, these areas are getting a paramount importance in understanding different dimensions of mental healthcare.

This book provides a comprehensive account of several aspects and developments from various South Asian countries that could determine the future directions for South Asian mental health services. The chapters provide an overview of the important dimensions of mental health and help in understanding and meeting the challenges that require a social psychiatry perspective, both in research and in the delivery of care. The book, indeed, adds a notable value to the current literature on this topic and will be helpful to mental health professionals for their future practices.

Altogether, this book gives an excellent overview of the topic. Different chapters are highly relevant to the changing regional landscape and policies in social psychiatry and can be useful for its relevance to other parts of the world as well.

Dr. S. M. Yasir Arafat and other editorial members are well acclaimed and much-admired psychiatrists in this region. They need appreciation for editing this book and including accounts from different countries from the region for documenting current trends in social psychiatry in this region. I hope that this book will have a significant impact on regional as well as global psychiatry.

Dr. Afzal Javed *Sitara-i-Imtiaz (Pakistan)*
M.B.B.S; M.C.P.S; D.Psych. (Lond.); Board Cert.Psych. (U.K); M.Phil. (Edin.); F.R.C.Psych. (UK); F.R.C.P (Ireland & Edinburgh), FCPS(Hon) Pakistan
Consultant Psychiatrist
Immediate Past President World Psychiatric Association
Chairman Pakistan Psychiatric Research Centre, Fountain House, Lahore, Pakistan

# Preface

The bio-psychosocial approach has been well accepted and considered while formulating the risk factors and treatment strategy for mental disorders. It indicates the importance of social structure and social influence on mental health, psychiatric disorders, their treatment and rehabilitation. The social determinants of mental health including social networks, culture, norms, socio-economic conditions and healthcare systems in South Asia vary remarkably from the West. Also, societal changes under Western influence are noticeable in several sections leading to a change in the style people cope with adversities. Besides, the political and economic instability in these countries poses additional challenges to mental health. The impact of social structure in South Asia on psychiatric disorders and vice-versa have not been adequately addressed yet. Also, there are various new, state-run, social initiatives to advance mental health and manage mental illnesses in the region. We did not find any book focusing on the impact of social dimensions on the mental health of people living in the eight South Asian countries with about 2 billion populations. Therefore, we focused on the social dimensions and determinants of mental health in South Asia based on the available literature and expertise.

It has been started by overviewing the current status of social psychiatry, cultural expression of mental illness, the challenges of mental health in South Asia. Then we included country-wise chapters. For each country, there is an introduction emphasizing the historical development of the country, social structure, cultural norms, stigma towards mental health, heath-seeking behavior, community attitude towards mental health, disorders and treatment, alcoholism, and substance abuse, culture-bound syndromes, political and human rights conditions, mental health challenges for disorders of western cultures like eating disorders, gender identity issues, the role of the family as a risk factor and in treatment of mental illness, social security, mental health insurance, poverty, and mental health, income inequity and mental health services, gender, masculinity and mental health, local religion, and mental health, social media, social capital, homelessness, somatization, social prescribing, cross-religion heal seeking to faith healers, impact of migration and displacement on mental health, role of traditional healing practices and their integration with modern psychiatric care, challenges and opportunities in implementing community-based mental health interventions, the impact of rapid urbanization on mental health, mental health needs of specific vulnerable populations, such as women, children, and the elderly, mental health, disasters, trauma and resilience, available research and gaps. Then we included chapters discussing the social determinants of mental health, social interventions for mental illness in South Asian society, the traditional approach to mental health treatments in South Asia. We dedicated a chapter on culture-bound syndromes prevailing in the region considering its impact of shaping psychopathology and help-seeking for mental illness. We highlighted how marriage affect psychiatric care and differences of psychopathology based on marital status, religion and its effect on mental health and treatment of mental disorder, violence and mental health in the South Asian region and the role and status regional conflict on mental illness in South Asian countries.

It is the first of its kind to discuss social aspects of mental health in South Asia examining the social attribution of mental disorders in the region. It identifies research gaps and gives recommendations for culturally appropriate interventions for mental disorders in South Asia. It will be helpful for academics, researchers, NGO personnel and other stakeholders working with social and transcultural psychiatry. It will also be a valuable asset for postgraduate students, and doctoral and postdoctoral researchers in transcultural psychiatry, and global mental health.

We thank Springer for considering the book, *Social Psychiatry in South Asia,* as well as the series *South Asian Perspectives in Mental Health and Psychology* focusing the mental health priorities in South Asia. We hope the book and book series will contribute to a better mental health for people living in the region and will be considered as a benchmark effort with the possibilities of further advancement.

Dhaka, Bangladesh — S. M. Yasir Arafat
Lucknow, Uttar Pradesh, India — Amit Singh
Lucknow, Uttar Pradesh, India — Sujita Kumar Kar

# Contents

# About the Editors

**Dr. S. M. Yasir Arafat** is currently working as Associate Consultant of Psychiatry at Bangladesh Specialized Hospital, Dhaka, Bangladesh. He is affiliated with Frontier University Garowe, Somalia as an Associate Professor, Dnet as Honorary Research Fellow and with the Biomedical Research Foundation, Bangladesh as Senior Research Fellow. He is an Associate Fellow of the Bangladesh Academy of Science. He was affiliated with the University of Bristol, UK as Visiting Senior Research Associate, (August 2021–2023). He completed an MD in Psychiatry, MPH in Health Economics, MBA in Marketing and MBBS. Dr. Arafat has (co)authored more than 400 peer-reviewed articles and book chapters, and (co)edited more than ten books with Springer. He has been included in the global 2% researcher list in 2021, 2022 and 2023. He is acting as an editorial member in more than 10 leading journals in mental health published by Elsevier, Wiley, Springer, Taylor and Francis. His research focused on mental health, suicidal behavior, psychometrics, panic buying and psycho-sexual disorders.

**Dr. Amit Singh** is currently working as Assistant Professor of Psychiatry at King George's Medical University, Lucknow, Uttar Pradesh, India. He is the deputy editor of the Indian Journal of Social Psychiatry. He is MD in Psychiatry and has specialization (DM) in Addiction Psychiatry. He has (co)authored more than 30 peer-reviewed articles and book chapters. His research interests include addiction and cultural psychiatry.

**Dr. Sujita Kumar Kar** is currently working as Additional Professor of Psychiatry at King George's Medical University, Lucknow, Uttar Pradesh, India. He is the editor-in-chief of *Indian Journal of Health, Sexuality and Culture*. He is also the editorial board member and reviewer of various national and international journals. He had written 74 book chapters and more than 500 articles in various national and international journals and made 70 presentations at various national and international conferences. He has been included in the global 2% researcher list released by Stanford University in 2021, 2022, 2023 and 2024. His research interests include brain stimulation, neuropsychiatry and suicide prevention.

# List of Figures

# List of Tables

**Chapter 10**



**Chapter 13**



**Chapter 14**

# Chapter 1
# Social Psychiatry in South Asia: An Overview

**Amit Singh and Sujita Kumar Kar**

**Abstract** South Asia bears a substantial mental health burden, partly attributable to its large population. The unique socio-cultural fabric of this region, characterized by diverse traditions, cultural beliefs and religions, and strong family systems, plays a crucial role in shaping mental health outcomes. Widespread poverty, unemployment, gender inequality, rapid urbanization, climate change, environmental disasters, political instability, and the social stigma surrounding mental disorders exacerbate the mental health challenges. Additionally, limited access to mental health services, a shortage of trained professionals, and deeply ingrained cultural beliefs often hinder the delivery of effective interventions. Understanding these unique socio-cultural, economic, and healthcare challenges is important in planning interventions targeting mental disorders. Meanwhile, mental health has gained increasing recognition in South Asia over the past few decades, leading to the formulation of mental health policies and the implementation of targeted initiatives. Innovative community-based interventions, psychosocial support groups, and culturally sensitive approaches have shown promise in addressing mental health issues. A stronger collaboration among policymakers, mental health professionals, and local communities will be needed to improve the accessibility and quality of mental healthcare delivery. Expanding access to care, reducing stigma, and integrating mental health services into broader healthcare systems will be key to fostering a more inclusive and effective mental health framework in the region.

**Keywords** South Asia · Mental Health · Social Psychiatry · Suicide · Poverty · Religion

---

A. Singh (✉) · S. K. Kar
Department of Psychiatry, King George's Medical University, Uttar Pradesh, Lucknow, India
e-mail: amitsingh0612@gmail.com



S. M. Y. Arafat et al. (eds.), *Social Psychiatry in South Asia*, South Asian Perspectives in Mental Health and Psychology , https://doi.org/10.1007/978-981-96-8078-8_1

# 1 Introduction

Individuals are the fundamental building blocks of society. The other key elements include the networks of individuals, their patterns of interaction and shared culture, as well as established social systems and institutions. These elements are deeply interconnected, shaping and influencing one another to sustain societal structure and cohesion. For humans, the legendary Greek philosopher Aristotle said that they are "social animals," implying that being social and living in social groups are fundamental characteristics of humans. According to him, individuals who are not engaged in common social life must be substantially different, thus emphasizing the importance of society in human lives.

Social groups offer humans a secure environment to thrive. A supportive social group or society is a source of care and comfort (Glenn, 2000). It is also key to positive mental health and preventing mental illnesses. Societal norms shape the behavior of individuals within a community or culture and influence how people interact and function in society. They might be either explicit, such as rules and regulations or implicit, like customs and traditions. While norms play a crucial role in maintaining order and coherence within society by shaping values, attitudes, and social roles, they can also have adverse effects, such as suppressing individuality, reinforcing harmful stereotypes, and obstructing progress by upholding outdated beliefs (González, 2025). Furthermore, the norms can place undue pressure on individuals to adhere to societal norms, with any deviation often being perceived as abnormal or even a transgression against humanity. Consequently, those who fail to adhere to the norms or harbor distinct beliefs, including individuals affected by mental health problems, may be subjected to stigma and vilification. Apart from the social factors, closely associated economic and environmental factors greatly influence mental health and the presentation of mental disorders (World Health Organization & Calouste Gulbenkian Foundation, 2014).

South Asia is home to about two billion people, approximately a quarter of the world's population, making it the most populous geographical region (World Bank Group, 2025). The World Bank and UNICEF define South Asia as consisting of Afghanistan, Bangladesh, Bhutan, India, the Maldives, Nepal, Pakistan, and Sri Lanka (Table 1). Most of these are low- and middle-income countries (LMIC). These nations not only have physical proximities but also have socio-cultural similarities. The deep socio-cultural ties among these nation regions go back thousands of years. A large portion of South Asia, including the current India, Pakistan, Bangladesh, and Sri Lanka region, was under British colonial occupation and gained independence within a few years of World War II. Even after gaining autonomy, these geographies endured continuing challenges like poverty, illiteracy, population growth, economic instability, and political turmoil, which exacerbated existing inequalities and hindered the overall development of the healthcare infrastructure. Mental healthcare was even less of a priority, leading to a great deal of delay in the development of the modern mental healthcare system. Over the past few decades, South Asian nations have increasingly recognized the significance of mental health, leading to a shift in

**Table 1** Basic demography and health information of countries in South Asia

| | Afghanistan | Bangladesh | Bhutan | India | Maldives | Nepal | Pakistan | Sri Lanka |
|---|---|---|---|---|---|---|---|---|
| Population | 41,454,761 | 171,466,990 | 786,385 | 1,438,069,596 | 525,994 | 29,694,614 | 247,504,495 | 22,971,617 |
| World Bank income level | Low income | LMC | LMC | LMC | UMC | LMC | LMC | LMC |
| Life expectancy | 59.1 | 73.1 | 74.9 | 67.3 | 75.4 | 70 | 66 | 77.2 |
| Current health expenditure (% of GDP) | 21.83 (2021) | 2.36 (2021) | 3.85 (2021) | 3.28 (2021) | 10.03 (2021) | 5.42 (2021) | 2.91 (2021) | 4.07 (2021) |

(WHO, 2024)
*LMC* Lower-middle income, *UMC* Upper-middle income

focus among policymakers and relevant institutions. Initially, efforts were primarily directed at containing people with mental illnesses (PwMI) and treating the disorders. However, over time, the approach has evolved to encompass a more holistic perspective, emphasizing rehabilitation, the rights of PwMI, and comprehensive recovery that addresses both mental and social well-being.

Since social determinants can either promote resilience or contribute to distress and mental disorders, understanding societal dynamics and the social factors influencing psychological well-being is crucial from a mental healthcare perspective in South Asia. This knowledge enables the development of targeted interventions to address these factors effectively.

## 2 Social Epidemiology

### *2.1 Psychiatric Disorders*

South Asia has a significant burden of mental disorders, including depression, anxiety, schizophrenia, and substance abuse (Table 2). An umbrella review reported a pooled prevalence of 16.0% for depression, 12.0% for anxiety, and 14.0% for both among the general adult population (Vidyasagaran et al., 2023). Earlier, a meta-analysis reported a pooled prevalence of 14.2% for common mental disorders, which was higher compared to the global prevalence of 13.4% (Naveed et al., 2020). The depressive symptoms were estimated to be present in 26.4%, anxiety in 25.8%, and mixed anxiety and depression in 28.4% of the population. Besides, alcohol use, tobacco smoking, and tobacco chewing were prevalent in 12.9%, 18.6%, and 21.0%, respectively (Naveed et al., 2020).

### *2.2 Suicide*

Suicide is a challenge for any society. In South Asia, suicidal behavior has been reported in about 6.4% of the population. The suicidal ideations, suicide plans, and suicide attempts are reported to be 3.1–12.4%, 0.9–4.1%, and 0.7–4.7%, respectively (Naveed et al., 2020). The suicide rate differs significantly among countries based on their level of development (Table 3). The major risk factors for suicide include the presence of stressful life events and interpersonal conflicts. Other psychosocial and cultural factors have been implicated in suicide, including the presence of psychiatric disorders such as depression, poverty, gender inequality, and financial insecurity (Arafat et al., 2022). Infertility, family conflicts, intimate partner violence, domestic abuse, husband's alcohol misuse, child marriage, forced marriages, and dowry disputes are among the leading factors contributing to suicide among women

**Table 2** Prevalence of mental disorders in South Asia

| Countries | Study | Findings |
|---|---|---|
| Afghanistan | National Mental Health Survey 2017 (Kovess-Masfety et al., 2021; Sabawoon et al., 2022) | Prevalence in last 12 months<br>• Major depressive disorder—11.71<br>• Generalized anxiety disorder—2.78<br>• Post-traumatic stress disorder—5.34<br>• Any substance addiction—8.22%<br>• Past-year suicidal ideation—2.2%<br>• Lifetime suicidal ideation—7.1%<br>• Lifetime suicide attempt—3.4% |
| Bangladesh | National Mental Health Survey 2019 (Alam, 2019) | Depressive disorders—6.7%<br>Anxiety disorders—4.7%<br>Somatic symptoms and related disorders—2.3%<br>Schizophrenia spectrum disorders—1%<br>Bipolar disorder—0.5%<br>Substance related and addictive disorders—0.5% |
| Bhutan | Annual heath bulletin 2024 (Ministry of Health, 2024) | Number of people consulting health facilities<br>• Dementia—144<br>• Alcohol use disorder—2825<br>• Substance use disorder—871<br>• Psychosis—1109<br>• Depression—2687<br>• Anxiety—3765<br>• Other mental disorders—1708 |

(continued)

**Table 2** (continued)

| Countries | Study | Findings |
|---|---|---|
| India | National Mental Health Survey of India, 2015–16 (Gururaj et al., 2016) | Overall weighted prevalence of mental morbidity was 10.6% and 13.7% for lifetime prevalence<br>Lifetime prevalence (as per ICD-10 classification)<br>• Schizophrenia and psychotic disorders (F20–F29)—1.4%<br>• Depressive disorders (F32–F33)—5.1%<br>Current prevalence (as per ICD-10 classification)<br>• Epilepsy (generalized tonic–clonic seizures)—0.3%<br>• Schizophrenia and psychotic disorders (F20–F29)—0.4%<br>• Depressive disorders (F32–F33)—2.7%<br>• Bipolar (affective) disorder (F30–F31)—0.3%<br>• Neurotic and stress-related disorders (F40–F48)—3.5%<br>• Alcohol use disorder (F10)—4.6%<br>• Other substance use disorders (F11–F19 except F17)—0.6% |
| Maldives | Maldives Mental Health Survey, 2003<br>National Drug Use Survey, 2011–2012 (UNODC, 2013) | Overall prevalence of mental disorders—29.1%<br>Prevalence of current drug users<br>• Male—6.64%<br>• Atolls—2.02%<br>Mental Disorder<br>• Neurotic disorders—23.3%<br>• Anxiety & Depressive Disorder—5%<br>• Epilepsy—6.1%<br>• Somatic disorders—4%<br>• Psychotic Disorders—1% |

(continued)

**Table 2** (continued)

| Countries | Study | Findings |
|---|---|---|
| | WHO STEPS survey (Raheem & Moosa, 2022) | Moderate to severe depression—3.8% |
| Nepal | | Mood disorder<br>• Current 1.4%<br>• Lifetime 3.0%<br>Bipolaraffective disorder<br>• Current 0.1%<br>• Lifetime 0.2%<br>Major depressive disorder<br>• Current 1.0%<br>• Lifetime 2.9%<br>Schizophrenia and associated disorder<br>• Current 0.1%<br>• Lifetime 0.2%<br>Neurotic and stress-related disorders—3.0%<br>Suicide behavior disorder—0.9%<br>Alcohol use disorder—4.2%<br>Other substance use disorder—0.2% |

(continued)

**Table 2** (continued)

| Countries | Study | Findings |
|---|---|---|
| Pakistan | National Psychiatric Morbidity Survey of Pakistan (NPMS) 2022 (Rahman et al., 2024) | All Psychiatric disorders<br>• Lifetime—37.91<br>• Current—32.28<br>F10-F19 Substance use disorders—0.85<br>• F10 Alcohol use disorder—0.53<br>• F11-F19 Other substance use disorders (except F17)—0.37<br>F20-F29 Schizophrenia & other psychotic disorders—4.03<br>F30-F39 Mood (affective disorders)—19.62<br>F30-F31 Bipolar affective disorders—4.45<br>F32-F33 Depressive disorders—17.80<br>F40-F48 Anxiety and stress-related disorders—24.81<br>F41.1 Generalized anxiety disorder—4.48<br>F42 Obsessive–compulsive disorder—1.29<br>F43.1 Post-traumatic stress disorder—19.91<br>F60.2 Antisocial Personality—0.88 |
| Sri Lanka | National Mental Health Survey (NMHS), 2007 (Institute for Research and Development, 2008) | One-month prevalence of mental disorders—15%<br>Major Depression—2.1%<br>Other Depressive syndromes—7.1%<br>Somatoform Disorders—3%<br>Panic Syndrome—0.5%<br>Other Anxiety Syndromes—0.9%<br>Bulimia—0.03%<br>Binge eating—0.02%<br>Alcohol Abuse—2.8%<br>PTSD—1.7%<br>Psychotic symptoms—3.6% |

**Table 3** Suicide rates in South Asia

| Countries | Age-standardized suicide rates (per 100,000 population) |
|---|---|
| Afghanistan | 5.3 [3.0–9.4] |
| Bangladesh | 2.9 [1.8–5.1] |
| Bhutan | 5.1 [2.8–8.9] |
| India | 12.6 [9.5–15.2] |
| Maldives | 2.0 [1.5–3.3] |
| Nepal | 11.1 [6.4–17.6] |
| Pakistan | 6.5 [3.6–11.3] |
| Sri Lanka | 14.0 [8.3–20.0] |

(WHO, 2025)

in South Asia (Fastenau et al., 2024). Sexual violence substantially increases the risk of suicide attempts in women (Sabawoon et al., 2022).

## 2.3 *Gender-Based Violence*

Gender-based violence (GBV) is a global health challenge (Table 4). In South Asia, the lifetime and past-year prevalence of intimate partner violence was reported to be 35% (26–46%) and 19% (12–27%), respectively (Sardinha et al., 2022). It was higher than the global prevalence estimates of 27% (lifetime) and 13% (past year). The GBV have been broadly categorized into sexual, physical, verbal, psychological (emotional), or socioeconomic violence. However, these can co-exist and can take many forms, from threats and coercion to rape or murder. Although individuals of any gender can experience GBV, it disproportionately affects women, who are the most common targets. Additionally, sexual minorities, including LGBTQI + individuals, are also vulnerable to GBV and often face heightened risks of violence and discrimination (Council of Europe, 2025). Gender-based violence has both immediate and long-term consequences on the physical and mental health of women and their children. These effects include injuries, depression, anxiety, unwanted pregnancies, and sexually transmitted infections, among others. In severe cases, it can even result in death (Sardinha et al., 2022). Survivors of sexual assault or rape, domestic violence, and honor-based crimes often suffer from post-traumatic stress disorder (PTSD), depression, and suicidal ideations. Socioeconomic systems, patriarchal attitudes, and prevailing societal conventions that establish gender roles are some of the many contributing factors to gender-based violence. Besides, social stigma and victim-blaming prevent many from seeking mental health support.

**Table 4** Intimate partner violence in South Asia

| Countries | Lifetime | Past year |
|---|---|---|
| Afghanistan | 46% [32– 61%] | 35% [22–50%] |
| Bangladesh | 50% [37 – 62%] | 23% [15–34%] |
| Bhutan | 22% [14–33%] | 9% [5–14%] |
| India | 35% [23 – 47%] | 18% [11–28%] |
| Maldives | 19% [12–28%] | 6% [4–11%] |
| Nepal | 27% [18–39%] | 11% [7–19%] |
| Pakistan | 29% [19–40%] | 16% [10–25%] |
| Sri Lanka | 24% [14–38%] | 4% [2–9%] |

(WHO, 2024)

## 3 Stigma and Cultural Beliefs

Stigma is closely associated with mental illnesses and is prevalent worldwide (Vaishnav et al., 2023). A recent systematic review that evaluated self-stigma in patients with severe mental illness found that nearly one-third of patients (31.3%) suffering from severe mental illness experience high levels of self-stigma (Dubreucq et al., 2021). This same study reported that in the Southeast Asia region, the frequency of self-stigma is highest compared to other parts of the world (Dubreucq et al., 2021). Despite of differences in levels of stigma, it has been found that the causes of stigma in mental illnesses are very much similar in most of the countries as reported from the eight Asian countries (Singapore, Lebanon, Japan, Nepal, India, China, Philippines, Thailand) (Kudva et al., 2020). It has been seen that stigma is encountered at the individual (personal) level, organizational level, and societal level (Vaishnav et al., 2023). Maximal stigma is encountered by the vulnerable population (children, elderly, gender minorities, and underprivileged populations). Several initiatives have been taken in Asian countries and other LMICs to combat the stigma associated with mental illness. However, there is a lack of data regarding the outcome of the interventions against stigma associated with mental illnesses (Vaishnav et al., 2023). The majority of the anti-stigma initiatives in South Asia countries are limited to enhancing awareness about mental illness through mass educational campaigns or individual-level psychoeducation of the patients, caregivers, and mental health professionals (Vaishnav et al., 2023). Culture and societal beliefs play a pivotal role in maintaining stigma, and stigma-related interventions need to be delivered in a culture-sensitive manner to make them more acceptable and effective (Kaur et al., 2021). Studies from South Asian countries like Nepal report that the anti-stigma interventions were not adequately culturally adapted, resulting in significant implementation challenges (Gurung et al., 2022). Stigma is one of the major challenges in accessing mental healthcare in Afghanistan, Pakistan, Bangladesh, Nepal, India, Bhutan, Sri Lanka, and the Maldives (Arafat & Kar, 2024; Grover, 2023; Ministry of Public Health Afghanistan, 2019; Mohamed & Mansoor, 2024; Seeman et al., 2016; Sharma & Joshi, 2024).

## 4 Religion

South Asian culture is significantly influenced by the religious practices present in the region. The major religions practiced in South Asian countries include Buddhism, Christianity, Hinduism, Islam, and Sikhism. However, it is not confined to these religions. Numerous other faiths play a vital role in shaping beliefs and behaviors within South Asian culture.

The religio-cultural beliefs and attributions associated with mental illness significantly affect access to mental healthcare, and people due to such beliefs often seek help from traditional or faith healers (Arafat & Kar, 2024; Campion & Bhugra, 1998; Dein, 2020; Kar & Menon, 2024; Mishra & Kar, 2023). Religious and cultural beliefs also contribute to the development of culture-specific psychopathologies (culture-bound syndrome), for example, Dhat syndrome in South Asia (Chadda & Ahuja, 1990; Kar & Sarkar, 2015; Kar & Singh, 2016; Kar et al., 2024; Rajkumar, 2024). In the South Asia region, possession states (a subtype of dissociative disorder) are attributed to Gods, Goddesses, and Spirits (Ferrari Fabrizio M., 2011). Many people suffering from psychiatric illnesses are taken to religious places for healing and religious healers play a key role in providing care to patients with psychiatric illnesses in South Asia (Arafat & Kar, 2024; Ferrari Fabrizio M., 2011; Kar & Menon, 2024; Mohamed & Mansoor, 2024). Religion provides a feeling of togetherness and enhances social support (South Asian Health Hub, 2024). Religion offers a means to deal with life's stressors and challenges. Individuals who adopt a religious coping strategy either cope by framing their experiences in a positive or negative light according to their faith and God (Fatima et al., 2022). Yoga, Meditation, and mindfulness techniques have their root in the religions. People with religious beliefs accept these therapeutic recommendations easily. These techniques are found to be effective strategies in dealing with the common mental health issues, stress, and some specific severe mental health issues as well (Domingues, 2018; Falsafi, 2016; Gangadhar & Varambally, 2015; Thirthalli & Rao, 2016).

Religion can also strongly determine the substance-taking and self-harm behavior (Kaufman et al., 2023). An Indian study reported that the tribal communities from Arunachal Pradesh use alcohol as a part of religious and cultural practices (Chaturvedi et al., 2019). This study reported that the use of alcohol is more among the indigenous population and Hindus in comparison to Buddhists and Christians (Chaturvedi et al., 2019). Religion significantly influences suicidal behavior and attitude toward suicide (Teo et al., 2021). Overall, religion plays a protective role against suicide (Wu et al., 2015). As South Asia is a hub of cultural and religious diversity, it is expected that the differences in the prevalence of suicidal behavior in South Asia might be influenced by religion as well.

## 5 Family System and Community Support

Family systems and family values are important determinants of human behavior. South Asia is unique for retaining the value of a joint family system for a considerable time in comparison to the West. Earlier studies supported that South Asian families have good support for patients with severe mental illnesses, and the expressed emotions are less, which is responsible for better outcomes of schizophrenia than in Western countries (Hashemi & Cochrane, 2009; Leff et al., 1990). There has been a rapid change in family type, structure, and dynamics in South Asia over the past few decades (De Silva, 2005; Katbamna et al., 2004; Yeung et al., 2018). Several factors contribute to changing family systems in South Asia, of which the important ones are:

- Migration: People migrate abroad and within the country from rural to urban areas for jobs, higher studies, and several other reasons. As a result, the family size is reduced in size compromising the physical support system within the family (Lam & Yeoh, 2019; Story, 2010).
- War, natural calamities, and disasters: Natural and manmade disasters are common in South Asia. They result in the dissolution of the families, migration, and displacement, as a result of which the family system and community support are significantly disrupted (Azizi, 2023; Fernando, 2010; Fothergill & Squier, 2018; Khadka, 2021; Koser, 2022).
- Political conflict: Political conflict can result in war and the displacement of the population. The social and community harmony is significantly affected by communal violence and political conflicts. Many people leave their country and live the life of a refugee due to the geo-political conflicts (Alemi et al., 2014; Datta, 2016; George et al., 2016; Gorlick, 2019; Hassan, 2010; Kronenfeld, 2008; Parnini et al., 2013; Valatheeswaran & Rajan, 2011).
- Climate Change impact: Climate change-related adversities are common in South Asia. Rise in sea-water level and flooding results in displacement of families and disintegration of the social support system (Harrison et al., 2021; Mirza, 2011; Sivakumar & Stefanski, 2010). Scarcity of water and famine are other climatic adversities encountered in the South Asia region (Vinke et al., 2017).
- Marital conflicts: Marital conflict is a rapidly rising social issue. Divorce and social separation may break the family structure and the support system within the family (Yeung et al., 2018).

## 6 Marriage and Dowry

Marriage is a social milestone in an individual's life. As it is a social event, several socio-cultural and religious factors play an important role in marriage. In South Asian culture, marriage establishes an important social connection between two families (Jones & Yeung, 2014). Different cultures and religions follow different rituals in marriage. There are several contexts of marriage that have significance socially; they are-

- Early and late marriage
- Re-marriage
- Live-in relationship
- Divorce and social separation
- Marital conflict
- Extra-marital affairs
- Multiple marriages

It has been seen that early marriage is a common phenomenon in South Asia; however, recent years have witnessed a changing course of marriage shifting toward a late age in the majority of Asian countries (Jones & Yeung, 2014). In South Asia, still, a significant proportion of marriages are decided by the parents of the bride and groom. These arranged marriages are mostly determined by significant socio-cultural factors like—religion, caste, occupation, socioeconomic status, income, domicile (rural or urban), language, eating preferences (vegetarian/non-vegetarian), social status, and many other interpersonal factors. Again, within the Asian countries, there is a difference in the age of marriage and number (frequency of marriage) between the countries of Eastern Asia and Western Asia (Jones & Yeung, 2014; Jones et al., 2015; Raymo et al., 2015). It has also been reported that there has been a decline in marriage rates in Asia in recent years, which might be due to rising individualism and a change in family attitudes toward marriage. Despite the above fact, about a quarter of South Asian women were married before the age of 18 years, and about 45% of child marriages in the world are in South Asia (UNICEF South Asia, 2025). Child marriage results in increased maternal mortality, anemia, poor pregnancy outcomes, a dropout from school, and many more life adversities, which increase the risk of mental illness (Subramanee et al., 2022).

The dowry system is highly prevalent in South Asian society. As the South Asia society is predominantly patriarchal, the bride after marriage stays away from her parents (in the in-laws' house) with her husband. Usually, the parents of the bride give money and gifts to the groom's family during the marriage contract. Despite having laws to prevent the dowry system in many countries, it is still not completely eliminated. Demanding more dowry many times results in domestic violence, homicide, suicide, and many legal conflicts, which have potential mental health implications (Afzal & Subhani, 2007; Diamond-Smith et al., 2020; K. Khanal & Sen, 2020a, 2020b).

## 7 Socioeconomic Factors

### 7.1 Poverty

Poverty is a key issue in South Asia. People living below the poverty line of $2.15 per day, $3.65 per day and $6.85 per day are 7.6%, 34.3% and 78.8%, respectively. It constitutes about 40% of the global poor population and accounts for one-fifth of the global extreme poor (World Bank, 2024). Also, it is the region only behind sub-Saharan Africa in terms of the high prosperity gap (World Bank, 2024). The poverty in this region is not only monetary, but multidimensional, encompassing health, education, and living standards. Multidimensional poverty is far higher than monetary poverty in South Asia, primarily due to low educational enrollment and attainment, as well as limited access to sanitation (World Bank, 2024). Thus, reducing illiteracy should be a target area for policymakers (Li et al., 2022). Poverty and mental illnesses have a bidirectional causal relationship (Ridley et al., 2020). Poverty often leads to unstable income and fluctuating expenses, creating worries and uncertainty that negatively impact mental health. Moreover, poverty disproportionately increases the exposure of individuals to crime, including violent offenses, intimate partner violence, as well as trauma, such as the early loss of loved ones (Ridley et al., 2020). Exposure to pollution, temperature extremes, harsh working, living, and challenging sleep environments adversely impact mental health (Marmot, 2005; Ridley et al., 2020). Meanwhile, factors such as stigma and discrimination related to severe mental illnesses may also contribute to the multidimensional poverty, especially among women and socially disadvantaged groups (Trani et al., 2015). Also, poor access to mental healthcare due to financial constraints means that many PwMI living in poverty go untreated. The cash transfer programs have been shown to reduce depression and improve mental well-being in India (Powell-Jackson et al., 2016). BRAC, a Bangladeshi non-governmental organization (NGO) operating nationwide programs, led microfinancing initiatives for "ultra-poor" that have been shown to reduce poverty. Similar programs offering a comprehensive set of services to the poorest households, including providing a productive asset along with other support mechanisms, have been shown to enhance economic stability and improve mental well-being in other countries as well, including India and Pakistan (Banerjee et al., 2015). Current trends suggest a remarkable slowdown in global poverty reduction efforts (World Bank, 2024). This may further increase in mental health-related challenges in South Asia.

### 7.2 Unemployment

Unemployment has been linked to negative psychological outcomes and is a key predictor of poor mental health. In South Asia, the unemployment rate for 2023 was 4.61% (Macrotrends, 2025). The youth unemployment rates are even higher at 14.6% (in 2023) (Table 5). High youth unemployment leads to stress, anxiety,

**Table 5** Youth unemployment in South Asia

| Countries | Youth Unemployment (% of total labor force ages 15–24) |
|---|---|
| Afghanistan | 17.3 |
| Bangladesh | 10.9 |
| Bhutan | 14.9 |
| India | 15.7 |
| Maldives | 15.0 |
| Nepal | 20.6 |
| Pakistan | 9.7 |
| Sri Lanka | 26.3 |

and depression due to financial insecurity and a lack of purpose. Besides, substance use rates are higher in the unemployed population. There is also a stigma attached to unemployment in South Asian societies, which may exacerbate feelings of failure and hopelessness. Job loss and economic uncertainty are linked to increased suicide rates. Also, it results in poor help-seeking behavior for mental health concerns, despite the higher prevalence of mental health issues.

### *7.3 Political Instability and Conflict*

Political instability in South Asia, marked by frequent government transitions, conflict, and violence, creates an atmosphere of uncertainty and fear, significantly impacting mental health. In countries like Pakistan, Afghanistan, Bangladesh, and Sri Lanka, political unrest has led to the economy taking major hits, food insecurity, and an alarming rise in mental health disorders such as anxiety, depression, and PTSD (David et al., 2017; Tol et al., 2010). Also, terrorism has a huge adverse impact on the mental health of people in South Asia. Pakistan, Afghanistan, and India rank among the top 15 nations severely impacted by terrorism (IEP, 2024). Exposure to violence, forced displacement, and persecution further intensifies emotional distress, particularly among vulnerable populations living in conflict zones.

Political instability not only worsens individual mental health outcomes but also disrupts broader economic and social systems, increasing unemployment and poverty. The compounding effects of war and environmental disasters, such as the earthquake in Afghanistan, added to the burden of a population already suffering from decades of war and economic instability, while inadequate mental health resources and deep-rooted stigma hindered effective intervention. Studies reveal that exposure to trauma in conflict-affected regions, particularly among women, significantly increases the risk of suicidal ideation and attempts, with PTSD, depression, and anxiety being strong predictors of self-harm (Hussaini et al., 2022; Sabawoon et al., 2022). Addressing the mental health impact of political instability requires not only improving access to care but also fostering political stability, economic recovery, and stronger community support systems (Hussaini et al., 2022).

## 7.4 Climate Change and Natural Disasters

Of the different World Bank regions, South Asia has the highest proportion of its population exposed to weather shocks such as floods, storms, droughts, and heat waves, at 88.1%. Also, it has the highest total population at risk (population that will struggle to recover) from extreme weather events, accounting for 32% of its population (World Bank, 2024). Air pollution in South Asia exceeds recommended levels by more than ten times (World Bank, 2022). In fact, the region hosts 37 of the world's 40 most polluted cities (World Bank. South Asia Regional Office, 2023). An estimated 2 million premature deaths occur annually as a result of air pollution, and the financial implications are high. The health costs in terms of mortality and morbidity caused by $PM_{2.5}$ air pollution exposure amounted to 10.3% of GDP in 2019 (World Bank, 2022). Displaced workers often struggle to transition to new employment due to skill mismatches, wage differences, and geographic barriers (World Bank. South Asia Regional Office, 2023).

Also, South Asian countries frequently experience natural disasters like tsunamis, floods, earthquakes, and cyclones. These extreme weather events often lead to significant trauma and loss, such as the destruction of homes, jobs, and disconnection from loved ones and communities, which can contribute to a range of mental health disorders like stress, anxiety, depression, and PTSD (Patwary et al., 2024). Studies conducted on affected populations in Southeast Asia show a wide prevalence of mental health issues, with mental health disorder rates ranging from 6.4% to 80.4% (Majumder et al., 2024). Anxiety was present in 0.4% to 100% of the respondents across 36 studies, while depression was found in 0.9% to 98.1% in 57 studies. Stress prevalence was documented to range from 0.6% to 93.8% in eight studies, and PTSD ranged from 0 to 100% in 83 studies. Intrusive symptoms were observed in 23.68% to 71.4% of cases, with avoidance behaviors seen in 1.5% to 62.8% of individuals.

Suicidal tendencies were reported in 1.1% to 24% of participants across 15 studies, with rates varying based on the timing of the studies. Suicidal ideation was lower (1.1–9.6%) within 12 months of the event but higher (2–24%) beyond a year. Insomnia, particularly among local populations, ranged from 8.3% to 62.5% in eight studies. The prevalence of disaster-related memories in children and adolescents (ages 5–19) ranged from 17.5% to 85%. Additionally, fear, particularly fear of recurrence, was prevalent in 11% to 94.3% of participants. Nightmares were reported in 17.2% to 83.1% of participants, with cyclone and tsunami survivors particularly affected (Majumder et al., 2024). These findings highlight the profound and lasting impact of extreme weather events on mental health, with varied prevalence of psychological distress across different types of disasters and affected populations.

### *7.5 Migration*

Migration can broadly be classified as internal and international migration. However, based on the motive for migration, it can be classified into voluntary or forced migration. In South Asia, the total refugee population by territory of asylum is 3.6 million (Migration Data in Southern Asia, 2025). Also, the region has the largest number of emigrants worldwide, with approximately 43.4 million people living outside their country of origin, making it the sub-region with the highest emigration rate. Conflicts and natural disasters, including floods and earthquakes, lead to massive internal displacement in South Asian countries (IDMC, 2020).

Migrants are at a higher risk of mental health issues due to a combination of trauma related to situations leading to migration, stress from relocation, social isolation, economic hardships, and limited access to healthcare (Virupaksha et al., 2014). Many are forced to flee their home countries due to conflict, persecution, or extreme poverty, often experiencing violence, displacement, and family separation, which can lead to PTSD, depression, and anxiety (WHO, 2021a). South Asian migrants to the West are found to suffer from higher health issues (Karasz et al., 2019). Upon arrival in a new country, they face cultural shock, language barriers, and discrimination, making it difficult to integrate and build a support system. Economic struggles, including unemployment, exploitative labor conditions, and financial insecurity, add to their psychological distress. Additionally, migrants often encounter significant barriers to mental health services, such as stigma, lack of culturally competent care, and legal uncertainties, preventing them from receiving the help they need (Kapilashrami & John, 2023). The cumulative effect of these challenges makes migrants particularly vulnerable to mental health disorders, highlighting the need for inclusive policies and accessible support systems.

## 8 Mental Healthcare System and Services

### *8.1 Regional Mental Health Policies*

All the South Asian nations have adopted standalone legislation for mental health (Table 6). However, there is a scope for improvement in some of the national policies, including those of Bhutan and Nepal, which are not entirely in line with the human rights instruments (WHO, 2021b). Also, there is a gap in the allocation of resources for their implementation. Bhutan, the Maldives and Nepal have yet to formulate a standalone law for mental health; however, some of the components related to the rights of PwMI are covered through other legislations, including those related to disability rights (Khanal et al., 2023).

National mental health programs in South Asian countries vary in scope and effectiveness, often facing challenges due to limited resources, stigma, and insufficient mental health infrastructure. Countries like India, Bangladesh, Sri Lanka,

**Table 6** Mental health policies and legislation in South Asia

| | Policy | Stand-alone Legislation for Mental Health | Suicide prevention strategy/ policy/plan |
|---|---|---|---|
| Afghanistan | Yes (2019) | Yes (2019) | Yes (2019) |
| Bangladesh | Yes (2020) | Yes (2018) | Yes (2020) |
| Bhutan | Yes (2015) | No | Yes (2018) |
| India | Yes (2014) | Yes (2017) | Yes (2022) |
| Maldives | Yes (2017) | No | No |
| Nepal | Yes (2020) | No | No |
| Pakistan | Yes (2024) | Yes (2001) | No |
| Sri Lanka | Yes (2020) | Yes (2017) | Yes (1996) |

and Pakistan have implemented national mental health policies to integrate mental healthcare into primary health services. India's National Mental Health Programme (NMHP) focuses on community-based interventions, training healthcare professionals, and increasing access to psychiatric care. Bangladesh has developed the National Mental Health Strategy 2020–2030, aiming to improve mental health services and reduce stigma. Sri Lanka has a decentralized approach, integrating mental health services into district hospitals, while Pakistan's mental health efforts remain fragmented due to political instability and resource constraints.

Nepal, Bhutan, and the Maldives have also taken steps to strengthen mental healthcare, with Bhutan emphasizing Gross National Happiness (GNH) as a framework that includes mental well-being. Despite these efforts, South Asia continues to struggle with inadequate funding, a shortage of trained professionals, and deeply rooted cultural barriers that hinder mental health awareness and treatment. Expanding community-based services, strengthening policy implementation, and addressing social stigma remain critical for improving mental healthcare across the region.

## *8.2 Healthcare Infrastructure*

The Mental Health Atlas 2020 highlighted the severe shortage of mental health professionals (psychiatrists, psychologists, and social workers) in many South Asian countries (Table 7). However, there is a recent push toward amending this situation. Despite that, the situation continues to be grim, considering the huge service gap. Mental healthcare is often concentrated in urban centers, leaving rural and remote populations underserved. To address the situation, decentralization of mental health services has been recommended for a long time, and is part of the mental health programs of most of the South Asian nations. The doctors and healthcare staff at primary care centers have been trained to provide mental healthcare. However, the dispensation of comprehensive psychiatric services through this system remains challenging. And it will need continuous skill-building and inspiring the staff to enhance the quality of services. In this regard, WHO has been actively promoting community-based mental healthcare as a more accessible and effective alternative to institutional care, aiming to reduce stigma, close treatment gaps, and protect human rights. The focus is on shifting mental health services from psychiatric hospitals to community-based settings. To accelerate progress, the member nations adopted the Paro Declaration in 2022, reaffirming their commitment to universal access to people-centered mental healthcare and services. Tele-mental health initiatives have been adopted in India to provide counseling services to people with mental health issues (Hossain et al., 2025; Hussain et al., 2023; MoHFW, 2025). Other South Asian nations can adopt similar initiatives.

**Table 7** Mental healthcare manpower in South Asia

| | Afghanistan | Bangladesh | Bhutan | India | Maldives | Nepal | Pakistan | Sri Lanka |
|---|---|---|---|---|---|---|---|---|
| Number of Psychiatrists | 129 | 270 | 3 | – | 17 | 183 | 300 | 123 |
| Psychiatrists per 100,000 population | 0.34 | 0.17 | 0.39 | 0.29 | 3.2 | 0.64 | 0.14 | 0.58 |
| Mental Health Nurses | 26 | 700 | 9 | – | 0 | 123 | 200 | 624 |
| Mental health nurses per 100,000 population | 0.07 | 0.43 | 1.18 | 0.80 | 0 | 0.43 | 0.09 | 2.93 |
| Psychologists | 133 | 565 | 0 | – | 7 | 31 | 100 | 61 |
| Psychologists per 100,000 population | 0.35 | 0.35 | 0 | 0.07 | 1.32 | 0.11 | 0.05 | 0.29 |
| Social Workers | 48 | 3 | 0 | – | 2 | – | 600 | 72 |
| Social workers per 100,000 population | 0.13 | 0.002 | 0 | 0.06 | 0.38 | – | 0.28 | 0.34 |

(WHO, 2021b)

## 9 Challenges and Service Gap

Mental health in South Asia is significantly impacted by socioeconomic challenges such as unemployment, poverty, gender-based violence, and political instability. These factors contribute to mental illnesses and also limit access to mental healthcare. Also, stigma remains a major barrier, resulting in delayed treatment seeking and mental health issues remaining underreported and untreated (Seeman et al., 2016). Poor mental healthcare infrastructure, limited facilities, shortage of trained professionals, high treatment costs, and inadequate government support are other key hurdles. The migration of mental health professionals to countries with better opportunities has led to a "brain drain," while limited training institutions result in the training of a low number of qualified professionals each year (Dorji, 2023).

The region's mental health policies are underfunded and poorly implemented. Geographic disparities, financial barriers, and a lack of political stability hinder the consistent enforcement of mental health initiatives. In many South Asian countries, mental health services receive a minimal portion of national health budgets. For example, in Pakistan, only 0.4% of total healthcare expenditure is allocated to mental health, resulting in inadequate support for those in need (Alvi et al., 2023). In India, the mental health budget share is 1.11% of the total health budget. Yet, considering the huge treatment gap for mental disorders, ranging from 70 to 92%, this budget may still be inadequate (Research Unit, 2025).

## 10 Future Directions

Mental health disorders are prevalent across South Asia, affecting diverse geographies and population groups, with some segments being more vulnerable. There should be a collective and dedicated effort of the stakeholders to improve accessibility and the quality of services. Psychiatry must expand beyond specialized hospitals to primary healthcare. Thus, the efforts to decentralize mental healthcare services should continue. Addressing the persistent stigma surrounding mental illness is crucial. Therefore, awareness generation and sensitization efforts for mental disorders should be initiated and promoted in schools to achieve a lasting impact. Community-based awareness programs and workplace education can promote mental well-being, reduce discrimination, and build resilience.

Efforts must prioritize holistic recovery and rehabilitation rather than just treatment. Legislative reforms and effective implementation of welfare programs are necessary to ensure the rights of individuals with mental illness. Strengthening legal protections for survivors of violence and economic challenges is also important. Addressing mental health impacts from natural disasters and political conflicts requires integrated mental health services. The rise in substance use disorders poses significant public health challenges, necessitating the equipping of community health facilities with adequate resources. Vulnerable groups such as women, children, sexual minorities, migrants, and displaced populations would require targeted support. Technological solutions like telepsychiatry, mobile apps, and online counseling can aid significantly in early identification and intervention, especially in remote areas. Advocacy and culturally tailored interventions are vital in alleviating the mental health burden. Legislative shortcomings, such as weak emphasis on human rights and lack of community-based approaches, must be addressed. Furthermore, future research in South Asia must adopt standardized diagnostic tools and broader community-based studies to generate more accurate prevalence estimates and inform effective interventions. Strengthening mental health infrastructure and fostering collaboration between policymakers, professionals, and local communities will be essential in creating a more accessible and inclusive mental health framework in South Asia.

## 11 Conclusions

The socio-cultural, environmental, and economic factors substantially influence mental health. In South Asia, the prevalence of mental disorders is high, with significant impacts on various population groups. Widespread poverty, unemployment, gender inequality, rapid urbanization, climate change, environmental disasters, political instability, and the social stigma surrounding mental disorders exacerbate the mental health challenges. Additionally, limited access to mental health services, a shortage of trained professionals, and deeply ingrained cultural beliefs often hinder the delivery of effective interventions. Addressing this challenge requires comprehensive strategies, including increasing awareness, reducing stigma, improving access to mental health services, and allocating adequate resources to mental healthcare. Collaborative efforts from governments, healthcare providers, and communities are essential to mitigate the impact of mental health disorders in the region.

## References

Afzal, S., & Subhani, M. I. (2007). Determinants of dowry: A case study of rural south Asia. *IUB Journal of Social Sciences and Humanities, 5*(1). https://papers.ssrn.com/sol3/papers.cfm?abstract_id=1927167

Alam, M. F. (2019). *National mental health survey 2019*. National Institute of Mental Health. https://nimh.gov.bd/wp-content/uploads/2021/11/Mental-Health-Survey-Report.pdf

Alemi, Q., James, S., Cruz, R., Zepeda, V., & Racadio, M. (2014). Psychological distress in afghan refugees: A mixed-method systematic review. *Journal of Immigrant and Minority Health, 16*(6), 1247–1261. https://doi.org/10.1007/s10903-013-9861-1

Alvi, M. H., Ashraf, T., Kiran, T., Iqbal, N., Gumber, A., Patel, A., & Husain, N. (2023). Economic burden of mental illness in Pakistan: An estimation for the year 2020 from existing evidence. *Bjpsych International, 20*(3), 54–56. https://doi.org/10.1192/bji.2023.4

Arafat, S. M. Y., & Kar, S. K. (Eds.). (2024). *Access to mental health care in south Asia: current status, Potential Challenges, and Ways Out*. Springer Nature. https://doi.org/10.1007/978-981-99-9153-2

Arafat, S. M. Y., Saleem, T., Menon, V., Ali, S.A.-Z., Baminiwatta, A., Kar, S. K., Akter, H., & Singh, R. (2022). Depression and suicidal behavior in south Asia: A systematic review and meta-analysis. *Global Mental Health, 9,* 181–192. https://doi.org/10.1017/gmh.2022.20

Azizi, M. A. (2023). War, conflict, climate change and internal displacement in Afghanistan. *Living with the Weather: Climate Change, Ecology and Displacement in south Asia,* 173–209.

Banerjee, A., Duflo, E., Goldberg, N., Karlan, D., Osei, R., Parienté, W., Shapiro, J., Thuysbaert, B., & Udry, C. (2015). A multifaceted program causes lasting progress for the very poor: Evidence from six countries. *Science, 348*(6236), 1260799. https://doi.org/10.1126/science.1260799

Campion, J., & Bhugra, D. (1998). Religious and indigenous treatment of mental illness in South India—A descriptive study. *Mental Health, Religion & Culture, 1*(1), 21–29. https://doi.org/10.1080/13674679808406494

Chadda, R. K., & Ahuja, N. (1990). Dhat syndrome. A sex neurosis of the Indian subcontinent. *The British Journal of Psychiatry: THe Journal of Mental Science, 156,* 577–579. https://doi.org/10.1192/bjp.156.4.577

Chaturvedi, H. K., Bajpai, R. C., & Tiwari, P. (2019). Association of religion and cultural tradition with alcohol use among some tribal communities of Arunachal Pradesh, India. *Journal of Ethnicity in Substance Abuse, 18*(2), 296–308. https://doi.org/10.1080/15332640.2017.1355766

Council of Europe. (2025). *Types of gender-based violence—Gender Matters—www.coe.int*. Gender Matters. https://www.coe.int/en/web/gender-matters/types-of-gender-based-violence

Datta, A. (2016). Dealing with dislocation: Migration, place and home among displaced Kashmiri Pandits in Jammu and Kashmir. *Contributions to Indian Sociology, 50*(1), 52–79. https://doi.org/10.1177/0069966715615024

David, S., Gazi, R., Mirzazada, M. S., Siriwardhana, C., Soofi, S., & Roy, N. (2017). Conflict in south Asia and its impact on health. *BMJ,* j1537. https://doi.org/10.1136/bmj.j1537

De Silva, W. I. (2005). Family transition in south Asia: Provision of social services and social protection. *Asia Pacific Population Journal, 20*(2), 13.

Dein, S. (2020). Religious healing and mental health. *Mental Health, Religion & Culture, 23*(8), 657–665. https://doi.org/10.1080/13674676.2020.1834220

Diamond-Smith, N. G., Dahal, M., Puri, M., & Weiser, S. D. (2020). Semi-arranged marriages and dowry ambivalence: Tensions in the changing landscape of marriage formation in south Asia. *Culture, Health & Sexuality, 22*(9), 971–986. https://doi.org/10.1080/13691058.2019.1646318

Domingues, R. B. (2018). Modern postural yoga as a mental health promoting tool: A systematic review. *Complementary Therapies in Clinical Practice, 31,* 248–255. https://doi.org/10.1016/j.ctcp.2018.03.002

Dorji, C. (2023). Addressing Mental Health in Bhutan. *The Druk Journal, 9*(1), 4–14.

Dubreucq, J., Plasse, J., & Franck, N. (2021). Self-stigma in serious mental Illness: A systematic review of frequency, correlates, and consequences. *Schizophrenia Bulletin, 47*(5), 1261–1287. https://doi.org/10.1093/schbul/sbaa181

Falsafi, N. (2016). A randomized controlled trial of mindfulness versus yoga: Effects on depression and/or anxiety in college students. *Journal of the American Psychiatric Nurses Association, 22*(6), 483–497. https://doi.org/10.1177/1078390316663307

Fastenau, A., Willis, M., Penna, S., Yaddanapudi, L., Balaji, M., Shidhaye, R., & Pilot, E. (2024). Risk factors for attempted suicide and suicide death among south-east Asian women: A scoping review. *International Journal of Environmental Research and Public Health, 21*(12), Article 12. https://doi.org/10.3390/ijerph21121658

Fatima, H., Oyetunji, T. P., Mishra, S., Sinha, K., Olorunsogbon, O. F., Akande, O. S., & Srinivasan, & Kar, S. K. (2022). Religious coping in the time of COVID-19 Pandemic in India and

Nigeria: Finding of a cross-national community survey. *The International Journal of Social Psychiatry, 68*(2), 309–315. https://doi.org/10.1177/0020764020984511
Fernando, N. (2010). *Forced relocation after the Indian Ocean tsunami, 2004* [PhD Thesis, Universitäts-und Landesbibliothek Bonn]. https://bonndoc.ulb.uni-bonn.de/xmlui/handle/20.500.11811/4548
Ferrari Fabrizio M. (2011). *Health and religious rituals in south Asia: Disease, possession and healing* (1st ed.). Routledge. https://www.routledge.com/Health-and-Religious-Rituals-in-South-Asia-Disease-Possession-and-Healing/Ferrari/p/book/9781138784796
Fothergill, A., & Squier, E. (2018). Women and children in the 2015 earthquake in Nepal. In J. H. Kruhl, R. Adhikari, & U. E. Dorka (Eds.), *Living under the threat of earthquakes* (pp. 253–271). Springer International Publishing. https://doi.org/10.1007/978-3-319-68044-6_16
Gangadhar, B. N., & Varambally, S. (2015). Integrating yoga in mental health services. *The Indian Journal of Medical Research, 141*(6), 747–748. https://doi.org/10.4103/0971-5916.160685
George, M., Vaillancourt, A., & Rajan, S. I. (2016). Sri Lankan Tamil refugees in India: Conceptual framework of repatriation success. *Refuge, 32,* 73.
Glenn, E. N. (2000). Creating a caring society. *Contemporary Sociology, 29*(1), 84–94. https://doi.org/10.2307/2654934
González, R. (2025). The role of norms as promoters of social change. *Political Psychology, 46*(2), 455–481. https://doi.org/10.1111/pops.13025
Gorlick, B. (2019). The Rohingya refugee crisis: Rethinking solutions and accountability. *Refugee Studies Centre, Working Paper Series, 131.* https://papers.ssrn.com/sol3/papers.cfm?abstract_id=3506638
Grover, S. (2023). Status of mental health in south Asian countries. *Journal of SAARC Psychiatric Federation, 1*(1), 1–5. https://journals.lww.com/jspf/fulltext/2023/01000/status_of_mental_health_in_south_asian_countries.1.aspx
Gurung, D., Poudyal, A., Wang, Y. L., Neupane, M., Bhattarai, K., Wahid, S. S., Aryal, S., Heim, E., Gronholm, P., Thornicroft, G., & Kohrt, B. (2022). Stigma against mental health disorders in Nepal conceptualised with a 'what matters most' framework: A scoping review. *Epidemiology and Psychiatric Sciences, 31,* Article e11. https://doi.org/10.1017/S2045796021000809
Gururaj, G., Varghese, M., Benegal, V., Rao, G. N., Pathak, K., Singh, L. K., Mehta, R. Y., Ram, D., Shibukumar, T. M., & Kokane, A. (2016). *National mental health survey of India, 2015–16: Prevalence, patterns and outcomes* (p. 129). National institute of mental health and neuro sciences, Nimhans publication.
Harrison, B. J., Daron, J. D., Palmer, M. D., & Weeks, J. H. (2021). Future sea-level rise projections for tide gauge locations in south Asia. *Environmental Research Communications, 3*(11), Article 115003.
Hashemi, A. H., & Cochrane, R. (2009). Expressed emotion and schizophrenia: A review of studies across cultures. *International Review of Psychiatry, 11*(2–3), 219–224. https://doi.org/10.1080/09540269974401
Hassan, K. W. (2010). *Migration of Kashmiri pundits: Kashmiriyat Challenged?* Bangalore, India. http://103.154.2.116/~max233devisec/wp-content/uploads/2023/07/WP-237-Khalid_2.pdf
Hossain, A. T., Rahman, M. H., Manna, R. M., Akter, E., Islam, S. M. H., Hossain, M. A., Ara, T., Usmani, N. G., Chandra, P., Khan, M. A., Rahman, S. M. M., Ahmed, H. U., Mozumder, M. K., Juthi, J. M., Shahrin, F., Shams, S. A., Afroze, F., Banu, M. J., Ameen, S., … Rahman, A. E. (2025). Enhancing access to mental health services for antepartum and postpartum women through Telemental health services at wellbeing centers in selected health facilities in Bangladesh: Implementation research. *JMIR Pediatrics and Parenting, 8,* e65912. https://doi.org/10.2196/65912
Hussain, A., Kumar, B., Kumar, M., & Roub, F. (2023). Reducing the mental health treatment gap in Kashmir: Scaling up to maximise the potential of telepsychiatry. *eClinicalMedicine, 59.* https://doi.org/10.1016/j.eclinm.2023.101972

Hussaini, S. J., Ali, S. H., Rahmat, Z. S., Islam, Z., & Tharwani, Z. H. (2022). Mental health impacts of earthquake on Afghans amidst humanitarian crisis. *Annals of Medicine & Surgery, 81*. https://doi.org/10.1016/j.amsu.2022.104521

IDMC. (2020). *Global report on internal displacement*. Internal Displacement Monitoring Centre (IDMC). https://www.internal-displacement.org/global-report/grid2020/downloads/2020-IDMC-GRID-south-asia.pdf?v=1.17

IEP. (2024). *Institute for Economics & Peace. Global Terrorism Index 2024: Measuring the Impact of Terrorism,*. Institute for Economics & Peace. https://www.economicsandpeace.org/wp-content/uploads/2024/02/GTI-2024-web-290224.pdf

Institute for Research and Development. (2008). *National survey on mental health in Sri Lanka 2007*. institute for research and development. https://ird.lk/wp-content/uploads/2007/03/NMHS-Final-Report-15-10-2008.pdf

Jones, G. W., Hull, T. H., & Mohamad, M. (2015). *Changing marriage patterns in Southeast Asia*. Routledge. https://api.taylorfrancis.com/content/books/mono/download?identifierName=doi&identifierValue=10.4324/9780203813461&type=googlepdf

Jones, G. W., & Yeung, W.-J.J. (2014). Marriage in Asia. *Journal of Family Issues, 35*(12), 1567–1583. https://doi.org/10.1177/0192513X14538029

Kapilashrami, A., & John, E. A. (2023). Health beyond borders: Migration and precarity in south Asia. In S. I. Rajan (Ed.), *Migration in south Asia: IMISCOE regional reader* (pp. 201–213). Springer International Publishing. https://doi.org/10.1007/978-3-031-34194-6_14

Kar, S. K., Arafat, S. M. Y., & Menon, V. (Eds.). (2024). *Dhat syndrome: Medical, psychological and sociocultural aspects*. Springer Nature. https://doi.org/10.1007/978-981-99-8870-9

Kar, S. K., & Menon, V. (2024). Mental healthcare access in India: Models, trends, and challenges. In S. M. Y. Arafat & S. K. Kar (Eds.), *Access to mental health care in south Asia* (pp. 71–89). Springer Nature Singapore. https://doi.org/10.1007/978-981-99-9153-2_5

Kar, S. K., & Sarkar, S. (2015). Dhat syndrome: Evolution of concept, current understanding, and need of an integrated approach. *Journal of Human Reproductive Sciences, 8*(3), 130–134. https://doi.org/10.4103/0974-1208.165143

Kar, S. K., & Singh, A. (2016). Person centered management approach for the Dhat syndrome. *International Journal of Person Centered Medicine, 6*(4), Article 4. https://doi.org/10.5750/ijpcm.v6i4.615

Karasz, A., Gany, F., Escobar, J., Flores, C., Prasad, L., Inman, A., Kalasapudi, V., Kosi, R., Murthy, M., Leng, J., & Diwan, S. (2019). Mental health and stress among south Asians. *Journal of Immigrant and Minority Health, 21*(Suppl 1), 7–14. https://doi.org/10.1007/s10903-016-0501-4

Katbamna, S., Ahmad, W., Bhakta, P., Baker, R., & Parker, G. (2004). Do they look after their own? Informal support for south Asian carers. *Health and Social Care in the Community, 12*(5), 398–406. https://doi.org/10.1111/j.1365-2524.2004.00509.x

Kaufman, C. C., Pirutinsky, S., & Rosmarin, D. H. (2023). Spirituality/religion and self-harm among patients with alcohol/substance use versus other disorders. *The Journal of Nervous and Mental Disease, 211*(8), 566–571. https://doi.org/10.1097/NMD.0000000000001655

Kaur, A., Kallakuri, S., Kohrt, B. A., Heim, E., Gronholm, P. C., Thornicroft, G., & Maulik, P. K. (2021). Systematic review of interventions to reduce mental health stigma in India. *Asian Journal of Psychiatry, 55*, Article 102466. https://doi.org/10.1016/j.ajp.2020.102466

Khadka, S. (2021). Earthquake induced displacement and living arrangements in Nepal. *Voice of Teacher, 6*(1), 159–168.

Khanal, G., Selvamani, Y., & Sapkota, P. (2023). Insights on historical milestones of mental health in Nepal: Country profile. *Indian Journal of Psychiatry, 65*(11). https://journals.lww.com/indianjpsychiatry/fulltext/2023/65110/insights_on_historical_milestones_of_mental_health.5.aspx

Khanal, K., & Sen, R. (2020a). An institutional analysis of the dowry system in south Asia. In *The Gift in the Economy and Society* (pp. 141–159). Routledge. https://www.taylorfrancis.com/chapters/edit/https://doi.org/10.4324/9781003044567-10/institutional-analysis-dowry-system-south-asia-kalpana-khanal-ruchira-sen

Khanal, K., & Sen, R. (2020b). The dowry gift in south Asia: An institution on the intersection of market and patriarchy. *Journal of Economic Issues, 54*(2), 356–362. https://doi.org/10.1080/00213624.2020.1743145

Koser, K. (2022). 8. The migration-displacement nexus and security in Afghanistan. In K. Koser & S. Martin (Eds.), *The migration-displacement nexus* (pp. 131–144). Berghahn Books. https://doi.org/10.1515/9780857451927-011

Kovess-Masfety, V., Keyes, K., Karam, E., Sabawoon, A., & Sarwari, B. A. (2021). A national survey on depressive and anxiety disorders in Afghanistan: A highly traumatized population. *BMC Psychiatry, 21*(1), 314. https://doi.org/10.1186/s12888-021-03273-4

Kronenfeld, D. A. (2008). Afghan refugees in Pakistan: Not all refugees, not always in Pakistan, not necessarily Afghan? *Journal of Refugee Studies, 21*(1), 43–63.

Kudva, K. G., El Hayek, S., Gupta, A. K., Kurokawa, S., Bangshan, L., Armas-Villavicencio, M. V. C., Oishi, K., Mishra, S., Tiensuntisook, S., & Sartorius, N. (2020). Stigma in mental illness: Perspective from eight Asian nations. *Asia-Pacific Psychiatry: Official Journal of the Pacific Rim College of Psychiatrists, 12*(2), Article e12380. https://doi.org/10.1111/appy.12380

Lam, T., & Yeoh, B. S. A. (2019). Parental migration and disruptions in everyday life: Reactions of left-behind children in Southeast Asia. *Journal of Ethnic and Migration Studies, 45*(16), 3085–3104. https://doi.org/10.1080/1369183X.2018.1547022

Leff, J., Wig, N. N., Bedi, H., Menon, D. K., Kuipers, L., Korten, A., Ernberg, G., & Day, R. (1990). Expressed emotion research in London, UK, Chandigarh, India and Aarhus, Denmark. *Mental Health Retrosight, 156*(3), 165.

Li, Y., Jin, Q., & Li, A. (2022). Understanding the multidimensional poverty in south Asia. *Journal of Geographical Sciences, 32*(10), 2053–2068. https://doi.org/10.1007/s11442-022-2036-z

Macrotrends. (2025). *south Asia Unemployment Rate 1991–2025.* https://www.macrotrends.net/global-metrics/countries/SAS/south-asia/unemployment-rate

Majumder, J., Saha, I., Bagepally, B. S., Kalita, M., Munikrishnappa, D., Ray, S., Saha, A., & Chakrabarti, A. (2024). Mental health burden following extreme weather events in South-east Asia: A systematic review and meta-analysis. *Indian Journal of Psychiatry, 66*(8), 683–694. https://doi.org/10.4103/indianjpsychiatry.indianjpsychiatry_348_24

Marmot, M. (2005). Social determinants of health inequalities. *The Lancet, 365*(9464), 1099–1104. https://doi.org/10.1016/S0140-6736(05)71146-6

*Migration data in Southern Asia.* (2025, January 31). Migration data portal. https://www.migrationdataportal.org/regional-data-overview/southern-asia

Ministry of Health. (2024). *Annual health bulletin.* Policy and Planning Division, Ministry of Mealth.

Ministry of Public Health Afghanistan. (2019). *Mental health guidelines.* General directorate of curative medicine directorate of central hospitals Kabul mental health hospital. https://moph.gov.af/sites/default/files/2019-09/Hospital%20Guidelines%20Mental%20Health%20English.pdf

Mirza, M. M. Q. (2011). Climate change, flooding in south Asia and implications. *Regional Environmental Change, 11*(S1), 95–107. https://doi.org/10.1007/s10113-010-0184-7

Mishra, S., & Kar, S. K. (2023). Perception of mental health and illness among North Indian population in the current era. *Odisha Journal of Psychiatry, 19*(2), 65–66.

Mohamed, A., & Mansoor, S. (2024). Challenges and opportunities in the mental health landscape of the Maldives. *Australasian Psychiatry.* https://doi.org/10.1177/10398562241289879

MoHFW. (2025). *National tele mental health programme (Tele MANAS).* https://telemanas.mohfw.gov.in/home

Naveed, S., Waqas, A., Chaudhary, A. M. D., Kumar, S., Abbas, N., Amin, R., Jamil, N., & Saleem, S. (2020). Prevalence of common mental disorders in south Asia: A systematic review and meta-regression analysis. *Frontiers in Psychiatry, 11,* Article 573150. https://doi.org/10.3389/fpsyt.2020.573150

Parnini, S. N., Othman, M. R., & Ghazali, A. S. (2013). The Rohingya refugee crisis and Bangladesh-Myanmar relations. *Asian and Pacific Migration Journal, 22*(1), 133–146. https://doi.org/10.1177/011719681302200107

Patwary, M. M., Bardhan, M., Haque, M. A., Moniruzzaman, S., Gustavsson, J., Khan, M. M. H., Koivisto, J., Salwa, M., Mashreky, S. R., Rahman, A. K. M. F., Tasnim, A., Islam, M. R., Alam, M. A., Hasan, M., Harun, M. A. Y. A., Nyberg, L., & Islam, M. A. (2024). Impact of extreme weather events on mental health in South and Southeast Asia: A two decades of systematic review of observational studies. *Environmental Research, 250,* Article 118436. https://doi.org/10.1016/j.envres.2024.118436

Powell-Jackson, T., Pereira, S. K., Dutt, V., Tougher, S., Haldar, K., & Kumar, P. (2016). Cash transfers, maternal depression and emotional well-being: Quasi-experimental evidence from India's Janani Suraksha Yojana programme. *Social Science & Medicine, 162,* 210–218. https://doi.org/10.1016/j.socscimed.2016.06.034

Raheem, R. A., & Moosa, S. (2022). *WHO step survey on risk factors for noncommunicable diseases Maldives 2020–2021.* The Maldives National University, Health Protection Agency, and World Health Organization.

Rahman, R., Sheehan, D., Javed, A., Ahmad, S. H., Shafiq, K., Kanwal, U., Afridi, M. I., Nizami, A. T., Rasool, G., Taj, R., Ansari, M., Naim, M., Farooq, S., Memon, A., Karim, M. S., Hana, Y., & Ayub, M. (2024). *The national psychiatric morbidity survey of Pakistan (2022): prevalence, socio-demographic and disability correlates* (p. 2024.07.08.24310056). medRxiv. https://doi.org/10.1101/2024.07.08.24310056

Rajkumar, R. P. (2024). The phenomenology of Dhat syndrome. In S. K. Kar, S. M. Y. Arafat, & V. Menon (Eds.), *Dhat syndrome: Medical, psychological and sociocultural aspects* (pp. 1–17). Springer Nature. https://doi.org/10.1007/978-981-99-8870-9_1

Raymo, J. M., Park, H., Xie, Y., & Yeung, W. J. (2015). Marriage and family in east Asia: Continuity and change. *Annual Review of Sociology, 41*(2015), 471–492. https://doi.org/10.1146/annurev-soc-073014-112428

Research Unit. (2025). *Advancing mental healthcare in India.* Ministry of Health and Family Welfare. https://static.pib.gov.in/WriteReadData/specificdocs/documents/2025/feb/doc202527497201.pdf

Ridley, M., Rao, G., Schilbach, F., & Patel, V. (2020). Poverty, depression, and anxiety: Causal evidence and mechanisms. *Science, 370*(6522), Article 6522.

Sabawoon, A., Keyes, K. M., Karam, E., & Kovess-Masfety, V. (2022). Associations between traumatic event experiences, psychiatric disorders, and suicidal behavior in the general population of Afghanistan: Findings from afghan national mental health survey. *Injury Epidemiology, 9*(1), 31. https://doi.org/10.1186/s40621-022-00403-8

Sardinha, L., Maheu-Giroux, M., Stöckl, H., Meyer, S. R., & García-Moreno, C. (2022). Global, regional, and national prevalence estimates of physical or sexual, or both, intimate partner violence against women in 2018. *The Lancet, 399*(10327), 803–813. https://doi.org/10.1016/S0140-6736(21)02664-7

Seeman, N., Tang, S., Brown, A. D., & Ing, A. (2016). World survey of mental illness stigma. *Journal of Affective Disorders, 190,* 115–121.

Sharma, P., & Joshi, D. (2024). Access to mental health care in Bhutan: Current status, potential challenges, and ways out. In S. M. Y. Arafat & S. K. Kar (Eds.), *Access to mental health care in south Asia* (pp. 57–69). Springer Nature Singapore. https://doi.org/10.1007/978-981-99-9153-2_4

Sivakumar, M. V. K., & Stefanski, R. (2010). Climate change in south Asia. In R. Lal, M. V. K. Sivakumar, S. M. A. Faiz, A. H. M. Mustafizur Rahman, & K. R. Islam (Eds.), *Climate change and food security in south Asia* (pp. 13–30). Springer Netherlands. https://doi.org/10.1007/978-90-481-9516-9_2

South Asian Health Hub. (2024, February 13). *Exploring the role of religion and spirituality in coping with mental illness in south Asia.* https://southasianhealth.co.uk/blog/exploring-the-role-of-religion-and-spirituality-in-coping-with-mental-illness-in-south-asia

Story, M. (2010). Displacement: Effect of Immigration on Families. *Caring For the south Asian Soul,* 9.

Subramanee, S. D., Agho, K., Lakshmi, J., Huda, Md. N., Joshi, R., & Akombi-Inyang, B. (2022). Child marriage in south Asia: A systematic review. *International Journal of Environmental Research and Public Health, 19*(22), 15138. https://doi.org/10.3390/ijerph192215138

Teo, D. C. L., Duchonova, K., Kariman, S., & Ng, J. (2021). Religion, spirituality, belief systems and suicide. In C. A. Alfonso, P. S. Chandra, & T. G. Schulze (Eds.), *Suicide by self-immolation: Biopsychosocial and transcultural aspects* (pp. 183–200). Springer International Publishing. https://doi.org/10.1007/978-3-030-62613-6_14

Thirthalli, J., & Rao, N. P. (2016). Special supplement: Yoga and mental health. *International Review of Psychiatry (Abingdon, England), 28*(3), 231–232. https://doi.org/10.1080/09540261.2016.1195975

Tol, W. A., Kohrt, B. A., Jordans, M. J. D., Thapa, S. B., Pettigrew, J., Upadhaya, N., & de Jong, J. T. V. M. (2010). Political violence and mental health: A multi-disciplinary review of the literature on Nepal. *Social Science & Medicine, 70*(1), 35–44. https://doi.org/10.1016/j.socscimed.2009.09.037

Trani, J.-F., Bakhshi, P., Kuhlberg, J., Narayanan, S. S., Venkataraman, H., Mishra, N. N., Groce, N. E., Jadhav, S., & Deshpande, S. (2015). *Mental illness, poverty and stigma in India: A case–control study*. https://doi.org/10.1136/bmjopen-2014-006355

UNICEF south Asia. (2025). *Child marriage | UNICEF south Asia*. https://www.unicef.org/rosa/what-we-do/child-protection/child-marriage

UNODC. (2013). *NATIONAL DRUG USE SURVEY MALDIVES - 2011 / 2012*. UNODC.

Vaishnav, M., Javed, A., Gupta, S., Kumar, V., Vaishnav, P., Kumar, A., Salih, H., Levounis, P., Ng, B., Alkhoori, S., Luguercho, C., Soghoyan, A., Moore, E., Lakra, V., Aigner, M., Wancata, J., Ismayilova, J., Islam, M. A., Da Silva, A. G., … Ashurov, Z. (2023). Stigma towards mental illness in Asian nations and low-and-middle-income countries, and comparison with high-income countries: A literature review and practice implications. *Indian Journal of Psychiatry, 65*(10), 995–1011. https://doi.org/10.4103/indianjpsychiatry.indianjpsychiatry_667_23

Valatheeswaran, C., & Rajan, S. I. (2011). Sri Lankan Tamil refugees in India: Rehabilitation mechanisms, livelihood strategies, and lasting solutions. *Refugee Survey Quarterly, 30*(2), 24–44.

Vidyasagaran, A. L., McDaid, D., Faisal, M. R., Nasir, M., Muliyala, K. P., Thekkumkara, S., Wright, J., Huque, R., Benkalkar, S., & Siddiqi, N. (2023). Prevalence of mental disorders in south Asia: A systematic review of reviews. *Cambridge Prisms: Global Mental Health, 10*, Article e78. https://doi.org/10.1017/gmh.2023.72

Vinke, K., Martin, M. A., Adams, S., Baarsch, F., Bondeau, A., Coumou, D., Donner, R. V., Menon, A., Perrette, M., Rehfeld, K., Robinson, A., Rocha, M., Schaeffer, M., Schwan, S., Serdeczny, O., & Svirejeva-Hopkins, A. (2017). Climatic risks and impacts in south Asia: Extremes of water scarcity and excess. *Regional Environmental Change, 17*(6), 1569–1583. https://doi.org/10.1007/s10113-015-0924-9

Virupaksha, H. G., Kumar, A., & Nirmala, B. P. (2014). Migration and mental health: An interface. *Journal of Natural Science, Biology, and Medicine, 5*(2), 233–239. https://doi.org/10.4103/0976-9668.136141

WHO. (2021a). *Mental health and forced displacement*. Mental Health and Forced Displacement. https://www.who.int/news-room/fact-sheets/detail/mental-health-and-forced-displacement

WHO. (2021b). *Mental health atlas 2020*. World Health Organization.

WHO. (2024). *Data*. Datadot. https://data.who.int/countries/004

WHO. (2025). *Indicators*. The Global Health Observatory. https://www.who.int/data/gho/data/indicators

World Bank. (2022). The Global health cost of pm2.5 air pollution: A case for action beyond. (2021). International development in focus. *World Bank*. https://doi.org/10.1596/978-1-4648-1816-5

World Bank. (2024). Poverty, prosperity, and planet report 2024: Pathways out of the Polycrisis. *World Bank*. https://doi.org/10.1596/978-1-4648-2123-3

World Bank Group. (2025). *World bank open data.* World Bank Open Data. https://data.worldbank.org

World Bank. south Asia Regional Office. (2023). *Striving for clean air: Air pollution and public health in south Asia.* International Bank for Reconstruction and Development/The World Bank.

World Health Organization, & Calouste Gulbenkian Foundation. (2014). *Social determinants of mental health.* World Health Organization. https://iris.who.int/bitstream/handle/10665/112828/9789241506809_eng.pdf

Wu, A., Wang, J.-Y., & Jia, C.-X. (2015). Religion and completed suicide: A meta-analysis. *PLOS ONE, 10*(6), Article e0131715. https://doi.org/10.1371/journal.pone.0131715

Yeung, W.-J.J., Desai, S., & Jones, G. W. (2018). Families in Southeast and south Asia. *Annual Review of Sociology, 44*(1), 469–495. https://doi.org/10.1146/annurev-soc-073117-041124

# Chapter 2
# Social Psychiatry in Afghanistan

**Mohammad Akbar Paiman**

**Abstract** The social epidemiology of mental illness in Afghanistan highlights the interplay of social, political, and economic factors that shape the burden and distribution of mental health disorders. Decades of armed conflict, displacement, poverty, and social inequality have contributed to a significant mental health crisis, with high prevalence and incidence rates of psychiatric disorders across various demographics. In Afghan society, mental illness is frequently misunderstood, which leads to significant stigmatization of individuals affected by psychiatric disorders. This stigma is rooted in traditional cultural beliefs, where mental health issues are often interpreted as personal weaknesses or moral failings, rather than medical conditions requiring professional treatment. As a result, individuals experiencing mental health challenges are often labeled as "crazy" or "possessed" by evil spirits, reinforcing harmful stereotypes. This misconception contributes to their marginalization, as they are subjected to social exclusion, verbal use, and even physical neglect. The collective nature of Afghan social structures means that mental health challenges are frequently interpreted as family or community concerns rather than individual medical conditions.

**Keywords** Mental health · Social psychiatry · Conflict · Illiteracy · Culture · Afghanistan

## 1 Introducing the Historical Development of Social Psychiatry

Afghanistan, a landlocked country in Central and South Asia, has a long and complex history marked by its geographical significance as a cultural and trade crossroads (Yar et al., 2023). The country has witnessed repeated invasions, wars, and shifting regimes that have influenced its social, cultural, and health structures, including

M. A. Paiman (✉)
UCN, WHO, Abuja, Nigeria
e-mail: paimanm@who.int

 
S. M. Y. Arafat et al. (eds.), *Social Psychiatry in South Asia*, South Asian Perspectives in Mental Health and Psychology , https://doi.org/10.1007/978-981-96-8078-8_2

mental health services (Rasool et al., 2024). Historically, Afghanistan was part of ancient empires such as the Achaemenid Empire, the Mauryan Empire, and later the Islamic caliphates. It became a significant trade and cultural exchange center during the Silk Road era. The emergence of Afghanistan as a modern nation-state in the eighteenth century under Ahmad Shah Durrani: unified fragmented regions, but instability persisted due to tribal divisions and external interference (Jalali, 2021).Please be aware that your name and affiliation and if applicable those of your co-author(s) will be published as presented in this proof. If you want to make any changes, please correct the details now. Please note that after publication corrections won't be possible. Due to data protection we standardly publish professional email addresses, but not private ones, even if they have been provided in the manuscript and are visible in this proof. If you or your co-author(s) have a different preference regarding the publication of your mail address(s) please indicate this clearly. If no changes are required for your name(s) and affiliation(s) and if you agree with the handling of email addresses, please respond with "Ok".Offical email ID added with new affliation Kindly check and verify that the author name(s) and the identification of the corresponding author(s) are correctly recognized and presented in the correct sequence order and spellings, i.e., given name, middle name/initial, and family name for the authors. In addition, please verify that the E-mail addresses and Affiliation(s) of the corresponding author(s) and co-author(s) shown on the metadata page are valid, and make any necessary amendments if required.Done

The socio-political landscape in Afghanistan has been shaped by colonial interests, particularly during the Anglo-Afghan Wars of the nineteenth century (Saikal, 2004). The twentieth century brought modernization efforts under King Amanullah Khan in the 1920s, but these were disrupted by conservative resistance. The Soviet invasion (1979–1989), subsequent civil war, Taliban rule (1996–2001), and two decades of conflict after the U.S.-led intervention (2001–2021) have significantly impacted Afghanistan's social and healthcare infrastructure (Saikal, 2004). The US-led collation government collapsed on 15 August 2021 and the Taliban took over the government for the second time in the past two decades. This prolonged instability has deeply influenced the population's mental health, leading to a high burden of trauma, depression, and anxiety (Alemi et al., 2023).

The historical landscape of mental health in Afghanistan is profoundly shaped by centuries of complex social, political, and cultural dynamics (Alemi et al., 2023). From the early modern period through successive waves of geopolitical transformation, Afghanistan's mental health trajectory reflects the intricate interplay between traditional societal structures, religious interpretations, and external political influences (Alemi et al., 2023; Barfield, 2022). Traditional Afghan cultural frameworks predominantly interpret mental illness through religious and supernatural lenses (Mustafaeva, 2015). Spiritual explanations, including possession by *Jinns* (supernatural entities), were common interpretations of psychological disturbances. Religious scholars and traditional healers, known as mullahs and hakims, played pivotal roles in addressing mental health challenges, often employing spiritual interventions and traditional healing practices (Mustafaeva, 2015).

The historical development of mental health services in Afghanistan from 1985–2019 is mentioned in Table 1, taken from the thematic review of four decades of research and interventions for Afghan mental health and psychosocial well-being (Alemi et al., 2023).

Islamic theological interpretations significantly influenced mental illness perceptions. The Quranic perspective generally viewed psychological suffering as a potential spiritual test or divine challenge, encouraging patience, prayer, and community support (Rassool, 2000). This theological framework simultaneously provided compassionate understanding and potential stigmatization of severe mental health conditions. The political landscape of Afghanistan profoundly impacted mental health structures and experiences (Eggerman & Panter-Brick, 2010). Successive

**Table 1** Historical development of mental health services in Afghanistan 1985–2019 (Alemi et al., 2023)

| Year | Milestones |
|---|---|
| 1985 | Department of Mental Health established in the Ministry of Public Health (MoPH), Kabul |
| 1987 | First Mental Health Act ratified by Parliament |
| 1988 | The First psychologists and social workers graduated from Kabul University |
| 1988 | Kabul Psychiatric Hospital (the first hospital dedicated to mental health) established with 100 beds |
| 1988 | The first mental health training manual (Mental Health for All) for general practitioners introduced |
| 1989 | The First drug treatment center in Afghanistan, established at the Khushal Khan Polyclinic, Kabul, supported by UNDCP and WHO |
| 1992 | Loosening of mental health facilities following the closure of the mental health department at the MoPH in Kabul |
| 2003 | Basic Package of Health Services introduced, with mental health as one of seven modules |
| 2004 | The mental health unit in the Ministry of Public Health re-established |
| 2005 | First published guideline for mental health in Afghanistan: "Mental Health in Primary Healthcare: Diagnosis and Treatment of Priority Mental Health Conditions in Afghanistan" |
| 2005 | Mental health included in the Essential Package of Hospital Services |
| 2005 | Directorate of Drug Demand Reduction established in the Ministry of Public Health |
| 2005 | Revision of the Basic Package of Health Services, which included psychosocial counseling as part of comprehensive health centers |
| 2011 | National Mental Health Strategy 2011–2015 launched |
| 2019 | Department of Counseling at Kabul University established |
| 2019 | The First National Suicide Prevention Strategy was developed |
| 2019 | National Mental Health Strategy 2019–2023 launched |
| 2019 | The first basic mental health training program for female school counselors, led by the Ghazanfar Institute of Health Science |

periods of conflict, including foreign invasions, internal civil wars, and prolonged international interventions, created complex psychological trauma landscapes. The Soviet-Afghan War (1979–1989) and subsequent civil conflicts generated extensive collective psychological trauma, disrupting traditional social support systems and exacerbating mental health challenges (Eggerman & Panter-Brick, 2010).

The Afghan society is organized around tribal, ethnic, and family-based structures, with Pashtuns, Tajiks, Hazaras, and Uzbeks being the major ethnic groups. Social cohesion revolves around extended families, and kinship plays a significant role in individual identity and decision-making (Yousaf, 2019). Afghan culture, rooted in Islam, emphasizes collectivism, modesty, and social harmony. Mental illness, however, remains a misunderstood and stigmatized topic in Afghan society (Saleem, 2015). Cultural norms often equate mental health disorders with moral or spiritual weakness, leading to individuals being ostracized or subjected to religious interventions, such as exorcisms and faith healing. Such beliefs delay professional help-seeking and exacerbate the burden of mental illness (Saleem, 2015). Common disorders such as post-traumatic stress disorder (PTSD), depression, and anxiety are often attributed to spiritual possession or divine punishment. For example, jinn possession is a common cultural belief associated with mental illness, and families may consult religious leaders before seeking medical intervention. Gender roles further shape mental health experiences (Mustafaeva, 2015). Women face higher rates of depression and anxiety due to pervasive gender-based violence, forced marriages, and lack of education. Traditional gender roles limit women's autonomy, compounding their vulnerability to mental health issues (Mustafaeva, 2015).

Human rights conditions, particularly concerning vulnerable populations like women and children, significantly influence mental health experiences. Patriarchal social structures, limited women's rights, and ongoing conflict created environments of chronic psychological stress and potential traumatization (Eggerman & Panter-Brick, 2010). The current de facto government of Afghanistan, the Taliban, has imposed a ban on education and employment for girls and women over the past three years. This has significantly worsened the mental health and well-being of Afghan women and girls. Such actions represent a clear violation of human rights, depriving millions of women and girls of their fundamental freedoms and opportunities (Hamidi, 2024). The lack of legal protections for individuals with mental illnesses further marginalizes them. There are few policies in place to address stigma or discrimination, and mental health remains a low priority in national agendas (Mustafaeva, 2015).

## 2 The Impact of Migration and Displacement on Mental Health

Migration and displacement in Afghanistan have had profound effects on the mental health of the population, driven largely by decades of armed conflict, political instability, natural disasters, and economic hardship (Saleem et al., 2021). These factors have created a context in which millions of Afghans are displaced internally or have sought refuge in other countries, significantly increasing the prevalence of mental health disorders such as depression, anxiety, and PTSD (Saleem et al., 2021). Repeated cycles of violence have forced families to leave their homes, often with little warning or resources (Saleem et al., 2021). Displacement is often prolonged, with many individuals living in camps or informal settlements for years, further exacerbating mental health challenges (Hosseini et al., 2024; Neyazi et al., 2024). Displacement often leads to the loss of livelihoods, social networks, and access to basic services, creating significant stress and anxiety. Studies show that up to 40–50% of displaced Afghans exhibit symptoms of mental health disorders, including PTSD, depression, and anxiety (Cardozo et al., 2004; Hosseini et al., 2024). The prevalence of PTSD is particularly high, with rates as high as 50–60% among those directly exposed to violence or forced to flee their homes (Jankovic-Rankovic & Panter-Brick, 2024; Saleem et al., 2021). Forced displacement disrupts community and familial bonds, critical sources of emotional and social support. Many displaced individuals report feelings of isolation, helplessness, and cultural disconnection. For refugees abroad, language barriers, discrimination, and lack of integration further amplify mental health challenges (Hosseini et al., 2024). Economic instability is a pervasive challenge for displaced populations (Saleem et al., 2021). In Afghanistan, internally displaced persons (IDPs) are often unable to secure stable jobs due to lack of documentation, skills, or discrimination. Refugees abroad frequently face similar challenges, with restricted access to work opportunities. Prolonged financial insecurity creates chronic stress and exacerbates symptoms of mental illness (Trani et al., 2016b). Access to mental healthcare for displaced populations is extremely limited. Afghanistan's under-resourced mental health system provides coverage for less than 10% of those in need (Hosseini et al., 2024). For refugees, mental health services are often inaccessible due to financial, cultural, and logistical barriers, leaving many untreated (Hosseini et al., 2024).

## 3 Social Epidemiology of Mental Illnesses in Afghanistan

The social epidemiology of mental illness in Afghanistan highlights the interplay of social, political, and economic factors that shape the burden and distribution of mental health disorders (Alemi et al., 2023; Mustafaeva, 2015). Decades of armed conflict, displacement, poverty, and social inequality have contributed to a significant mental health crisis, with high prevalence and incidence rates of psychiatric disorders across various demographics (Mustafaeva, 2015).

### 3.1 Prevalence of Mental Disorders

Research indicates that one in two Afghans experiences symptoms of mental health disorders, with rates particularly high among women, children, and displaced populations. According to a report by the World Health Organization (WHO), approximately 60–70% of Afghanistan's population suffers from symptoms of depression, anxiety, or PTSD (Aminullah, 2021). Studies conducted in Afghanistan further emphasize that about 50% of adults demonstrate signs of psychological distress, with women showing higher prevalence due to gender-based violence, societal restrictions, and lack of access to care (Trani et al., 2016a).

The prevalence of PTSD in Afghanistan is among the highest globally, with rates ranging from 35 to 40% among the general population (Cardozo et al., 2004). For women, especially widows and victims of violence, PTSD prevalence reaches up to 60%. Anxiety disorders are also widespread, affecting 45% of adults. Depression, often exacerbated by poverty and unemployment, affects approximately 30% to 40% of the population, with notable regional variations (Trani et al., 2016c). Mental health disorders are particularly high among displaced individuals, with PTSD rates exceeding 50%. Refugees and IDPs also suffer from depression and substance use disorders, driven by trauma, uncertainty, and loss of social networks (Morina et al., 2018). Social determinants, such as poverty, unemployment, violence, and displacement, play a central role in Afghanistan's mental health crisis. With 55% of the population living below the poverty line, chronic economic hardship fosters stress and hopelessness (Trani et al., 2016c). Unemployment, which affects 40% of Afghans, particularly the youth, contributes to substance use and increased risk of depression and suicide (Trani et al., 2016c).

In children, mental disorders are particularly alarming. A study conducted revealed that around 38% of Afghan children display symptoms of PTSD, depression, and other anxiety-related disorders due to exposure to violence, conflict, and displacement (Qamar et al., 2022). These conditions impair cognitive development and school performance, perpetuating cycles of poverty and ill health (Qamar et al., 2022).

### 3.2 Substance Use

Substance use represents a profound and escalating public health crisis in Afghanistan, intricately linked to complex social, economic, and psychological dynamics (Shaikh et al., 2024). The country's geopolitical landscape, characterized by prolonged conflict, economic instability, and global drug production networks, has created a multifaceted substance use environment with significant mental health implications (Shaikh et al., 2024). Epidemiological research reveals alarming substance use patterns. According to the United Nations Office on Drugs and Crime, approximately 11–12% of the Afghan population struggles with substance dependency, representing one of the highest addiction rates globally (Singh et al., 2024). Opioid use, particularly heroin and opium, constitutes the primary substance use challenge, with methamphetamine and cannabis usage emerging as secondary concerns (Nafeh et al., 2022). Substance use prevalence demonstrates significant regional variations. Urban centers like Kabul and Herat exhibit higher substance dependency rates compared to rural areas (Nafeh et al., 2022). Young male populations between 18 and 35 years represent the most vulnerable demographic, with socioeconomic marginalization and chronic trauma exposure contributing to increased addiction risks (Farook et al., 2022). Substance use in Afghanistan functions as a complex maladaptive coping mechanism. Chronic exposure to conflict, intergenerational trauma, economic instability, and psychological distress creates environments where substance use emerges as a potential emotional regulation strategy (Shaikh et al., 2024). Individuals experiencing prolonged psychological challenges frequently utilize substances as temporary relief mechanisms from anxiety, depression, and post-traumatic stress symptoms (Miller & Rasmussen, 2010; Shaikh et al., 2024). Afghanistan's role as a global opium producer creates unique substance use dynamics (Goodhand, 2005). The agricultural and economic infrastructure surrounding opium production generates complex socioeconomic networks that facilitate substance availability and normalization (Mansfield, 2016). Limited economic opportunities, particularly in rural regions, contribute to individuals' engagement in drug production and consumption ecosystems (Mansfield, 2016).

Gender represents a critical analytical lens in understanding substance use patterns. Male populations demonstrate significantly higher substance dependency rates, reflecting broader social structures and masculinity conceptualizations (Mukerji et al., 2023). Women's substance use experiences remain largely hidden due to stringent social norms and potential familial stigmatization (Mukerji et al., 2023). Substance use demonstrates profound comorbidity with various mental health conditions (Sullivan, 2022). Epidemiological studies indicate that approximately 60–65% of individuals with substance dependency experience concurrent mental health challenges, including major depressive disorder, PTSD, generalized anxiety disorder, and bipolar spectrum disorder (Sullivan, 2022). Cultural frameworks significantly influence substance use perceptions. Religious interpretations, community norms, and traditional healing practices create nuanced perspectives on addiction (Alemi et al., 2018). Some communities view substance dependency as a moral failing, while others interpret it through spiritual or supernatural lenses, complicating professional intervention strategies (Alemi et al., 2018).

## 4 Mental Health Literacy and Stigma

Mental health literacy in Afghanistan remains notably low, primarily due to a combination of deeply ingrained cultural beliefs, limited educational resources, and restricted access to reliable information (Alemi et al., 2023). In Afghan society, mental illness is frequently misunderstood, which leads to significant stigmatization of individuals affected by psychiatric disorders. This stigma is rooted in traditional cultural beliefs, where mental health issues are often interpreted as personal weaknesses or moral failings, rather than medical conditions requiring professional treatment (Alemi et al., 2023). As a result, individuals experiencing mental health challenges are often labeled as "crazy" or "possessed" by evil spirits, reinforcing harmful stereotypes. This misconception contributes to their marginalization, as they are subjected to social exclusion, verbal use, and even physical neglect (Alemi et al., 2023; Trani et al., 2016a). The stigma extends beyond the individual, impacting their families as well. In a culture where family honor and reputation are of paramount importance, having a family member with a mental illness is frequently viewed as a source of shame. This perception often leads to further isolation, as families may avoid seeking help to protect their social standing (Alemi et al., 2023). Such social stigma creates significant barriers to mental healthcare, discouraging individuals and families from seeking treatment or support. Many are reluctant to acknowledge mental health problems, fearing the shame and social ostracism that may follow. This cultural dynamic also discourages open discussion of mental health, making it even more difficult for individuals to access the necessary resources for coping with mental distress (Alemi et al., 2023). In response to these challenges, several international organizations and non-governmental organizations (NGOs) have launched efforts to improve mental health literacy in Afghanistan. These initiatives include community-based education programs designed to challenge misconceptions and raise awareness about mental health issues. By focusing on educating the public about the biological and psychological aspects of mental illnesses, these programs aim to reduce stigma and encourage a more compassionate understanding of mental health (Alemi et al., 2023). Despite these efforts, progress remains slow. Deep-seated cultural resistance to changing traditional beliefs about mental illness remains a significant obstacle. Many communities continue to view mental health issues through the lens of superstition or religious interpretation, which complicates the acceptance of modern psychiatric care (Alemi et al., 2023). Additionally, the ongoing political instability and conflict in Afghanistan, along with a lack of trained mental health professionals, further exacerbate the situation. While there have been some positive developments, such as the establishment of mental health services in certain regions, the overall impact on the country's mental health landscape has yet to reach the scale needed for widespread change (Alemi et al., 2023; Hamidi, 2024).

## 5 Health-Seeking Behavior and Community Attitude Toward Mental Health

The intricate landscape of mental health help-seeking in Afghanistan represents a complex interplay of deeply rooted cultural beliefs, socioeconomic constraints, and traditional healing practices (Mustafaeva, 2015). Health-seeking behaviors emerge from a sophisticated ecosystem of cultural interpretation, social hierarchy, and limited healthcare infrastructure that fundamentally shapes how mental health challenges are perceived and addressed. Traditional healing practices constitute the primary initial intervention for mental health concerns in Afghan communities. Spiritual healers, known as *mullahs and pirs,* are pivotal in interpreting psychological disturbances through religious and supernatural frameworks (Mustafaeva, 2015). These practitioners typically employ a combination of Quranic recitations, herbal treatments, and spiritual interventions deeply embedded in Islamic theological perspectives. The traditional healing often involves ritualistic practices such as *dam* (spiritual healing through Quranic recitations), amulet writing, and herbal remedies (Alemi et al., 2023). Families frequently view these interventions as holistic approaches that address both spiritual and physical dimensions of mental suffering. The belief that psychological challenges can be manifestations of spiritual trials or supernatural interventions remains prevalent across various Afghan ethnic communities (Alemi et al., 2023).

Gender represents a critical dimension in mental health help-seeking behaviors. Patriarchal social structures create significant barriers to women's access to mental health services (Mustafaeva, 2015). Women's medical consultations are frequently mediated through male family members, creating complex decision-making landscapes that delay or prevent appropriate interventions. Societal norms restrict women's independent movement and healthcare choices, necessitating male familial approval for medical consultations (Alemi et al., 2023). This structural constraint means that women's mental health challenges are often silenced, minimized, or addressed through familial and community-based mechanisms rather than professional medical interventions. Economic constraints significantly impede mental health help-seeking behaviors (Mustafaeva, 2015). Afghanistan's persistent economic challenges, exacerbated by prolonged conflict and political instability, create substantial barriers to accessing professional mental health services (Alemi et al., 2023). Rural communities face particularly challenging circumstances, with limited healthcare infrastructure and significant financial constraints preventing specialized psychiatric interventions. The economic burden of mental health treatment extends beyond direct medical costs (Alemi et al., 2023). Transportation expenses, potential loss of daily wage earnings, and indirect family support costs create substantial financial disincentives for seeking professional help. Many families prioritize immediate survival needs over specialized mental health interventions (Mustafaeva, 2015).

Social networks play a crucial role in mediating mental health help-seeking behaviors. Extended family structures, tribal affiliations, and community elder recommendations significantly influence treatment decisions (Alemi et al., 2023). Community perception and potential stigmatization create complex psychological landscapes where individuals must balance personal mental health needs with broader social expectations. The collective nature of Afghan social structures means that mental health challenges are frequently interpreted as family or community concerns rather than individual medical conditions (Alemi et al., 2023). This perspective can simultaneously provide supportive mechanisms and create potential barriers to specialized interventions. Limited trust in formal medical institutions, resulting from years of conflict and healthcare system disruptions, further complicates help-seeking behaviors (Miller & Rasmussen, 2010). Experiences of political instability, healthcare infrastructure collapse, and limited professional mental health resources have created generational skepticism toward formal medical interventions. Mental illness in Afghan contexts is frequently interpreted through multidimensional lenses that blend medical, spiritual, and social perspectives (Pirani, 2009). Psychological challenges are often understood as potential spiritual tests, supernatural interventions, or manifestations of broader familial or community challenges (Alemi et al., 2023). These interpretative frameworks create nuanced help-seeking pathways where individuals might simultaneously engage multiple healing mechanisms (Alemi et al., 2023). A family might consult a religious healer, seek traditional herbal treatments, and potentially explore limited professional medical interventions in a complex, layered approach to mental health management (Cardozo et al., 2004). Emerging generational shifts, particularly in urban centers like Kabul, demonstrate increasingly sophisticated approaches to mental health (Alemi et al., 2023). Younger, more educated populations show growing openness to professional psychiatric interventions, reflecting broader educational and societal transformations. Urban–rural divides create significant variations in help-seeking behaviors. Urban populations demonstrate relatively more progressive attitudes, greater access to information, and increased willingness to explore professional mental health services compared to more traditional rural communities (Alemi et al., 2023; Miller & Rasmussen, 2010).

## 6 Challenges and Opportunities in Community-Based Mental Health Interventions in Afghanistan

Community-based mental health interventions in Afghanistan offer a crucial pathway to addressing the country's significant mental health crisis (Trani et al., 2016a). However, implementing such initiatives faces various challenges, including cultural, logistical, and financial constraints. At the same time, the country's resilience and strong community networks present unique opportunities for integrating mental health services into community settings (Trani et al., 2016a).

## 6.1 Challenges in Community-Based Mental Health Interventions in Afghanistan

Addressing mental health in deteriorated environments requires tailored strategies that integrate community needs and cultural sensitivities. Mental health awareness campaigns delivered in local languages by government appointees can educate populations about behavioral health issues and the benefits of seeking psychiatric care. Strengthening primary care workers' mental health training—targeting nurses, midwives, and doctors—can bridge the gap until specialized mental health workers are more widely available (Sheikh Shoib et al, 2024). NGOs play a crucial role in improving access to quality mental health services, while psychiatric education reforms in medical schools and timely referrals by healthcare workers contribute to strengthening the mental health framework. Initiatives like the Basic Package of Health Services (2005) have introduced mental health education, case detection, and treatment as core elements (Sheikh Shoib et al, 2024). Partnerships with international NGOs and the use of telemedicine have enhanced service delivery and accessibility, particularly in urban areas and for vulnerable populations such as women and girls. However, further revisions to policies and legislation are needed to address emergency preparedness, law enforcement, and expanded access to mental health services (Sheikh Shoib et al., 2024).

### 6.1.1 Stigma and Cultural Barriers

Afghan society attaches a high degree of stigma to mental health issues, often viewing them as signs of personal weakness or spiritual failure. This perception discourages individuals from seeking professional care and leads families to rely on traditional or faith-based healers (Trani et al., 2016a). Moreover, cultural norms often marginalize discussions on mental illness, especially for women, due to gender roles and societal expectations (Gough & Novikova, 2020). The Taliban banned girls' and women's education and employment further exacerbating the mental health of girls and women and depriving them of their basic human rights in Afghanistan (Alemi et al., 2023).

### 6.1.2 Lack of Mental Health Infrastructure

The Afghan healthcare system is underfunded and overstretched, with less than 1% of the national health budget allocated to mental health. The availability of trained mental health professionals is minimal which hampers the scale and effectiveness of community-based mental health interventions in Afghanistan and a huge number of health professionals left the country after the collapse of the government on 15 August 2021(Alemi et al., 2023).

### 6.1.3 Poverty and Socioeconomic Challenges

High levels of poverty and unemployment—affecting over 50% of the population—divert priorities away from mental health. People often prioritize basic needs, such as food and shelter, over seeking mental health services. Financial constraints also make it difficult for communities to invest in health promotion and preventive care (Alemi et al., 2023; Shaikh et al., 2024).

## *6.2 Opportunities in Community-Based Mental Health Interventions in Afghanistan*

Afghanistan has made efforts to address mental health through national policies and programs, beginning with the enactment of its first mental health policy in 1987. This policy emphasized integrating mental health services into primary healthcare, reducing reliance on large psychiatric hospitals, and advocating for patient rights. Subsequent revisions in 1997 incorporated provisions for voluntary and involuntary treatment, judicial processes for individuals with mental illness, and improved accreditation of mental health professionals and facilities (WHO, 2010). In 2005, the Ministry of Public Health introduced the Basic Package of Health Services, which includes mental health education, case detection, and treatment, aimed at expanding access to mental healthcare across the country. Despite these initiatives, challenges persist in fully implementing these policies, particularly in rural and conflict-affected areas. Rehabilitation facilities in Afghanistan are limited and primarily concentrated in urban centers, where small groups of NGOs provide mental health support, particularly for vulnerable populations such as women and girls. These facilities offer services like counseling, psychotherapy, and psychosocial support to help individuals regain independence and improve their quality of life (Alemi et al., 2023). However, Afghanistan lacks a robust health insurance system to cover mental health services, leaving many patients to rely on international aid organizations and NGOs. Partnerships with groups like Health Net International and International Medical Corps have played a crucial role in filling gaps in service delivery. Expanding rehabilitation facilities and introducing mental health insurance schemes remain critical priorities to ensure equitable and sustainable mental healthcare for all Afghans (WHO, 2010).

### 6.2.1 Integration with Primary Healthcare

One of the most promising strategies for expanding mental health services is integrating mental health into primary healthcare (Alemi et al., 2023). Community health workers (CHWs) already operating in remote areas can be trained to provide basic mental health interventions, such as psychological first aid and referrals to higher-level care. This integration reduces stigma and improves accessibility (Alemi et al., 2023).

### 6.2.2 Utilizing Traditional and Religious Leaders

Afghanistan's community structure revolves around traditional leaders and religious clerics, who hold significant influence over societal norms. Partnering with these figures can help normalize mental health discussions and encourage people to seek appropriate care (Alemi et al., 2023).

### 6.2.3 Task-Shifting and Capacity Building

Given the shortage of mental health professionals, task-shifting—training CHWs and nurses to deliver evidence-based psychological interventions—is a viable solution. Programs like the Basic Package of Health Services (BPHS) have demonstrated success in incorporating mental health into community health delivery models (Alemi et al., 2023).

### 6.2.4 Role of NGOs and International Agencies

Several NGOs and international organizations, including WHO, UNICEF, and Médecins Sans Frontières, support mental health programs in Afghanistan. These organizations can provide technical expertise, training, and funding to strengthen Community-Based Mental Health Interventions in Afghanistan, especially in rural areas (Alemi et al., 2023).

### 6.2.5 Community Resilience and Social Networks

Afghan communities exhibit high levels of social cohesion and resilience. These networks can be leveraged to create peer support groups and community-based rehabilitation programs, which are cost-effective and culturally acceptable (Trani et al., 2016a). Coercion psychiatry refers to the use of involuntary measures to treat individuals with mental health disorders, often justified in cases where the person poses a danger to themselves or others. In Afghanistan, the concept of coercion psychiatry is fraught with ethical, cultural, and systemic challenges, rooted in the country's limited mental health infrastructure and social stigmas surrounding mental illness (Trani et al., 2016a).

Afghanistan lacks a comprehensive mental health act or legal framework to regulate involuntary psychiatric treatment. As a result, coercion practices often occur informally and without oversight, frequently driven by families seeking help for relatives with severe mental disorders, such as schizophrenia or psychosis. These individuals are sometimes confined in homes or religious shrines under the care of traditional healers, a practice influenced by cultural beliefs associating mental illness with spiritual afflictions (Trani et al., 2016a).

## 7 Telepsychiatry in Afghanistan

Telepsychiatry presents a significant opportunity to address Afghanistan's mental health challenges, particularly given the limited infrastructure and workforce. With fewer than 0.3 psychiatrists per 100,000 people, and mental health facilities concentrated in urban centers, vast rural populations lack access to care. Telepsychiatry, involving remote consultations through technology, can bridge this gap by providing mental health services to underserved regions.

### *7.1 Afghan Telemedicine Initiative*

The Afghan Telemedicine initiative (afghan-telemedicine.org) is focused on addressing the healthcare challenges in Afghanistan by utilizing telemedicine and e-learning platforms.

- Purpose: To improve access to healthcare, especially in rural and underserved areas, where the availability of mental health professionals is critically low.
- Programs: Includes telemedicine workshops, training for local healthcare providers, and e-learning modules to enhance medical knowledge and service delivery, including mental healthcare.
- Impact on Mental Health: The platform is instrumental in integrating telepsychiatry services to connect patients with psychiatric care providers, overcoming the barriers posed by geographical and infrastructural limitations.

### *7.2 Online Therapy Services by MantraCare*

MantraCare (mantracare.org) offers comprehensive online therapy solutions tailored to the needs of Afghan residents.

- Services Offered:

  Cognitive Behavioral Therapy (CBT): Effective for treating anxiety, depression, and trauma.
  Dialectical Behavior Therapy (DBT): Focused on managing emotional dysregulation and stress.

Eye Movement Desensitization and Reprocessing (EMDR): Specialized for trauma-related care.

- Accessibility: These services are designed to be affordable and accessible through virtual platforms, making it possible for individuals in remote areas to receive mental healthcare.
- Significance: The service bridges the gap for Afghans facing stigma around in-person mental health services by providing a private and secure alternative.

## 8 Recommendations

Interventions addressing mental health in Afghanistan must be culturally relevant and aligned with Afghan conceptualizations of well-being. This requires intensive consultation with local stakeholders, ensuring co-ownership and sustainability by incorporating cultural values such as faith, perseverance, and family relationships. Effective programs should focus on the social and physical manifestations of distress rather than over-medicalizing symptoms while addressing gender disparities within the framework of Afghan worldviews. Emphasizing the social embeddedness of psychosocial distress is critical for interventions to resonate with local populations. In Afghanistan, mental health challenges are deeply rooted in everyday stressors like economic hardship, family conflicts, and restrictive social norms. Refugees, while often demonstrating resilience and adaptability, face unique challenges, including economic exclusion, cultural bereavement, and shifts in social status and gender roles. Programs must address these interconnected issues, supporting both in-country populations and refugees through approaches that mitigate social stressors and promote hope, agency, and inclusion (Alemi et al., 2023).

Strengthening community-based psychosocial support and evidence-based psychological interventions in Afghanistan requires substantial investment. Equitable access to services must prioritize vulnerable groups, including women, ethnic minorities, children, and adolescents. Given the familial conflicts often underpinning mental health issues and the reluctance of some Afghans to seek professional help due to family resistance, interventions should focus on enhancing individual and family capacities to manage stress and support one another. Community-level approaches that normalize mental healthcare, rather than pathologize it, have shown feasibility and effectiveness, emphasizing the need for culturally and contextually adapted solutions. Further research is crucial to establish evidence-based psychological interventions tailored to Afghan languages and contexts. This includes assessing their effectiveness and understanding the mechanisms for scaling up interventions through implementation research. Using community-based participatory approaches ensures local voices guide the development of mental health and psychosocial support (MHPSS) programs, making them relevant and sustainable. Additionally, integrating mental health initiatives into broader strategies targeting poverty alleviation, social cohesion, peacebuilding, and reconciliation can amplify their impact and promote long-term well-being (Alemi et al., 2023).

Core mental health services must be integrated into primary health centers and general hospitals across Afghanistan to ensure accessibility. Sustained financial support is critical to prevent the collapse of the health system and to prioritize mental health within the broader healthcare framework. A minimally acceptable standard of psychiatric services, as outlined by the Ministry of Public Health, must be preserved despite resource constraints. This requires initiatives to address systemic barriers to care and efforts to reduce the stigma associated with mental illnesses through widespread psychoeducation. Additionally, urgent action is needed to prevent and address substance use, particularly among at-risk youth, as the rise in drug use poses significant public health challenges. This concern is compounded by the increasing prevalence of HIV/AIDS and widespread misconceptions about its transmission. Targeted interventions combining education, prevention, and treatment are essential to mitigate these interconnected issues and to promote mental and physical well-being within Afghanistan's vulnerable populations (Alemi et al., 2023).

Core mental health services in Afghanistan must be sustained at accessible points such as primary health centers and general hospitals. To prevent the collapse of the country's overstretched health system, urgent financial support is required, with explicit attention to mental health needs. Maintaining a minimally acceptable standard of psychiatric care, as outlined in Ministry of Public Health guidelines, is essential. This effort must be accompanied by initiatives to reduce healthcare access barriers and destigmatize mental illnesses through psychoeducation. Addressing the urgent issue of drug use among at-risk youth is also critical, given its link to the rising prevalence of HIV/AIDS, and widespread misconceptions about its transmission. The prevalence of HIV was highest in Iran (11.0%), followed by Pakistan (8.6%) and Afghanistan (3.1%). For HCV, Pakistan recorded the highest prevalence (54.4%), followed by Iran (47.7%) and Afghanistan (37.3%) (Shayan et al., 2021). These findings highlight the substantial risk posed by needle sharing among injecting drug users in these countries. To address this, heightened awareness and targeted interventions are necessary to reduce the spread of HIV and HCV among this vulnerable group. Public health strategies, including harm reduction programs, needle exchange initiatives, and education campaigns, are recommended to curb the dual epidemics in this population (Shayan et al., 2021).

Humanitarian efforts should focus on building sustainable mental healthcare systems that integrate community-based psychosocial support, psychotherapeutic interventions, and clinical care into a cohesive framework. Capacity-building initiatives must engage the remaining mental health and psychosocial support (MHPSS) professionals in supervisory and training roles within Afghanistan. In countries hosting Afghan refugees, efforts should prioritize reinforcing social support systems and enhancing access to mental health services. This includes involving Afghan refugees in service provision, fostering community-based approaches, and creating culturally relevant programs to meet the mental health needs of displaced populations (Alemi et al., 2023).

# 9 Conclusion

The social epidemiology of mental illness in Afghanistan reveals the profound impact of social, political, and economic factors on mental health. Decades of armed conflict, displacement, poverty, and inequality have created a widespread mental health crisis, with high rates of psychiatric disorders across various demographics. However, mental illness remains highly stigmatized, as traditional Afghan cultural beliefs often perceive it as a moral failing or personal weakness rather than a medical condition requiring professional care. This stigma leads to social exclusion, discrimination, and neglect, with affected individuals frequently labeled as "crazy" or "possessed" by evil spirits. The collectivist nature of Afghan society further complicates mental health recognition, as psychological distress is often viewed as a family or community issue rather than an individual health concern. Addressing mental health challenges in Afghanistan requires culturally relevant interventions that align with local values and beliefs. Programs should be community-driven and incorporate traditional concepts of well-being, such as faith, perseverance, and family support, to ensure acceptance and sustainability. Collaboration with local stakeholders, religious leaders, and healthcare professionals is essential to destigmatize mental illness and integrate mental health services into existing social structures. Additionally, awareness campaigns, training for healthcare workers, and accessible mental health services can bridge the gap between traditional perceptions and modern psychiatric care, ultimately reducing the burden of mental disorders in Afghan society.

# References

Alemi, Q., Panter-Brick, C., Oriya, S., Ahmady, M., Alimi, A. Q., Faiz, H., Hakim, N., Hashemi, S. A. S., Manaly, M. A., Naseri, R., Parwiz, K., Sadat, S. J., Sharifi, M. Z., Shinwari, Z., Ahmadi, S. J., Amin, R., Azimi, S., Hewad, A., Musavi, Z., … Siddiqi, A. M. (2023). Afghan mental health and psychosocial well-being: Thematic review of four decades of research and interventions. *BJPsych Open, 9*(4), e125. https://doi.org/10.1192/bjo.2023.502

Alemi, Q., Stempel, C., Koga, P. M., Montgomery, S., Smith, V., Sandhu, G., Villegas, B., & Requejo, J. (2018). Risk and protective factors associated with the mental health of young adults in Kabul, Afghanistan. *BMC Psychiatry, 18*,, 1–10. https://doi.org/10.1186/s12888-018-1648-4

Aminullah, A. (2021). *The impact of physical disability on psychological status like anxiety and depression of Afghani people on Paktia province Afghanistan* Bangladesh Health Professions Institute, Faculty of Medicine, the University …]. https://doi.org/10.1177/0022146520921371

Barfield, T. J. (2022). Afghanistan: A cultural and political history. https://www.jstor.org/stable/j.ctt7sqkc

Cardozo, B. L., Bilukha, O. O., Crawford, C. A. G., Shaikh, I., Wolfe, M. I., Gerber, M. L., & Anderson, M. (2004). Mental health, social functioning, and disability in postwar Afghanistan. https://doi.org/10.1001/jama.292.5.575.

Eggerman, M., & Panter-Brick, C. (2010). Suffering, hope, and entrapment: Resilience and cultural values in Afghanistan. *Social Science & Medicine, 71*(1), 71–83. https://doi.org/10.1001/jama.292.5.575

Farook, M. İ, İlhan, M. N., & Koçak, C. (2022). Determination of epidemiological characteristics of addicts treated in drug addiction clinics in Kabul. *Journal of Ethnicity in Substance Abuse, 21*(3), 1063–1082. https://doi.org/10.1080/15332640.2020.1824842

Goodhand, J. (2005). Frontiers and wars: The opium economy in Afghanistan. *Journal of Agrarian Change, 5*(2), 191–216. https://doi.org/10.1080/15332640.2020.1824842; https://doi.org/10.1111/j.1471-0366.2005.00099.x

Gough, B., & Novikova, I. (2020). *Mental health, men and culture: how do sociocultural constructions of masculinities relate to men's mental health help-seeking behaviour in the WHO European Region?* WHO. https://www.ncbi.nlm.nih.gov/books/NBK559706/

Hamidi, A. B. (2024). Restriction Policy on Afghan Girls' Education and its Consequences. *Edukasiana: Jurnal Inovasi Pendidikan, 3*(2), 228–243. https://doi.org/10.56916/ejip.v3i2.691

Hosseini, Z., Syed, H., Raza, Z., Mansouri, M., Magan, I. M., & Awaad, R. (2024). A Systematic Review of Evidence-Based Interventions for Afghan Refugee Mental Health: A Cultural Adaptation Analysis. *Journal of Cross-Cultural Psychology, 55*(1), 25–46. https://doi.org/10.1177/00220221231213884

Jalali, A. A. (2021). Afghanistan: A military history from the ancient empires to the great game. *University Press of Kansas*. https://doi.org/10.2307/j.ctv264f9qw

Jankovic-Rankovic, J., & Panter-Brick, C. (2024). Physiological and genomic signatures of war and displacement: a comprehensive literature review and future directions. *Psychoneuroendocrinology,* 107084. https://doi.org/10.1016/j.psyneuen.2024.107084

Mansfield, D. (2016). *A state built on sand: How opium undermined Afghanistan.* Oxford University Press. https://www.hurstpublishers.com/book/a-state-built-on-sand/

Miller, K. E., & Rasmussen, A. (2010). War exposure, daily stressors, and mental health in conflict and post-conflict settings: Bridging the divide between trauma-focused and psychosocial frameworks. *Social Science & Medicine, 70*(1), 7–16. https://doi.org/10.1016/j.socscimed.2009.09.029

Morina, N., Akhtar, A., Barth, J., & Schnyder, U. (2018). Psychiatric disorders in refugees and internally displaced persons after forced displacement: A systematic review. *Frontiers in Psychiatry, 9,* 433. https://doi.org/10.5167/uzh-158377

Mukerji, R., Saboor, L., Paphitis, S., Devakumar, D., & Mannell, J. (2023). How does domestic violence stigma manifest in women's lives in Afghanistan? A study of survivors' lived experiences of help-seeking across three provinces. *Global Public Health, 18*(1), 2212035. https://doi.org/10.1080/17441692.2023.2212035

Mustafaeva, S. (2015). *The cultural shaping of depression: A qualitative investigation into afghan women's perspectives on depression.* The University of Regina (Canada). file:///C:/Users/akbar/Downloads/Mustafaeva_Shahlo_200241238_PhD_ClinPSYC_Spring2016.pdf

Nafeh, F., Fusigboye, S., & Sornpaisarn, B. (2022). Understanding injecting drug use in Afghanistan: A scoping review. *Substance Abuse Treatment, Prevention, and Policy, 17*(1), 65. https://doi.org/10.1186/s13011-022-00491-1

Neyazi, A., Mohammadi, A. Q., Razaqi, N., Rahimi, B. A., Sifat, S., Rahimy, N., Tareen, Z., Mehmood, Q., Satapathy, P., & Griffiths, M. D. (2024). Health survey on anxiety, depression, and stress in Afghanistan: A large-scale cross-sectional study amid ongoing challenges. *Discover Mental Health, 4*(1), 38. https://doi.org/10.1007/s44192-024-00090-5

Pirani, F. (2009). *Therapeutic encounters at a Muslim shrine in Pakistan: an ethnographic study of understandings and explanations of ill health and help-seeking among attenders.* Middlesex University.

Qamar, K., Rija, A., Vohra, L. I., Nawaz, F. A., & Essar, M. Y. (2022). Mental health implications on Afghan children: An impending catastrophe. *Global Mental Health, 9,* 397–400.

Rasool, G., Mukhtarova, K., & Jan, B. N. (2024). The role of Afghanistan in central Asia: risks and future prospects overview. *International Relations & International Law Journal/Seriâ Meždunarodnye Otnošeniâ & Meždunarodnoe Pravo, 106*(2). https://doi.org/10.26577/IRILJ.2024.v106.i2-06

Rassool, G. H. (2000). The crescent and Islam: healing, nursing and the spiritual dimension. Some considerations towards an understanding of the Islamic perspectives on caring. *Journal of Advanced Nursing, 32*(6), 1476–1484. https://doi.org/10.1046/j.1365-2648.2000.01614.x
Saikal, A. (2004). *Modern Afghanistan: A history of struggle and survival.* Bloomsbury Publishing. https://www.booktopia.com.au/modern-afghanistan-amin-saikal/book/9781780761220.html
Saleem, F. (2015). *Muslim mental health service providers reflect on working with Muslim women* University of Saskatchewan].https://harvest.usask.ca/server/api/core/bitstreams/fdfb8ffd-57d8-46d9-8a41-55d14b901c82/content
Saleem, S. M., Shoib, S., Dazhamyar, A. R., & Chandradasa, M. (2021). Afghanistan: Decades of collective trauma, ongoing humanitarian crises, Taliban rulers, and mental health of the displaced population. *Asian Journal of Psychiatry, 65,* Article 102854. https://doi.org/10.1016/j.ajp.2021.102854
Shaikh, O. A., Shoib, S., Saeed, F., & Nazari, S. K. (2024). Current perspectives on substance use disorders in Afghanistan. *Current Perspectives on Substance Use Disorders in South Asia: Public Mental Health Aspects,* 19-35. https://doi.org/10.1007/978-981-97-6619-2_2
Shayan, S. J., Nazari, R., & Kiwanuka, F. (2021). Prevalence of HIV and HCV among injecting drug users in three selected WHO-EMRO countries: A meta-analysis. *Harm Reduction Journal, 18*(1), 59. https://doi.org/10.1186/s12954-021-00505-4
Shoib, S., Hussaini, S.S., Nazari, S.K., Saeed, F. (2024). Mental Healthcare in Afghanistan. In: Arafat, S.M.Y., Kar, S.K. (eds) Access to Mental Health Care in South Asia. Springer, Singapore. https://doi.org/10.1007/978-981-99-9153-2_2
Singh, A., Joshi, M., & Parmar, A. (2024). Substance use disorder among women and children in South Asia. In *Current perspectives on substance use disorders in South Asia: Public mental health aspects* (pp. 279–303). Springer. https://doi.org/10.1007/978-981-97-6619-2_14
Sullivan, M. A. (2022). Drug use and mental health: Comorbidity between substance use and psychiatric disorders. *Substance and non-substance related addictions: A global approach,* 3-17. https://doi.org/10.1007/978-3-030-84834-7_1
Trani, J.-F., Ballard, E., Bakhshi, P., & Hovmand, P. (2016a). Community based system dynamic as an approach for understanding and acting on messy problems: A case study for global mental health intervention in Afghanistan. *Conflict and Health, 10,* 1–11. https://doi.org/10.1186/s13031-016-0089-2
Trani, J.-F., Ballard, E., & Peña, J. B. (2016b). Stigma of persons with disabilities in Afghanistan: Examining the pathways from stereotyping to mental distress. *Social Science & Medicine, 153,* 258–265. https://doi.org/10.1016/j.socscimed.2016.02.024
Trani, J.-F., Kuhlberg, J., Cannings, T., & Chakkal, D. (2016c). Multidimensional poverty in Afghanistan: Who are the poorest of the poor? *Oxford Development Studies, 44*(2), 220–245. https://doi.org/10.1080/13600818.2016.1160042
WHO. (2010). *WHO-AIMS: Mental health systems in selected low-and middle-income countries: a WHO-AIMS cross-national analysis.* World Health Organization. https://www.who.int/publications/i/item/9789241547741
Yar, F. G. M., Zahid, S., & Miakhil, J. M. (2023). Afghanistan's geopolitical and geo-economic significance in regional connectivity and development. *Journal of Political and Legal Sovereignty, 1*(2), 78–86. https://www.researchgate.net/publication/374813370_Afghanistan's_Geopolitical_and_Geo-Economic_Significance_in_Regional_Connectivity_and_Development_Corresponding_Author
Yousaf, F. (2019). https://docslib.org/doc/4577686/tribes-and-intrastate-conflict-using-indigenous-methods-for-conflict-resolution-in-pakistan-s-tribal-frontier

# Chapter 3
# Social Psychiatry in Bangladesh

**S. M. Yasir Arafat and Atiqul Haq Mazumder**

**Abstract** The etiopathological explanations of psychiatric disorders shifted from the biological to the biopsychosocial model. However, social determinants of psychiatric disorders have been poorly researched in South Asian countries like Bangladesh. Social psychiatry is yet to be developed as a separate entity with a lack of specialized degrees and training. In the current chapter, we discuss various aspects of social psychiatry in Bangladesh like social epidemiology of mental illness, mental health literacy and stigma toward mental health, health-seeking behavior, community attitude toward mental health, disorders and treatment, substance abuse, culture-bound syndromes, different social determinants of mental illness, mass media representation of mental illness, somatization, social prescribing, the role of traditional healing practices and their integration with modern psychiatric care, challenges and opportunities in implementing community-based mental health interventions, Mental Health Act and social rights, suicidal behavior, and prison mental health. We presented it based on available evidence from Bangladesh and to some extent our personal experience.

**Keywords** Social psychiatry · Social determinants · Bangladesh · Mental health · Health-seeking behavior

## 1 Introduction

Bangladesh is a lower-middle-income country with an area of 147,570 square kilometers in South Asia. It has a shared border with India on three sides and the Bay of Bengal lies on its South (Fig. 1). It has about 170 million people with a heavy

S. M. Y. Arafat (✉)
Department of Psychiatry, Bangladesh Specialized Hospital, Dhaka, Bangladesh
e-mail: arafatdmc62@gmail.com

Biomedical Research Foundation, Dhaka, Bangladesh

A. H. Mazumder
Department of Psychiatry, Faculty of Medicine, Research Unit of Clinical Medicine, University of Oulu, Oulu, Finland



S. M. Y. Arafat et al. (eds.), *Social Psychiatry in South Asia*, South Asian Perspectives in Mental Health and Psychology , https://doi.org/10.1007/978-981-96-8078-8_3

base population pyramid. The life expectancy was about 75 years which was slightly more in females. About 10% of the population was aged from 10 to 15 years, 28.6% were below 15 years, 56.4% were under 30 years, and 90.7% were under 60 years (Bangladesh Bureau of Statistics, 2024). Among the population, about 65% were married and about 30% were never married. The mean age of marriage was above 25 years for males and above 19 years for females. More than 90% of this population are Muslims. The male-to-female ratio was 0.98 and about 1.4% populations had disabilities. About 70% of the populations with aged 15 years and above use mobile phone, among them about 37% use internet, more than 25% had bank account and about 39% use mobile banking services. About 59% of the dwellers live in kancha house-holds, about 22% live in pucca house-holds, and about 18% lives in semi-pucca house-holds. Predominantly, Bangladesh has a male-dominant agro-based society with joint family culture in place with gradual shift in nuclear one. Generally, males are the major bread winners and females manage child rearing the household activities. Parents bear the financial supports for their children till they become economically productive. There are concerns of early marriage and parental decisions dominates the events in majority of the cases. There are high stigma toward mental illness and low mental health literacy. Psychiatric disorders are attributed to supernatural powers like Jinn, black magic, and evil eye (Arafat et al., 2024a).

Bangladesh got independence from Pakistan in 1971 which was a part of the British Empire till 1947. Constitutionally Bangladesh is a democratic country; however, the transition of power has been struggled to date. Military took the power several times. Moreover, in recent days, an authoritarian regime has grown in the country. Mass uprisings happened in 1990 and 2024 against authoritarian regimes protesting corruption (United Nations, 2025). There has been rampant corruption, money laundering, human rights violations, forced disappearance, extra-judicial killing, and political oppression over the years (Ahasan, 2023; Amnesty International, 2024; United Nations, 2025).

Despite these issues, after the independence Bangladesh experienced significant economic growth. The per capita income was 172 USD in 1974 which has raised to 2688 USD in 2022 (macrotrend, 2024). There is rise in urban population (9% in 1974; >31% in 2021), literacy rate (29% in 1974; 75% in 2021), unemployment (20% in 1974; 30% in 2021), and reduction of floating populations, population growth, dependency ratio (Bangladesh Bureau of Statistics, 2024).

Mental health is a neglected component of people living in Bangladesh. During the British period (before 1947), the establishment of asylum was noted in Dhaka (Murlibazar/Muralibazar) in 1815. During the Pakistan period (1947–71), a mental hospital was established in Pabna in 1957. After liberation, hospital set up was gradually expanded throughout the country (Arafat, 2024a; Arafat et al., 2024a). Although the services have been expanded the quantity is inadequate when compared to the services burden. There are extremely low budgetary allocation, inadequate and inequitably distributed human resources, high stigma, and supernatural causation of mental disorders persists in the country.

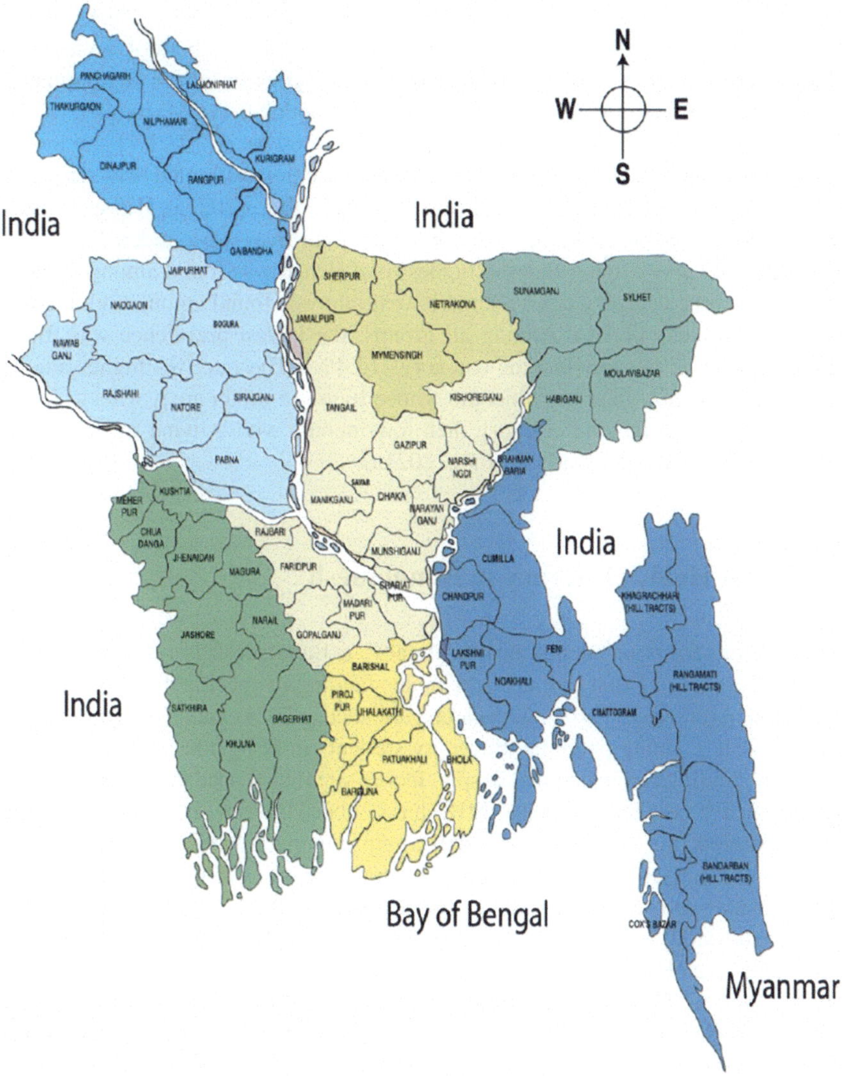


**Fig. 1** Map of Bangladesh (Adapted from Arafat et al., 2024a)

## 2 Social Epidemiology of Mental Illness

The latest nationwide community-based survey revealed the prevalence of psychiatry disorder among adults was 18.7 and among children (7–17 years) was 12.6% (Alam et al., 2024; Ministry of Health and Family Welfare, 2021a). The prevalence among adults was about 16% found in the previous study (Firoz et al., 2006). It revealed prevalence of mental illness was associated with socioeconomic deprivation (Firoz et al., 2006). The prevalence was significantly higher among females (2019, females 21.5%, males-15.7%; 2003–05, females-19%, males 12.9%) in both of the national mental health survey (Alam et al., 2024; Firoz et al., 2006). This female predominance has also been reported in other studies among adult populations (Mazumder, 2024). The rate was highest among the elderly age group (≥60 years) [28.1%] and lowest among young persons (18–29 years) [14.6%]. No variation was noted between urban and rural population (Ministry of Health and Family Welfare, 2021a). However, other studies indicate that the prevalence was higher in urban areas (Mazumder, 2024). The latest national survey found that the highest prevalence was found among females with high income category (24.4%) and lowest rate was found among high income category of males (14.5%). Among all groups, the lowest prevalence was found among females in the low-income category (13.4%). The rate was higher among low-income category than high income whose living in urban areas whistle it was higher among high income category then low-income whose living in rural areas (Ministry of Health and Family Welfare, 2021a).

## 3 Mental Health Literacy in Bangladesh

The academic focus on mental health literacy in Bangladesh is relatively recent. Research is emerging that evaluates the understanding of specific disorders such as depression (Arafat et al., 2019). A research published in 2024 examined mental health literacy (MHL) among potential university students in Bangladesh (Mamun et al., 2024). The findings indicated that despite facing significant academic pressures and psychological challenges, students' MHL has not been thoroughly investigated. The study identified four key aspects of MHL: help-seeking behaviors, stigma, mental health knowledge, and comprehension of mental illnesses. Furthermore, it unveiled notable gender and sociodemographic disparities in MHL.

A research study involving 2036 university students in Bangladesh evaluated their understanding and awareness of mental health (Siddique et al., 2022). The findings indicated that 62.1% of the participants had a strong knowledge of mental health, while 85.1% demonstrated high awareness. Female students and those with personal income and family backing exhibited greater knowledge levels. Additionally, older students tended to have higher awareness. Although awareness was high, knowledge levels were lacking, indicating a need for educational initiatives to bridge these gaps. The study recommends the development of national programs and policies aimed at integrating mental health services and enhancing community awareness through collaborative efforts from various disciplines and non-governmental organizations (NGOs).

There is a lack of content related to mental health in school curriculums, which contributes to low mental health literacy throughout the country. One important assessment of science books of primary and secondary schools (up to grade 10) and found that content on mental health was almost absent (Uddin, 2020).

## 4 Stigma Toward Mental Health in Bangladesh

Mental health remains a widespread stigmatized issue in the country. Both rural and urban populations harbor misconceptions about mental illness. Additionally, there is some bias against this topic, even among doctors of other specialities (Arafat et al., 2024a).

A cross-sectional survey revealed that various factors such as gender, age, geographical location, socioeconomic status, and occupation significantly impact the levels of stigma (Faruk et al., 2023). The research also highlighted a significant treatment gap, suggesting that many people avoid seeking the mental healthcare they need due to the stigma associated with mental illness.

A cross-sectional survey investigated the perspectives of mental health professionals (MHP) and media professionals (MP) regarding the reduction of mental illness stigma in Bangladesh involving 174 participants (Qusar et al., 2022). Both groups acknowledged that stigma is a critical issue and agreed on the necessity of improving public perceptions of psychiatry. The study recommends implementing reciprocal training and awareness programs to bridge the gaps between MHP and MP. Additionally, it suggests that further research with larger and more homogeneous samples is needed to enhance understanding and address these issues effectively.

Another research by Sifat et al., 2022 involved a survey of 350 university students in Bangladesh to evaluate their knowledge of mental health, awareness, and utilization of services. The findings revealed that the perceived need for mental health support was the most significant factor predicting the use of clinical services (Sifat et al., 2022). Additionally, favorable attitudes toward these services were associated with their usage, shaped by social influences and mental health knowledge. The study underscores the necessity of educational campaigns to enhance mental health literacy and diminish stigma, stressing the importance of culturally sensitive approaches and improved support systems within universities.

A research carried out at a hospital in Dhaka, examined family support and stigma experienced by 151 mental health patients (Jahan et al., 2017). The diagnoses represented included schizophrenia (56.3%), bipolar disorder (23.8%), and substance-related disorders (6.6%). A majority of the patients (66.2%) reported feeling supported by their families, yet 57.6% expressed fears of stigma if their condition were to be disclosed. The study emphasizes the importance of improving communication among patients, their families, and healthcare providers to help mitigate stigma. Limitations of the study include potential selection bias and issues with generalizability. The researchers suggest conducting further large-scale studies for more comprehensive insights.

Giasuddin and his colleagues conducted a study at *Faridpur Medical College* evaluated the stigma that medical students hold toward persons with mental disorders (PMDs) and their attitudes toward the field of psychiatry (Giasuddin et al., 2015). The findings indicated that older age, advanced years in medical school, and specific socioeconomic factors were associated with heightened stigma. Conversely, more positive attitudes toward psychiatry were linked to being female and belonging to a middle socioeconomic status. Even though attitudes toward psychiatry improved in the later years of study, the stigma against PMDs increased, emphasizing the necessity for anti-stigma initiatives and strategies to be incorporated into the medical curriculum.

## 5 Community Attitude Toward Mental Health in Bangladesh

Community attitudes toward mental health in Bangladesh are complex and influenced by various factors like literacy, stigma, and enduring beliefs about mental health. A 2008 study examined how mental illness was perceived in a village in Bangladesh, focusing on local terminology such as "*paglami*" and the beliefs surrounding the causes of illness, which included supernatural influences. Through observations, interviews, and focus groups, it was found that certain conditions were regarded as lifelong and untreatable from birth, while others were associated with substance abuse. Urban mental health services were not easily accessible (Selim & Satalkar, 2008). The research underscored the importance of combining traditional knowledge with current mental health systems in Bangladesh and advocated for more research to fill in the gaps and clarify these perceptions.

A cross-sectional survey was conducted among different indigenous groups to explore the stigma associated with mental illness in indigenous communities located in the Chattogram Hill Tracts of Bangladesh (Faruk & Rosenbaum, 2023). The study showed that women experienced higher levels of stigma compared to men. The stigma was linked to factors such as age, gender, socioeconomic status, and income. The results underscore the importance of implementing targeted anti-stigma initiatives and mental health strategies. These findings can help guide policymakers and stakeholders in creating effective programs aimed at reducing stigma and enhancing mental health literacy among indigenous populations in the area.

A study conducted in Narail, Bangladesh, evaluated mental health awareness, knowledge, and help-seeking behaviors among 2425 adults (Uddin et al., 2019). The findings indicated that awareness of mental health conditions (MHCs), such as depression and anxiety, was quite limited, particularly among older adults and women. Better awareness was associated with higher education levels and financial stability. Nevertheless, individuals who had some knowledge of MHCs showed a willingness to seek help. The study recommends focused interventions aimed at women, older adults, and individuals from low socioeconomic backgrounds to enhance mental health literacy and support in rural Bangladesh.

Community-based rehabilitation (CBR) can enhance service access for people with psychosocial or intellectual disabilities, epilepsy, or other cognitive impairments (Koly et al., 2022). Stigma, discrimination, and human rights abuses persist in Bangladesh, worsened by gender inequality. These factors act as barriers to access mental health in terms of cost, distance, and frequency of visits to mental health professionals.

Mental healthcare in Bangladesh faces challenges due to insufficient facilities, staff, skilled professionals, financial resources, and widespread stigma. Effective governance and mental health policies are lacking, exacerbating these issues. Stigma hinders help-seeking behavior, leading to social isolation and high psychiatric morbidity. Mass media interventions, like the Meena program, have shown success in reducing stigma related to autism and could be adapted for other mental illnesses (Hasan & Thornicroft, 2018). Political commitment, adequate funding, and international support are essential for effective stigma reduction programs.

## 6 Help-Seeking Behavior for Mental Illness in Bangladesh

Several factors need to be considered while considering the help-seeking behavior. Importantly, there is no functioning referral system and epidemiological catchment area. Additionally, psychiatrists are only posted at tertiary care level of health system. Thus, in a pluralistic health system with government, non-government, private, donor participants, people can visit any level of healthcare delivery and any level psychiatrist (Fig. 2). Due to the enduring stigma and misconceptions such as supernatural causation of mental disorder, sometimes it takes years to reach a mental health professionals and few percent reach mental health professionals directly (Arafat et al., 2024a; Arafat, 2024a; Giasuddin et al., 2012; Nuri et al., 2018). Traditional healers, religious leaders, village doctors are the first contacts for a good portion of patients. Traditional healers are available in several names like "Palli cikitsak or village doctors," alternate medicine practitioners, herbal practitioners, "Ojha," "Kabiraz," "Baba," "Pirr," "Sufi," "Fakir," "Huzur," "Samans," and "Homeopathy" (Giasuddin et al., 2012; Nuri et al., 2018; World Health Organization, 2015). The practice is so intense that cross-religion help-seeking to faith healers has been noted. There are incidences that Hindus visit Muslim faith healers for psychiatric symptoms and use "Tabiz" (Talisman) for treatment purposes of psychiatric illness. They expressed that they do it to relieve them from the suffering (personal experience).

One study found that only 16% of the patients with mental illness visited mental health professionals as their first contact (Giasuddin et al., 2012). Among the rest of the patients, 44% consulted general physicians, 22% consulted religious leaders, and 12% attended village doctors (Giasuddin et al., 2012). Another research conducted by Nuri et al. (2018) found that 30% of psychiatric consulted non-medical caregivers and 42.5% visited non-psychiatric doctors as their first service contact point. More than one in four patients (26.3%) consulted traditional healers, religious leaders, and herbal practitioner (Islam et al., 2001). The national mental health survey among children found that 30% of the guardians of child(ren) with mental illness visited traditional healers (Ministry of Health & Family Welfare, 2021). Available evidence suggests the extent of availing traditional services for mental illness could be up to 50% (Arafat et al., 2024a).

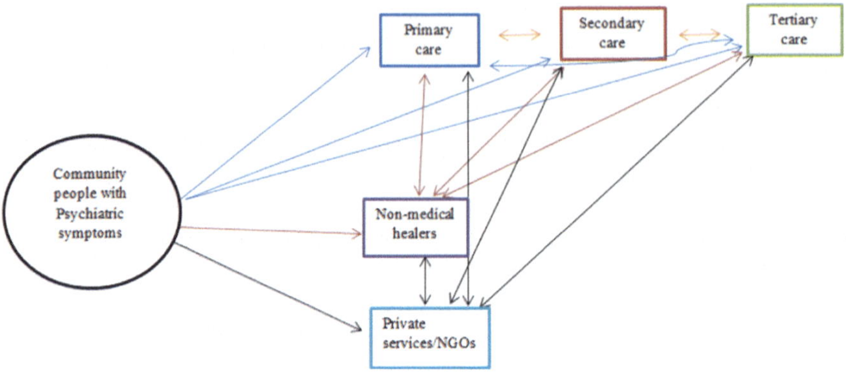


**Fig. 2** Potential help-seeking options for mental symptoms in Bangladesh (Adapted from Arafat et al., 2024a)

## 7 Culture-Bound Syndromes

### *7.1 Dhat Syndrome*

It is the most common psychosexual syndrome prevailed in Bangladesh related to anxiety in response to semen loss (Kar et al., 2021; Arafat & Ahmed, 2017; Miah et al., 2015; Mullick et al., 1995; Maruf et al., 2022; Maruf et al., 2024a). Hence, it has been considered as a sexual neurosis. A wide range of symptoms like somatic symptoms, psychiatric symptoms, and sexual dysfunctions are presented by the patients with Dhat syndrome. All the symptoms are attributed to the loss of semen through masturbation, nocturnal emission, and other natural ways. Generally, it is found in young, unmarried, less educated persons living in rural areas with low socioeconomic conditions. Semen has been considered as a valuable substance of soul and it should be preserved. Loss of semen causes loss of energy. However, it is also reported in females, married persons, and educated persons living in cities.

### *7.2 Jinn Possession*

The concept of Jinn is rooted in Islam. As more than 90% of inhabitants are Muslims, all most all mental symptoms are attributed to Jinn possession. Similar issues have been noted in Pakistan and other Islamic countries (Zulfiqar et al., 2019). Any psychological symptoms have been attempted to explain by Jinn possession. One study identified that, 61% of the respondents attributed mental disorder to Jinn possession (Mullick et al., 2013). Another study found that 22% of the psychiatric patients visited religious or traditional healers as first line caregiver (Giasuddin et al., 2012). The first national mental health survey found that about half of community participants believed the supernatural causation of mental disorder (Firoz et al., 2006).

### *7.3 Black Magic (Kalajadu) and Evil Eye (Bodnojor)*

It is also a culturally prevailed belief (Selim & Satalkar, 2008). People think that neighbors or enemies can produce psychiatric illness by black magic and evil eye. Surrounding people, neighbors, in-laws may become jealous and they can perform black magic to turn into mad. Their evil eye can also produce psychiatric illness. Traditional healers like Kabiraj convey similar message to the persons with psychiatric symptoms that someone (known or unknown) did black magic that produced the illness. It is also found in Pakistan (Zulfiqar et al., 2019). One study in Bangladesh found that 50% of respondents believed in black magic and 44% believed in evil eye (Mullick et al., 2013).

## 8 Somatization

Psychiatric patients can present with physical symptoms which is shaped by mental health literacy, stigma toward mental illness in the society, perception of mental disorders, available services for psychiatric disorders. Somatization has been found in about 50% of cases in developed countries even though the prevalence is higher in low- and middle-income countries (Lloyd, 1986). Somatization is common in Bangladesh in clinical practice. However, a limited number of studies have been revealed on it. Somatic presentation of depression has been studied in some studies (Nahar et al., 1995; Qusar et al., 2019; Selim, 2010). The earliest study assessed 52 patients with depression and found about 79% of respondents had somatic symptoms. The symptoms were burning sensation of whole body, headache, discomfort in head, body ache, and abdominal symptoms (Nahar et al., 1995). Another study noted somatic symptoms such as dizziness, body ache, pain, burning sensation, weakness, breathing difficulties, chest discomfort (Selim, 2010). Another study assessed 105 patients with depression in a tertiary care hospital and found that 36% of the patients had somatic symptoms. The revealed symptoms were headache, weakness, body ache, hearing difficulties, chest discomfort, and gastro-intestinal symptoms (Qusar et al., 2019).

## 9 Social Prescribing

It is an emerging way of improving mental well-being by addressing complex needs in the community specially in primary and secondary care level by voluntary and community participants through encouraging self- and personalized care (Calderón-Larrañaga et al., 2022). In Bangladesh, mental health services in the community and community participation for mental healthcare have been in the rudimentary stage (Karim et al., 2024; Arafat, 2024a; Arafat et al., 2024a). At this background, social prescribing is yet to be initiated in the country (Khan et al., 2024).

## 10 Mental Health Insurance

There is no available mental health insurance facility in Bangladesh for psychiatric care (Giasuddin et al., 2012; Arafat, 2024a; Arafat et al., 2024a). Mental healthcare gets <0.5% of total health budget, the majority of which has been used of hospital facilities. The per person expenditure on mental health is 0.1 USD per year (World Health Organization, 2022). Therefore, the out-of-pocket expense is high in the country. Although there is an extreme dearth of study assessing the issue, available evidence suggests that the out-of-pocket expense is more than 70% (Alamgir, 2024; World Bank, 2023).

## 11 Mental Health Act and Social Rights

The Mental Health Act has been passed in 2018 that supersedes the Lunacy Act, 1912 (Mental Health Act, 2018). It mentions about rights of health, property, dignity, education, and other rights in the Sect. 6. It also mentions the conditions of establishing the mental hospital, and their licensing. In the Sect. 17, the rights for health of the persons with mental illness have been mentioned. It declared that a persons with mental illness without guardians or relatives or without address shall be handed over to the nearest government mental hospital by the representative of the local government institution. If the person has mental illness and seems to be dangerous then local police will take over the person and send to the mental hospital. It is important to mention that to admit a patient at government mental hospital, it is mandatory to have at least an accompanying person. These ambiguity needs to be resolved.

Section 18 discusses the rehabilitation of persons with mental illness. It mentions that after the recovery of the mentally ill person without guardian or relative or without address, the concerned mental hospital shall transfer the said person to the concerned district or nearest social service institution or rehabilitation center along with his fitness certificate.

## 12 Coercion Psychiatry

The *Mental Health Act* categories hospitalizations of mentally ill patients in three different ways named as voluntary, non-protesting, and involuntary (Mental Health Act, 2018). Involuntary hospitalizations can be attempted with the application or consent of the guardian or relative of the person suffering from mental illness or the police officer working in the local jurisdiction or the medical officer in charge after completing a prescribed form. Emergency admission up to 72 h can be done based on the recommendation of the medical officer; admission for treatment or assessment for up to 28 days is permitted by recommendations of a psychiatrist. The admission can be extended based on the assessment and recommendations of the Mental Health Review and Monitoring Committee (Mental Health Act, 2018). Unfortunately, there is no services available at public level for forceful hospitalizations. Some private hospitals have such services named as emergency medical services (EMS) for picking up patients from home settings for involuntary admission (Arafat et al., 2016).

## 13 Prison Mental Health

It is a neglected area of mental health services in Bangladesh. There are 42,887 occupancies in 68 Jails (central Jail-13, district Jails-55). The occupancy rate is about 200%. As of 15 October 2024, there were 53,831 prisoners with an incarceration rate of 44 per 100,000 population, and the occupancy rate was about 125.5% (Arafat et al., 2024b; World Prison Brief, 2025). There was a release of more than 300,000 prisoners after the ousting of the authoritarian regime, followed by a mass uprising. According to the previous estimate (2023), the occupancy rate was about 200% which has reduced to 125.5%. The situation indicates the overall condition and mental health crisis in the prisons due to the political situation. The prevalence of psychiatric disorders ranged from 66.4 to 100% based on different studies, methods, and sample size in different time (see Ahmed et al., 2024; Arafat et al., 2024b; Arafat, 2025a). There is no nationwide study assessing the prevalence of psychiatric disorders among prisoners, no publicly available data on suicidal behavior among prisoners in the country, no existing mental health services in the prisons, no facility to visit prisoners by mental health professionals. There are 15 inpatient beds at the *National Institute of Mental Health (NIMH)*, Dhaka for Forensic Psychiatry services. Liaising with the legal bodies, disability assessment, diagnosis and management of prisoners with mental illness, and provision of mental health reports to government and autonomous bodies are the main domains of Forensic Psychiatry in Bangladesh (see Ahmed et al., 2024; Arafat et al., 2024b; Arafat, 2025a).

## 14 Tele-Psychiatry

Tele-psychiatry and tele-counselling are the emerging modes of psychiatric services for persons unable to attend chambers in person due to physical illness, distance, and environmental issues. It gets popularity during the COVID-19 pandemic. It is also an option for expatriates of Bangladesh. When they feel a psychological issue, then their relatives visit mental health professionals, arrange tele consultancy with the person, arrange medications, and send them to them. Psychiatrists, psychologists, counsellors use electronic modes frequently for these services. Private organizations also arrange it along with traditional services. At public level, it has been practiced at NIMH, Dhaka. Other institutions are yet to start it (Arafat, 2024a; Arafat et al., 2024a). *WhatsApp*, *Messenger*, *IMO*, and *FaceTime* are the widely used applications for the services. Tele-psychiatry services through Skype where medication names are mentioned in Bangla has also been noted in the country. It ensures better compliance.

## 15 Substance Abuse

The rate of substance abuse has been increasing over the last two decades (Maruf et al., 2024b). There are about 6 million persons with different forms of substance abuse (Department of Narcotics Control, 2023). The national community-based study found the prevalence was 3.3% among adults (Ministry of Health and Family Welfare, 2021b). It was 1.5% among 12–17 years of age and 0.2% among 7–11 years. Cannabis, methamphetamine (Yaba), and opioids as mostly used drugs in Bangladesh (Kamal et al., 2018; Maruf et al., 2024b). Alcohol use disorder is not common in the country like the Western countries.

## 16 Suicidal Behavior in Bangladesh

Likewise, the rest part of the world, suicidal behavior is a public health problem in Bangladesh. However, there is lack of political will to prevent it as evident by there is not national suicide prevention initiative, well-accepted suicide estimates, and nationwide study on suicidality. Additionally, there are concerns of misclassification and underreporting of suicide as it is a criminal offense in Bangladesh. Suicides have been noted in a wide range of age (8–78 years); however, the majority of suicides happened among persons aged up to 30 years. Suicides happen more in females than their male counterparts. Psychiatric disorders, life-events, unemployment, past non-fatal attempts, and marital and sexual relationship problems are important risk factors for suicide. Hanging and poisoning are the two prominent methods of suicide whereas superficial cut injury and sedative overdose are the prominent methods of self-harm. Suicidal behavior has been irresponsibly reported in news portals, newspapers, and cinema and movies with high proportions of harmful reporting characteristics and without potentially helpful reporting characteristics. There are high stigma toward suicidality and low literacy of suicide. There are sporadic, irregular, and inadequate suicide prevention initiatives in the country. Strong political will, professional participation and collaboration, and decriminalization of suicidal behavior could be some potential macro-level changes in favor of suicide prevention in Bangladesh (see Arafat & Saleem, 2025; Arafat, 2025b; Arafat & Khan, 2024, 2023; Arafat, 2023, 2024b; Kabir et al., 2023).

## 17 Marriage, Family, and Mental Illness

Family members have significant influence as a risk factor (predisposing, precipitating, and perpetuating) and management of psychiatric illness. Importantly, in Bangladesh, there is no epidemiological catchment area, well-functioning referral system family influences the patients to seek help from non-medical caregivers like traditional healers, may affect compliance in either way. Usually, family members are supportive and take care about the treatment of other members (Arafat et al., 2022). A marriage after an affair has not been well-accepted by the in laws in most of the situations that causes a lots of adjustment issues within the family. Additionally, a good portion of wives wants to live separately leaving the in laws apart that creates social issues and adjustment problems in the family. However, studies assessing the social parameters are warranted to dictate the direction precisely.

## 18 Social Security, Social Capital, Unemployment, and Mental Health in Bangladesh

Bangladesh made remarkable progress in poverty reduction since its independence. Poverty has been reduced from about 50% to 25% in 2015. The National Social Security Strategy (NSSS) of 2015 prioritized poverty, vulnerable groups, and marginalized population with an approach of considering "Life Cycle Risks" and about 2% allocation of *Gross Domestic Product (GDP)* (Government of the People's Republic of Bangladesh, 2015).

One cross-sectional study was conducted in Narsingdi among elderly population assessing the association of social capital and mental health [measured by *General Health Questionnaire* (GHQ-12) (Islam & Alam, 2014). It revealed that a mental health status was positively associated with cohesion with neighbors, social network, norms of reciprocity and social trust. A case–control study with 420 geriatric persons aged 60 years and above assessed the association between social capital and depression in a rural area (Islam et al., 2024). It revealed that geriatric depression was associated with sex, nuptiality, educational attainment, occupation, family dynamics (type, size, monthly income, interpersonal trust and reciprocity). It indicates cognitive social capital affects depression among elderly persons (Islam et al., 2024). One study with 824 youths (18–29 years) living in urban slum assessed the association between social network and psychiatric morbidity (measured by GHQ-12) (Rabbani et al., 2018). It revealed that social connections provide buffering effects to anxiety and stress that improves mental well-being. Another study assessed the association between social capital and perceived stress among 485 women (with and without employment) and found that social capital is negatively associated with perceived stress (Masoom, 2024). The finding was specially noted among unmarried and women without employment. There were no significant variations in social capital based on nuptiality and income. One study assessed the impact of smart phone addition and social capital among 384 university students (Mahmud et al., 2020). It found that smart phone addiction reduces social capital by reducing emotional sharing and responsibility toward family members (Mahmud et al., 2020).

Unemployment has been found as a contributing factor for mental disorders among unemployed educated job seekers (Mamun et al., 2020; Islam & Amanullah, 2024; Rafi et al., 2019).

## 19 Masculinity and Mental Health

Bangladeshi society is a male dominated culture where sometimes masculinity revealed as hegemonic while justifying tortures toward wives (Anwary, 2015; Yount et al., 2016). The prevalence of intimate partner violence was 15.5–82.7% and violence against women can play a complex interaction with mental illness (Bakchi et al., 2018; Islam et al., 2018; Esie et al., 2019). Common mental disorders were more than two times (2–2.3, AOR = 2.09) higher among women exposed to IPV in Bangladesh (De & Murshid, 2018; Tran et al., 2020). IPV was significantly associated with the development of maternal depression after childbirth between 6 and 8 months (Kabir et al., 2014), postpartum depression (Islam et al., 2017; Tasnim et al., 2021).

## 20 Migration and Displacement on Mental Health in Bangladesh

There are about one million Rohingya refugees in Bangladesh since 2017 (Jahan et al., 2024; UNHCR, 2024). Being forcefully displaced, these populations faced life-threatening trauma that made them vulnerable to develop different psychiatric disorder. The prevalence of mental disorders was around 90% among the Rohingya refugee in Bangladesh (Hossain et al., 2021; Riley et al., 2017). The Rohingya refugee rush creates an additional burden to mental health services as well as it causes an increase in local crime and drug abuse in the camps.

## 21 Disasters, Pandemics, and Mental Health in Bangladesh

Bangladesh is a coastal country affected by multiple disasters like floods, cyclones, droughts, fire, earthquakes affecting physical and mental health (Wahid et al., 2024; Siddik et al., 2024; Fatema et al., 2023). Depressive disorders, problems due to distress, and post-traumatic stress disorder were noted among adolescents affected by flood (Siddik et al., 2024). Exposure to floods was associated with poor psychological health notably anxiety, depression, stress, and PTSD (Wahid et al., 2024; Rahman et al., 2023; Mahmud et al., 2021). About two-thirds of the populations had mental trauma where females were more affected than males during disaster (Choudhury et al., 2006). Climate change also affects women due to their gender roles and household duties (Goudet et al., 2024). Poorer mental health conditions were noted among disaster affected women who experienced injuries, demised family members, and relocated during disasters (Fatema et al., 2023).

The COVID-19 pandemic affected mental health in Bangladesh. The prevalence of depression, anxiety, and stress was 47% and 44%, respectively (Hosen et al., 2021). Studies assessed loneliness, depression, anxiety, and sleep disturbances among general populations (Banna et al., 2022; Das et al., 2021), depression, anxiety, stress, fear among physicians (Ali et al., 2023; Rahman et al., 2021a, 2021b), COVID-19 survivors (Kibria et al., 2024), and among students (Faisal et al., 2022) and revealed higher rates of mental illnesses.

## 22 Disorders of Western Cultures

Eating disorders and gender identity issues are clinically under-researched in Bangladesh. Studies are coming out assessing different eating disorders university students with screening tools and highlighting the risk of developing eating disorders (Banna et al., 2025). However, we did not find any study conducted in clinical settings, across the country, and using diagnostic tools.

Research on gender dysphoria is scant. There are persons with gender dysphoria and there are 4504–8882 transgenders in the country (Hia and Mozumdar, 2024). There is a negative attitude toward the gender diverse populations in Bangladesh as Bangladesh is a Muslim-majority country and homosexuality is prohibited in Islamic laws (Islam, 2024; Rafiq, 2022). The enduring legal system also contradicts the homosexuality (Hia and Mozumdar, 2024). There is evidence of violence and homicidal attack on gender diverse activist that creates as sense of insecurity and intimidation (Hia & Mozumder, 2024; Barua & Khan, 2023). There is also evidence of social media movements of anti-homosexuality. However, one study revealed that sensitivity and tolerance for usual life style of gender diverse populations is increasing among the youths (Anjum et al., 2021).

# 23 Social and Mass Media Representation of Mental Illness in Bangladesh

Mental illness is a major public health concern worldwide, including in Bangladesh (Bai, Parvin & Kabir, 2024). How mental illness is depicted in social and mass media significantly influences public perceptions and attitudes. This section looks at the portrayal of mental illness in Bangladeshi social and mass media, assessing how these representations affect stigma, public awareness, and mental health outcomes.

## *23.1 Social Media Representation*

Social media is a strong tool for talking about mental health. In Bangladesh, many people use Facebook, Twitter, and Instagram to share their personal stories and spread awareness (Muhammad and Arafat, 2024). Social media's extensive reach allows governments to connect with the public, ensuring safety, communication, and support during crises (Nandy, Biswas & Das, 2024). It fosters a sense of belonging and care, crucial for maintaining social cohesion and humanity, especially during epidemics where social distancing is vital. While sharing these experiences can help reduce stigma and build support, it can also sometimes lead to negative reactions or misinformation.

### 23.1.1 Positive Effects

Sharing personal stories about mental health on social media can help reduce stigma by making these conversations more common. Research shows that when people see others openly discussing their mental health struggles, it can lead to more understanding and less judgment (Zhang et al., 2024). Studies suggest that public mental illness disclosures on social media can reduce stigma. Future research should explore different types of messengers and messages to tailor anti-stigma campaigns effectively, involving celebrities and influencers for maximum impact.

This is especially crucial in Bangladesh, where stigma often prevents people from seeking the mental healthcare they need. Mental health stigma is widespread in both rural and urban Bangladesh, contributing to a significant treatment gap. Factors like age, socioeconomic status, and education level predict stigma (Faruk et al., 2023). These findings can help develop targeted mental health programs to reduce stigma and improve care availability and adequacy. Social media campaigns and personal stories help create a supportive community, encouraging people to seek help and share their experiences. This fosters understanding and reduces stigma, making it easier for individuals to talk about their mental health issues.

### 23.1.2 Negative Effects

Social media's influence on mental health perceptions is complex. Social networking site use has been found to be related to loneliness, depression, anxiety, and sleep disturbances in young Bangladeshis (Islam et al., 2024). While offering platforms for sharing experiences and fostering support networks, anonymity, and widespread reach can also fuel misinformation and harmful stereotypes. Individuals bravely sharing their struggles may encounter cyberbullying and negative feedback, worsening their conditions. This highlights the need for responsible online behavior and the creation of supportive, moderated online communities that prioritize empathy and understanding. The potential for both positive and negative impacts underscores the necessity for media literacy and proactive measures to combat online harassment and misinformation surrounding mental health (Zhang et al., 2024). Sensationalized or inaccurate depictions of mental illness in media perpetuate damaging stereotypes, hindering understanding and empathy. Such portrayals often focus on extreme behaviors, ignoring the diverse realities of mental health conditions. This fuels stigma, preventing individuals from seeking help, and contributing to isolation and discrimination. Responsible and accurate representations are crucial to fostering a supportive and inclusive environment for those experiencing mental health challenges. Balanced portrayals showing both the challenges and resilience of individuals are essential to counteract harmful stereotypes.

## *23.2 Mass Media Representation*

Mass media, including television, newspapers, and radio, also plays a significant role in shaping public perceptions of mental illness in Bangladesh. The representation of mental illness in mass media can influence societal attitudes and contribute to either the reduction or perpetuation of stigma.

### 23.2.1 Positive Representation

Efforts to use mass media to reduce stigma and promote mental health awareness have been significant. Campaigns and programs that accurately portray mental illness and highlight stories of recovery and resilience can help change public perceptions. For example, mass media campaigns in Bangladesh have been used to educate the public about mental health, aiming to reduce stigma and promote understanding. These initiatives often include television, radio, and social media platforms to reach a broad audience, providing information, sharing personal stories, and encouraging open discussions about mental health issues. This approach helps to normalize mental health conversations and fosters a more supportive community (Hasan & Thornicroft, 2018).

These campaigns often collaborate with mental health professionals and utilize diverse media formats to reach a wide audience. By incorporating expert insights and leveraging television, radio, and social media, they effectively disseminate information, share personal stories, and foster open discussions. This multifaceted approach helps to normalize mental health conversations and build a more supportive community.

### 23.2.2 Negative Representation

Despite ongoing efforts to promote mental health awareness, negative portrayals of mental illness remain common in Bangladeshi mass media. These portrayals often sensationalize mental illness, emphasizing extreme cases or violent behavior. Such representations can perpetuate fear and misunderstanding, reinforcing the stigma surrounding mental health issues. This can hinder progress in changing public perceptions and discourage individuals from seeking help or discussing their mental health openly (Hasan et al., 2021).

Inaccurate and unsympathetic portrayals of mental illness can deter individuals from seeking help, reinforcing stigma and discrimination. This perpetuates a harmful cycle, where fear and misunderstanding prevent open discussions and access to necessary support, ultimately hindering efforts to improve mental health awareness and acceptance.

The representation of mental illness in Bangladeshi social and mass media significantly influences public perceptions and stigma. Despite positive initiatives to use media for reducing stigma and promoting mental health awareness, negative depictions remain prevalent. It's essential to enhance the accuracy and empathy in these representations. By doing so, we can foster a more supportive and understanding society, encouraging individuals to seek help and improving overall mental health outcomes. Continued efforts in this direction are vital for creating an environment where mental health issues are openly discussed and addressed with compassion and understanding.

## 24 Training and Education in Social Psychiatry

Social psychiatry contents have been included in postgraduate psychiatry courses as part of psychiatry in Bangladesh. However, there is no specialized degree, training, or courses on social psychiatry in the country.

## 25 Challenges and Opportunities in Implementing Community-Based Mental Health Interventions in Bangladesh

There are multiple obstacles in Bangladesh to design and implement community-based mental health interventions. Lack of local evidence and research is an important obstacle (Karim et al., 2024). There is also lack of community mental health guidelines even though some NGOs are working on the issue (Faruk, 2022). There are inadequate psychiatrists, psychologist, psychiatric nurses, and psychiatric social workers in the country [0.2, 0.3, and 0.4 psychiatrists, psychologists and mental health nurses respectively per 100,000 population (Arafat, 2024a; Faruk, 2022). One psychiatrist for 93,500 persons with mental illness (Arafat et al., 2024a)]. Additionally, there is no allocation of psychiatrist in primary and secondary care level and distribution of psychiatrist are mostly city based (Arafat, 2024a). There is inadequate budgetary allocation for the development of community-based mental health interventions (Arafat, 2024a; Faruk, 2022). High stigma and low mental health literacy are other potential challenges (Arafat et al., 2018).

Integration of mental health services into the primary health facility could be an important way out (Arafat et al., 2018; Faruk, 2022). Bangladesh has a well-functioning community clinic system with 13,000 community clinics (usually 1 for 6000 persons) (Faruk, 2022) that can be utilized incorporating mental health components. Training and supervision should be important endurances to community service providers. Integrating the traditional healers with adequate training in mental health could be a potential option. There is no alternative to adequate funds, research, and political will.

## 26 Integration of Traditional Healers into Modern Psychiatric Care

We discussed about the health-seeking behavior and role of traditional healers in management of psychiatric disorders in Bangladesh. Based on the scenario, it is important to integrate traditional healers into the modern psychiatric practices. Enduring collaboration, adequate, and structured training focusing mental health literacy, making aware of potential referral pathways could reduce the treatment gap. There are some notable initiatives at public level. The Islamic Foundation Ban *Islamic Foundation, Bangladesh* (http://www.islamicfoundation.gov.bd/) arranges regular training for Imams working in different parts of the country. The contents include health where mental health could be reinforced (Islam et al., 2024). At personal level, we found evidence that one previous psychiatry leader (Prof. Dr. A H M Firoz) practiced it by arranging a monthly meeting on Friday and educating the Islamic religious leaders about the psychiatric disorders and managements (Chowdhury et al., 2024).

## 27 Available Research and Gaps

Research in social psychiatry is scanty in Bangladesh. The WHO-ATLAS data (2022) mentioned that there were about 35 published articles in 2020 on mental health in Bangladesh (World Health Organization, 2022). Therefore, domains of social psychiatry have been grossly under-researched. The prevalence of psychiatric disorders has been studied among in general population which is the major accomplishment in social psychiatry in the country (Ministry of Health and Family Welfare, 2021a, b; Alam et al., 2024; Firoz et al., 2006). The rest of the aspects of social psychiatry need academic attention.

## 28 Conclusions

Social determinants of mental health have been poorly studied in Bangladesh even though there are enduring challenges like disaster, poverty, income inequality, high stigma, low literacy, inadequate human resource, and low budgetary allocation along with some emerging challenges like immigration, climate change, and conflict. Integration of mental health services at community level through community clinics could be a potential area to consider. Policy level attention is warranted to improve the status quo of social psychiatry in the country.

## References

Ahasan, N., 2023. Body count. *Netranews*. https://interactive.netra.news/extrajudicial-killings-bangladesh/ (Accessed on October 07, 2024).

Ahmed, A., Bose, P. K., & Arafat, S. M. Y. (2024). Forensic psychiatry in Bangladesh. In S. M. Y. Arafat (Eds.), *Mental Health in Bangladesh*. Springer. https://doi.org/10.1007/978-981-97-0610-5_10

Alam, M. F., Ahmed, H. U., Alam, M. T., Sarkar, M., Khan, N. M., Uddin, M. J., & Sarkar, A. A. (2024). Community prevalence of psychiatric disorders: Findings from a nationwide survey in Bangladesh. *Asian Journal of Psychiatry, 92*, 103897. https://doi.org/10.1016/j.ajp.2023.103897

Alamgir, H.A., (2024). Rising out-of-pocket health expenditure in Bangladesh. The Financial Express. https://thefinancialexpress.com.bd/views/rising-out-of-pocket-health-expenditure-in-bangladesh (Accessed on October 20, 2024).

Ali, M. M., Naharin, N. E., Hossain, S. E., & Manjur, M. (2023). Psychological status of healthcare professionals of Bangladesh during the COVID-19 Pandemic. *Journal of Monno Medical College, 9*(1), 15–19. https://doi.org/10.3329/jmomc.v9i1.69022

Amnesty International, 2024. Bangladesh 2023. https://www.amnesty.org/en/location/asia-and-the-pacific/south-asia/bangladesh/report-bangladesh/ (Accessed on October 07, 2024).

Anwary, A. (2015). Construction of hegemonic masculinity: Violence against wives in Bangladesh. *Women's studies international forum, 50*, 37–46. https://doi.org/10.1016/j.wsif.2015.02.011

Anjum, H., Tamanna, R., Reza, S., Kamol, S., & Khan, T. (2021). Ensuring human rights for the gender diverse population in Bangladesh: The protection perspectives. *Beijing Law Review, 12*, 342–378. https://doi.org/10.4236/blr.2021.122020

Arafat, S. M. Y. (2025a). Forensic psychiatry and prison mental health in Bangladesh. In A. Parmar, S. K. Kar, & S. M. Y. Arafat (Eds.), *Forensic psychiatry and prison mental health in South Asia*. Springer. https://doi.org/10.1007/978-981-96-7206-6_2

Arafat, S. M. Y. (2025b). Suicide prevention in Bangladesh: The role of police. *The Lancet. Psychiatry, 12*(3), 173. https://doi.org/10.1016/S2215-0366(24)00443-7

Arafat, S. M. Y., & Saleem, T. (2025). Suicide in Bangladesh: An ecological systems analysis. *Brain and Behavior, 15*(1), Article e70233. https://doi.org/10.1002/brb3.70233

Arafat, S. M. Y. (2024a). Mental health services in Bangladesh. In S. M. Y. Arafat (Ed.), *Mental health in Bangladesh*. Springer. https://doi.org/10.1007/978-981-97-0610-5_3

Arafat, S. M. Y. (2024b). Suicidal behavior and suicide prevention in Bangladesh. In S. M. Y. Arafat (Ed.), *Mental health in Bangladesh*. Springer. https://doi.org/10.1007/978-981-97-0610-5_11

Arafat, S. M. Y., Giasuddin, N. A., & Mazumder, A. H. (2024a). Access to mental health care in Bangladesh. In S. M. Y. Arafat & S. K. Kar (Eds.), *Access to mental health care in South Asia*. Springer. https://doi.org/10.1007/978-981-99-9153-2_3

Arafat, S. M. Y., Kar, S. K., Abhayanayake, C., Sharma, P., & Marthoenis, M. (2024b). Prison mental health in South-East Asia: A narrative review. *Brain and Behavior, 14*(8), Article e70004. https://doi.org/10.1002/brb3.70004

Arafat, S. M. Y., & Khan, A. R. (2024). Suicidal behavior in Bangladesh. In S. M. Y. Arafat, M. Rezaeian, M. M. Khan (Eds.), *Suicidal behavior in Muslim majority countries*. Springer. https://doi.org/10.1007/978-981-97-2519-9_4

Arafat, S. M. Y., & Khan, M. M. (Eds.). (2023). *Suicide in Bangladesh: Epidemiology, risk factors, and prevention*. Springer Nature. https://doi.org/10.1007/978-981-99-0289-7

Arafat, S. M. Y. (2023). Mental health and suicide in Bangladesh. In S. M. Y. Arafat & M. M. Khan (Eds.), *Suicide in Bangladesh*. Springer. https://doi.org/10.1007/978-981-99-0289-7_3

Arafat, S. M. Y., Saleem, T., Edwards, T. M., Ali, S. A., & Khan, M. M. (2022). Suicide prevention in Bangladesh: The role of family. *Brain and Behavior, 12*(5), Article e2562. https://doi.org/10.1002/brb3.2562

Arafat, S. M. Y., Al Mamun, M. A., & Uddin, M. S. (2019). Depression literacy among first-year university students: A cross-sectional study in Bangladesh. *Global Psychiatry, 2*(1), 31–36. https://doi.org/10.2478/gp-2019-0002

Arafat, S. Y., Roy, S., & Huq, N. (2018). Integrating mental health into primary health care in Bangladesh: Problems and prospects. *Mental Health and Addiction Research, 3*(2), 1–2. https://doi.org/10.15761/MHAR.1000158

Arafat, S. M. Y., & Ahmed, S. (2017). Burden of misconception in sexual health care setting: A cross-sectional investigation among the patients attending a psychiatric sex clinic of Bangladesh. *Psychiatry Journal,* 9827083.https://doi.org/10.1155/2017/9827083

Arafat, S. M. Y., Uddin, M. S., Chowdhury, E. Z., Huq, N., Chouudhury, S. R., & Chowdhury, M. H. R. (2016). Demography and diagnosis of patients received emergency medical service from two private psychiatric hospital in Dhaka City. *International Journal of Neurorehabilitation, 3*(6), 240. https://doi.org/10.4172/2376-0281.1000240

Bai, A. C. M., Parvin, S., Kabir, R. (2024). Public mental health in Bangladesh. In S. M. Y. Arafat (Eds.), *Mental health in Bangladesh*. Springer. https://doi.org/10.1007/978-981-97-0610-5_14

Bakchi, J., Kundu, S., Ghosh, S., & Akter, S. (2018). Intimate partner violence in Bangladesh: A scoping review. *Bangladesh Journal of Bioethics, 9*(3), 15–27.

Bangladesh Bureau of Statistics, (2024). Population & housing census 2022. https://bbs.gov.bd/site/page/47856ad0-7e1c-4aab-bd78-892733bc06eb/Population-&-Housing (Accessed on 28 September 2024).

Banna, M. H. A., Kundu, S., & Arafat, S. M. Y. (2025). Eating disorders in Bangladesh: A narrative review. *Health Science Reports, 8,* Article e70537. https://doi.org/10.1002/hsr2.70537

Banna, M. H. A., Sayeed, A., Kundu, S., Christopher, E., Hasan, M. T., Begum, M. R., Kormoker, T., Dola, S. T. I., Hassan, M. M., Chowdhury, S., & Khan, M. S. I. (2022). The impact of the COVID-19 pandemic on the mental health of the adult population in Bangladesh: A nationwide cross-sectional study. *International Journal of Environmental Health Research, 32*(4), 850–861. https://doi.org/10.1080/09603123.2020.1802409

Barua, A., & Khan, S. A. (2023). Addressing violence against transgender people in Bangladesh: A call for policy intervention. *Frontiers in Sociology, 7,* Article 995448. https://doi.org/10.3389/fsoc.2022.995448

Calderón-Larrañaga, S., Greenhalgh, T., Finer, S., & Clinch, M. (2022). What does the literature mean by social prescribing? A critical review using discourse analysis. *Sociology of Health & Illness, 44*(4–5), 848–868. https://doi.org/10.1111/1467-9566.13468

Choudhury, W. A., Quraishi, F. A., & Haque, Z. (2006). Mental health and psychosocial aspects of disaster preparedness in Bangladesh. *International Review of Psychiatry (Abingdon, England), 18*(6), 529–535. https://doi.org/10.1080/09540260601037896

Chowdhury, N. F., Fariduzzaman, A. M., Arafat, S. M. Y. (2024). Prominent figures in psychiatry in Bangladesh. In S. M. Y. Arafat (Eds.), *Mental health in Bangladesh.* Springer. https://doi.org/10.1007/978-981-97-0610-5_1

Das, R., Hasan, M. R., Daria, S., & Islam, M. R. (2021). Impact of COVID-19 pandemic on mental health among general Bangladeshi population: A cross-sectional study. *British Medical Journal Open, 11*(4), Article e045727. https://doi.org/10.1136/bmjopen-2020-045727

Department of Narcotics Control. (2023). Annual report 2022–23. Dhaka: Ministry of home, Bangladesh. Retrieved November 9, 2023, from https://dnc.gov.bd/site/view/annual_reports/

De, P. K., & Murshid, N. S. (2018). Associations of intimate partner violence with screening for mental health disorders among women in urban Bangladesh. *International Journal of Public Health, 63*(8), 913–921. https://doi.org/10.1007/s00038-018-1139-x

Esie, P., Osypuk, T. L., Schuler, S. R., & Bates, L. M. (2019). Intimate partner violence and depression in rural Bangladesh: Accounting for violence severity in a high prevalence setting. *SSM—Population Health, 7,* 100368. https://doi.org/10.1016/j.ssmph.2019.100368

Faruk, M. O. (2022). Community-based mental health services in bangladesh: Prospects and challenges. *World Social Psychiatry, 4*(3), 187–192. https://doi.org/10.4103/wsp.wsp_7_22

Faruk, M. O., & Rosenbaum, S. (2023). Mental illness stigma among indigenous communities in Bangladesh: A cross-sectional study. *BMC Psychology, 11*(1), 216. https://doi.org/10.1186/s40359-023-01257-5

Faruk, M. O., Khan, A. H., Chowdhury, K. U. A., Jahan, S., Sarker, D. C., Colucci, E., & Hasan, M. T. (2023). Mental illness stigma in Bangladesh: Findings from a cross-sectional survey. *Global Mental Health (Cambridge, England), 10,* Article e59. https://doi.org/10.1017/gmh.2023.56

Faisal, R. A., Jobe, M. C., Ahmed, O., & Sharker, T. (2022). Mental health status, anxiety, and depression levels of Bangladeshi university students during the covid-19 pandemic. *International Journal of Mental Health and Addiction, 20*(3), 1500–1515. https://doi.org/10.1007/s11469-020-00458-y

Fatema, S. R., Rice, K., Rock, A., Islam, M. S., East, L., & Usher, K. (2023). Physical and mental health status of women in disaster-affected areas in Bangladesh. *Natural Hazards, 117*(3), 2715–2733. https://doi.org/10.1007/s11069-023-05964-5

Firoz, A. H. M., Karim, M. E., Alam, M. F., Rahman, A. H. M. M., & Zaman, M. M. (2006). Prevalence, medical care, awareness and attitude towards mental illness in Bangladesh. *Bangladesh Journal of Psychiatry, 20*(1), 9–32.

Giasuddin, N. A., Levav, I., & Gal, G. (2015). Mental health stigma and attitudes to psychiatry among Bangladeshi medical students. *The International Journal of Social Psychiatry, 61*(2), 137–147. https://doi.org/10.1177/0020764014537237

Giasuddin, N. A., Chowdhury, N. F., Hashimoto, N., Fujisawa, D., & Waheed, S. (2012). Pathways to psychiatric care in Bangladesh. *Social Psychiatry and Psychiatric Epidemiology, 47*(1), 129–136. https://doi.org/10.1007/s00127-010-0315-y

Government of the People's Republic of Bangladesh, (2015). National social security strategy. https://socialprotection.gov.bd/wp-content/uploads/2018/09/National-Social-Security-Strategy-English.pdf (Accessed on November 06, 2024).

Goudet, J. M., Binte Arif, F., Owais, H., Uddin Ahmed, H., & Ridde, V. (2024). Climate change and women's mental health in two vulnerable communities of Bangladesh: An ethnographic study. *PLOS Global Public Health, 4*(6), Article e0002080. https://doi.org/10.1371/journal.pgph.0002080

Hasan, M. T., & Thornicroft, G. (2018). Mass media campaigns to reduce mental health stigma in Bangladesh. *The Lancet Psychiatry, 5*(8), 616. https://doi.org/10.1016/S2215-0366(18)30219-0

Hasan, M. T., Anwar, T., Christopher, E., Hossain, S., Hossain, M. M., Koly, K. N., Saif-Ur-Rahman, K. M., Ahmed, H. U., Arman, N., & Hossain, S. W. (2021). The current state of mental healthcare in Bangladesh: Part 2 - setting priorities. *Bjpsych International, 18*(4), 82–85. https://doi.org/10.1192/bji.2021.42

Hia, M. S., & Mozumder, M. K. (2024). Mental health of vulnerable populations in Bangladesh. In S. M. Y. Arafat (Eds.) Mental health in Bangladesh. Springer. https://doi.org/10.1007/978-981-97-0610-5_17

Hosen, I., Al-Mamun, F., & Mamun, M. A. (2021). Prevalence and risk factors of the symptoms of depression, anxiety, and stress during the COVID-19 pandemic in Bangladesh: A systematic review and meta-analysis. *Global Mental Health (Cambridge, England), 8,* Article e47. https://doi.org/10.1017/gmh.2021.49

Hossain, A., Baten, R. B. A., Sultana, Z. Z., Rahman, T., Adnan, M. A., Hossain, M., Khan, T. A., & Uddin, M. K. (2021). Predisplacement abuse and postdisplacement factors associated with mental health symptoms after forced migration among rohingya refugees in Bangladesh. *JAMA Network Open, 4*(3), Article e211801. https://doi.org/10.1001/jamanetworkopen.2021.1801

Islam, J., (2024). The spread of transgender ideology in Bangladesh: A critique from Islamic perspective. (2024). *Islami Ain O Bichar, 20*(78), 109–134. https://doi.org/10.58666/iab.v20i78.276

Islam, M. K., Maruf, M. M., Saeed Khan, M. A., & Arafat, S. M. Y. (2024). Literacy and stigma of suicide among Islamic religious leaders (Imams) in Bangladesh: A cross-sectional study. *International Review of Psychiatry (Abingdon, England), 36*(4–5), 535–542. https://doi.org/10.1080/09540261.2023.2252507

Islam, M. M., Ali, M., & Fenonia, P. (2001). Care seeking behavior of mentally ill: A qualitative and quantitative approach. *Bangladesh Journal of Psychiatry, 15,* 13–18.

Islam, M. S., & Alam, M. S. (2014). Social capital and mental health: Results from a cross-sectional study in Bangladesh. *Asian Social Science, 10*(2), 118–125. https://doi.org/10.5539/ass.v10n2p118

Islam, S. A., & Md. Amanullah. (2024). The effect of unemployment on mental health: A study on the university graduates of Bangladesh. *Khulna University Studies,* 300–312. https://doi.org/10.53808/KUS.2024.21.01.1074-mb

Islam, M. M., Jahan, N., & Hossain, M. D. (2018). Violence against women and mental disorder: A qualitative study in Bangladesh. *Tropical Medicine and Health, 46,* 5. https://doi.org/10.1186/s41182-018-0085-x

Islam, M. J., Broidy, L., Baird, K., & Mazerolle, P. (2017). Intimate partner violence around the time of pregnancy and postpartum depression: The experience of women of Bangladesh. *PLoS ONE, 12*(5), Article e0176211. https://doi.org/10.1371/journal.pone.0176211

Islam, M. R., Jannath, S., Moona, A. A., Akter, S., Hossain, M. J., & Islam, S. M. A. (2021). Association between the use of social networking sites and mental health of young generation in Bangladesh: A cross-sectional study. *Journal of Community Psychology, 49*(7), 2276–2297. https://doi.org/10.1002/jcop.22675

Jahan, R., Amin, R., & Arafat, S. M. Y. (2024). Practical challenges for mental health services among Rohingya refugee in Bangladesh. *Asian Journal of Psychiatry, 97,* Article 104069. https://doi.org/10.1016/j.ajp.2024.104069

Jahan, N., Maruf, M. M., Sultana, B., Habib, S. H., Khan, M. Z. R., & Begum, A. (2017). Family Support and Stigma among Patients Attending a Tertiary Care Hospital in Bangladesh. *BIRDEM Medical Journal, 7*(2), 148–154. https://doi.org/10.3329/birdem.v7i2.32454

Kabir, R., Hasan, M. R., & Arafat, S. M. Y. (2023). Epidemiology of suicide and data quality in Bangladesh. In S. M. Y. Arafat & M. M. Khan (Eds.), *Suicide in Bangladesh.* Springer. https://doi.org/10.1007/978-981-99-0289-7_1

Kabir, Z. N., Nasreen, H. E., & Edhborg, M. (2014). Intimate partner violence and its association with maternal depressive symptoms 6–8 months after childbirth in rural Bangladesh. *Global Health Action, 7,* 24725. https://doi.org/10.3402/gha.v7.24725

Khan H., Giurca B. C., Sanderson J., et al. (2024). Social prescribing around the world. London: National Academy for Social Prescribing. [cited 2024 October 25] Available from: https://socialprescribingacademy.org.uk/media/thtjrirn/social-prescribing-around-the-world-2024.pdf

Kamal, M., Huq, N., Mali, B., Akter, H., & Arafat, S. M. Y. (2018). Epidemiology of substance abuse in Bangladesh: A narrative review. *Journal of Mental Disorders and Treatment, 4,* 165. https://doi.org/10.4172/2471-271X.1000165

Kar, S. K., Menon, V., Arafat, S. Y., Singh, A., Das, A., Shankar, A., Sharma, P., & Perera, S. (2021). Dhat syndrome: Systematic review of epidemiology, nosology, clinical features, and management strategies. *Asian Journal of Psychiatry, 65,* Article 102863. https://doi.org/10.1016/j.ajp.2021.102863

Karim, M. E., Islam, R., Mazumder, A. H., Arafat, S. M. Y. (2024). Community psychiatry in Bangladesh: development and current status. In: S. M. Y. Arafat (Eds.), *Mental health in Bangladesh.* Springer. https://doi.org/10.1007/978-981-97-0610-5_8

Kibria, M. G., Kabir, R., Rahman, U. S., Ahmed, S., Amin, S. S., Rahman, M. M., & Arafat, S. Y. (2024). Prevalence and factors associated with depression and anxiety among COVID-19 survivors in Dhaka city. *Frontiers in Psychiatry, 15,* 1280245. https://doi.org/10.3389/fpsyt.2024.1280245

Koly, K. N., Abdullah, R., Shammi, F. A., Akter, T., Hasan, M. T., Eaton, J., & Ryan, G. K. (2022). Mental health and community-based rehabilitation: A qualitative description of the experiences and perspectives of service users and carers in Bangladesh. *Community Mental Health Journal, 58*(1), 52–66. https://doi.org/10.1007/s10597-021-00790-0

Lloyd, G. G. (1986). Psychiatric syndromes with a somatic presentation. *Journal of Psychosomatic Research, 30*(2), 113–120. https://doi.org/10.1016/0022-3999(86)90039-5

macrotrend, (2024). Bangladesh GDP per capita 1960–2024. https://www.macrotrends.net/global-metrics/countries/BGD/bangenhagen/gdp-per-capita (Accessed on October 16, 2024).

Mahmud, A., Adnan, H. M., & Islam, M. R. (2020). Smartphone addiction and bonding social capital among university students of youth community in Bangladesh. *Global Social Welfare, 7,* 315–326. https://doi.org/10.1007/s40609-020-00177-1

Mahmud, K. H., Ahmed, R., & Tuya, J. H. (2021). Geographic variability of post-disaster mental health: case study after the 2017 flood in Bangladesh. *Geospatial Health, 16*(2). https://doi.org/10.4081/gh.2021.1018

Mamun, M. A., Al-Mamun, F., Ikram, T., Trisha, M. K., Limon, M. H., Mostofa, N. B., Chowdhury, T. B. K., Shanto, N. P., & ALmerab, M. M., Apou, A. C., Roy, N., Hossain, Md. B., & Hossain, Md. S. (2024). Exploring mental health literacy among prospective university students using GIS techniques in Bangladesh: An exploratory study. *Cambridge Prisms: Global Mental Health, 11,* Article e92. https://doi.org/10.1017/gmh.2024.115

Mamun, M. A., Akter, S., Hossain, I., Faisal, M. T. H., Rahman, M. A., Arefin, A., Khan, I., Hossain, L., Haque, M. A., Hossain, S., Hossain, M., Sikder, M. T., Kircaburun, K., & Griffiths, M. D. (2020). Financial threat, hardship and distress predict depression, anxiety and stress among the unemployed youths: A Bangladeshi multi-city study. *Journal of Affective Disorders, 276,* 1149–1158. https://doi.org/10.1016/j.jad.2020.06.075

Maruf, M.M., Saleem, T., Arafat, S. M. Y. (2024a). Dhat syndrome: A fact or myth. In S. K. Kar, S. M. Y. Arafat, & V. Menon (Eds.), *Dhat syndrome.* Springer. https://doi.org/10.1007/978-981-99-8870-9_15

Maruf, M. M., Chowdhury, A., & Islam, M. R. (2024b). Substance use and mental health conditions: Co-existence of dual problems in Bangladesh. In S. M. Y. Arafat (Eds.), *Mental health in Bangladesh.* Springer. https://doi.org/10.1007/978-981-97-0610-5_7

Maruf, M. M., Khan, M. Z. R., Jahan, N., Ahmed, A. U., Sadiq, M. S., & Ferdush, R. (2022). Sociodemographic profile and co-morbid symptoms among individuals with semen loss. *Bangladesh Journal of Medicine, 33*(1), 64–69. https://doi.org/10.3329/bjm.v33i1.56792

Masoom, M. R. (2024). The effect of social capital on perceived stress: A comparative analysis of employed and non-employed women of Bangladesh. *Human Affairs, 34*(1), 38–55. https://doi.org/10.1515/humaff-2023-0033

Mazumder, A.H. (2024). Epidemiology and burden of mental disorders in Bangladesh. In S. M. Y. Arafat (Eds.), *Mental health in Bangladesh.* Springer. https://doi.org/10.1007/978-981-97-0610-5_2

Mental Health Act. (2018). Bangladesh. [Online] [Accessed on 14.10.2024] Available from. http://bdlaws.minlaw.gov.bd/act-1273.html

Miah, M. A. A., Al-Mamun, M. A., Khan, S., & Mozumder, M. K. (2015). Sexual myths and behavior of male patients with psychosexual dysfunction in sexual myths and behavior of male patients with psychosexual dysfunction in Bangladesh. *Dhaka University Journal of Psychology, 39,* 89–100.

Ministry of Health and Family Welfare. (2021a). National mental health survey 2019. https://nimh.gov.bd/wp-content/uploads/2021/11/Mental-Health-Survey-Report.pdf (Accessed on October 17, 2024).

Ministry of Health and Family Welfare. (2021b). Prevalence and associated factors of substance use in Bangladesh. (Project report). Dhaka: Ministry of health and family welfare, Bangladesh. Retrieved October 29, 2023, from https://nimh.gov.bd/english/wp-content/uploads/2021/11/Substance-Use-Full.pdf

Muhammad, F., Arafat, S. M. Y. (2024). Technology-based interventions for mental health support in Bangladesh. In S. M. Y. Arafat (Eds.), *Mental health in Bangladesh.* Springer. https://doi.org/10.1007/978-981-97-0610-5_16

Mullick, M. S. I., Karim, M. E., Islam, M. S., Chowdhury, S., Rahman, M., & Islam, M. R. (1995). Clinical pattern of Dhat syndrome. *Bangladesh Medical Journal, 24,* 3–7.

Mullick, M. S. I., Khalifa, N., Nahar, J. S., & Walker, D.-M. (2013). Beliefs about Jinn, black magic and evil eye in Bangladesh: The effects of gender and level of education. *Mental Health, Religion & Culture, 16*(7), 719–729. https://doi.org/10.1080/13674676.2012.717918

Nahar, J. S., Mullick, M. S. I., & Maliha, G. A. (1995). Symptom presentation of major depressive disorder. *Bangladesh Journal of Psychiatry, 8,* 14–18.

Nandy, A., Biswas, M., & Das, J. (2022). Social media & mental health: A narrative study on Bangladesh during the Lockdown time of COVID-19 Pandemic. *International Journal of Research and Innovation in Social Science, VI,* 680–689. https://doi.org/10.47772/IJRISS.2022.6142

Nuri, N. N., Sarker, M., Ahmed, H. U., Hossain, M. D., Beiersmann, C., & Jahn, A. (2018). Pathways to care of patients with mental health problems in Bangladesh. *International Journal of Mental Health Systems, 12,* 39. https://doi.org/10.1186/s13033-018-0218-y

Qusar, M. S., Arafat, S. M., Chowdhury, M. R., Ahmed, S., Morshed, N. M., & Rahman, W. (2019). Cultural variations in symptom presentations of depression: A cross-sectional observation in a tertiary care hospital of Bangladesh. *Mymensingh Medical Journal: MMJ, 28*(2), 410–417.

Qusar, M. M. A. S., Hossain, R., Sohan, M., Nazir, S., Hossain, M. J., & Islam, M. R. (2022). Attitudes of mental healthcare professionals and media professionals towards each other in reducing social stigma due to mental illness in Bangladesh. *Journal of Community Psychology, 50*(7), 3181–3195. https://doi.org/10.1002/jcop.22823

Rabbani, A., Biju, N. R., Rizwan, A., & Sarker, M. (2018). Social network analysis of psychological morbidity in an urban slum of Bangladesh: A cross-sectional study based on a community census. *British Medical Journal Open, 8*(7), Article e020180. https://doi.org/10.1136/bmjopen-2017-020180

Rafiq, T. (2022). Gender dysphoria and Islamic perspective of gender-related issues. *JIHĀT-UL-ISLĀM, 16,* 16–32.

Rafi, M. A., Mamun, M. A., Hsan, K., Hossain, M., & Gozal, D. (2019). Psychological implications of unemployment among Bangladesh civil service job seekers: A pilot study. *Frontiers in Psychiatry, 10,* 578. https://doi.org/10.3389/fpsyt.2019.00578

Rahman, M. M., Alam Shobuj, I., Tanvir Hossain, M., & Tasnim, F. (2023). Impact of disaster on mental health of women: A case study on 2022 flash flood in Bangladesh. *International Journal of Disaster Risk Reduction, 96,* Article 103935. https://doi.org/10.1016/j.ijdrr.2023.103935

Rahman, A., Deeba, F., Akhter, S., Bashar, F., Nomani, D., Koot, J., Koly, K. N., Salah, F. B., Haverlag, K., & Anwar, I. (2021a). Mental health condition of physicians working frontline with COVID-19 patients in Bangladesh. *BMC Psychiatry, 21*(1), 615. https://doi.org/10.1186/s12888-021-03629-w

Rahman, M. A., Rahman, S., Wazib, A., Arafat, S. M. Y., Chowdhury, Z. Z., Uddin, B. M. M., Rahman, M. M., Bahar Moni, A. S., Alif, S. M., Sultana, F., Salehin, M., Islam, S. M. S., Cross, W., & Bahar, T. (2021b). COVID-19 Related Psychological Distress, Fear and Coping: Identification of High-Risk Groups in Bangladesh. *Frontiers in Psychiatry, 12,* Article 718654. https://doi.org/10.3389/fpsyt.2021.718654

Riley, A., Varner, A., Ventevogel, P., Taimur Hasan, M. M., & Welton-Mitchell, C. (2017). Daily stressors, trauma exposure, and mental health among stateless Rohingya refugees in Bangladesh. *Transcultural Psychiatry, 54*(3), 304–331. https://doi.org/10.1177/1363461517705571

Selim, N., & Satalkar, P. (2008). Perceptions of mental illness in a Bangladesh village. *BRAC University Journal, V,* 47–57.

Selim, N. (2010). Cultural dimensions of depression in Bangladesh: A qualitative study in two villages of Matlab. *Journal of Health, Population, and Nutrition, 28*(1), 95–106. https://doi.org/10.3329/jhpn.v28i1.4528

Siddique, M. A. B., Ovi, M. R., Ahammed, T., Chowdhury, M. A. B., & Uddin, M. J. (2022). Mental health knowledge and awareness among university students in Bangladesh. *Heliyon, 8*(10). https://doi.org/10.1016/j.heliyon.2022.e11084

Siddik, M.A.B., Munmun, M.S., Ahmed, Z., Nabil, K. & Mubin, N. (2024). Climate change, natural disasters, and mental health of adolescents: A qualitative study from Bangladesh. *International Journal of Population Studies, 10*(2), 0339. https://doi.org/10.36922/ijps.0339

Sifat, M. S., Tasnim, N., Hoque, N., Saperstein, S., Shin, R. Q., Feldman, R., Stoebenau, K., & Green, K. M. (2022). Motivations and barriers for clinical mental health help-seeking in Bangladeshi university students: A cross-sectional study. *Global Mental Health, 9,* 211–220. https://doi.org/10.1017/gmh.2022.24

Tasnim, F., Rahman, M., Islam, M. M., Hasan, M., Mostofa, M. G., & Rahman, M. M. (2021). Exposure to domestic violence and the risk of developing depression within 6 months postpartum in Bangladesh. *Social Psychiatry and Psychiatric Epidemiology, 56*(7), 1189–1200. https://doi.org/10.1007/s00127-020-01998-3

Tran, L. M., Nguyen, P. H., Naved, R. T., & Menon, P. (2020). Intimate partner violence is associated with poorer maternal mental health and breastfeeding practices in Bangladesh. *Health Policy and Planning, 35*(Supplement_1), i19–i29. https://doi.org/10.1093/heapol/czaa106

Uddin, M. S. (2020). Mental health content in school science textbooks in Bangladesh. *The Lancet Psychiatry, 7*(3), Article e10. https://doi.org/10.1016/S2215-0366(20)30008-0

Uddin, M. N., Bhar, S., & Islam, F. M. A. (2019). An assessment of awareness of mental health conditions and its association with socio-demographic characteristics: A cross-sectional study in a rural district in Bangladesh. *BMC Health Services Research, 19*(1), 562. https://doi.org/10.1186/s12913-019-4385-6

UNHCR. (2024). Country—Bangladesh. https://data.unhcr.org/en/country/bgd (Accessed on November 09, 2024).

United Nations. (2025). Human rights violations and abuses related to the protests of July and august 2024 in Bangladesh. https://www.ohchr.org/sites/default/files/documents/countries/bangladesh/ohchr-fftb-hr-violations-bd.pdf (Accessed on February 21, 2025).

Wahid, S. S., Islam, M. N., & Raza, W. A. (2024). Climate change and mental health in Bangladesh: vulnerability, inequality, and the crucial need for intervention on the frontlines of the climate crisis. In S. M. Y. Arafat (Eds.), *Mental Health in Bangladesh*. Springer. https://doi.org/10.1007/978-981-97-0610-5_15

World Bank. (2023). Out-of-pocket expenditure (% of current health expenditure)—Bangladesh. Retrieved from April 04, 2023, https://data.worldbank.org/indicator/SH.XPD.OOPC.CH.ZS?locations=BD

World Health Organization. (2015). Bangladesh health system review. *Health Systems in Transition, 5,* 1–214.

World Prison Brief. (2025). Bangladesh. https://www.prisonstudies.org/country/Bangladesh (Accessed on April 04, 2025).

World Health Organization. (2022). Mental health atlas 2020 country profile: Bangladesh. Retrieved from March 30, 2023, https://www.who.int/publications/m/item/mental-health-atlas-bgd-2020-country-profile

Yount, K. M., Miedema, S. S., Martin, C. C., Crandall, A., & Naved, R. T. (2016). Men's coercive control, partner violence perpetration, and life satisfaction in Bangladesh. *Sex Roles, 74,* 450–463. https://doi.org/10.1007/s11199-016-0584-3

Zhang, Z., Morgan, A., Armstrong, G., Campbell, A., & Reavley, N. (2024). *Public mental illness disclosure on social media and the effects on stigma toward people with mental illness: A systematic review*. Advance online publication. https://doi.org/10.1037/sah0000531

Zulfiqar, L., Idrees, N., & Rafiq, M. (2019). Culture bound syndromes in Pakistan: Implications and strategic vision for health management. *Pakistan Journal of Neurological Sciences (PJNS), 14*(4), 52–59.

# Chapter 4
# Social Psychiatry in India-Heralding a Paradigm Shift

**Roy Abraham Kallivayalil and P. N. Suresh Kumar**

**Abstract** Social psychiatry in India is heralding a paradigm shift in mental healthcare. The traditional Western-based model has become unavailable, unaffordable and inaccessible to large sections of the population—especially the marginalized, in India and many of the Low and Middle Income (LAMI) countries. This calls for a paradigm shift in our approach to medicine and psychiatry with greater focus on social factors and social determinants of health. Mental health is of low priority in most countries with poor investment, poor infrastructure and inadequate personnel. Social psychiatry has started receiving greater attention in India and the world heralding a new approach to mental healthcare, which is inclusive of all. This paper discusses the roots of social psychiatry in India, its history and relevance, the contributions to the Indian Association for Social Psychiatry, milestone studies, stigma, suicides, the role of spirituality and religion and other related social psychiatry topics from India, which is relevant to Asia and the rest of the world.

**Keywords** Social Psychiatry · India · History · Studies · Stigma · Suicides · Spirituality paradigm shift

## 1 Introduction

Modern medical care in India has often tried to imitate the Western model with an emphasis on sophisticated technology, advances in pharmacological treatment and high-tech hospitals. However, the large majority of the population remains left behind, especially those who cannot afford costly medical treatments and those without medical insurance. This calls for a paradigm shift in our approach to medicine and psychiatry with a greater focus on social factors and social determinants of health.

R. A. Kallivayalil (✉)
Pushpagiri Institute of Medical Sciences, Thiruvalla & Mar Sleeva Medicity, Palai, India
e-mail: roykalli@gmail.com

P. N. S. Kumar
Chethana Centre for Neuropsychiatry, Kozhikode, India

 
S. M. Y. Arafat et al. (eds.), *Social Psychiatry in South Asia*, South Asian Perspectives in Mental Health and Psychology , https://doi.org/10.1007/978-981-96-8078-8_4

Mental health has long been neglected in India and most of the Low and Middle Income (LAMI) countries. Psychiatry and mental health have remained out of the focus of governments, policymakers and administrators for far too long. At the same time, the burden of disease due to mental illness in these countries, as everywhere else, has been huge. Social psychiatry must receive greater attention in India and the world, heralding a new approach to mental healthcare which is inclusive of all.

## 1.1 Roots of Social Psychiatry in India

Social psychiatry is a discipline that focuses on the social dimension of mental health, mental illness and mental healthcare. Social psychiatry uses concepts and methods of social sciences, including psychology and anthropology, to investigate social factors in influencing and relevant to the occurrence, expression, course and care of mental disorders. The roots of social medicine can be found in the ancient Indian civilizations. The earliest roots of social medicine can be found in the ancient texts of Ayurveda. The focus of the physician in Ayurveda is on the patient's health rather than the disease. There is often a stipulated harmonious framework for health and life. There is a greater emphasis on quality of life rather than just the curative aspect of disease. The treatment approach in Ayurveda is person-centred and often takes into consideration the person as a whole. The same would apply to ancient Greek philosophy. Socrates, Plato, Aristotle and Hippocrates talked about the importance of the social paradigm of health. The concept is summarized in Socrates's quote, "If the whole is not well, it is impossible for the part to be well" (Mezzich, 2007).

In India, Hinduism encourages people to achieve a certain life purpose, often closely tied to fulfilment in the afterlife. The objective of earthly life is to respect the laws of Dharma and gain benefit from the cycle of life and reincarnation. In the same fashion, religious rites give expression to communal beliefs, and everyone's self-perceived role becomes a physical manifestation of these beliefs.

## 1.2 History of Social Psychiatry in India

The Indian Association for Social Psychiatry (IASP) completed its 40th year of existence in 2024. The Association was registered on 6 June 1984 (Regn. No. 1178/84) under the Societies Act of India. It has a membership of more than 1000. Members include mental health professionals from different fields, including psychiatrists, clinical psychologists, psychiatric social workers and psychiatric nurses.

The association supports continued medical education through its yearly national conference—The National Conference of Indian Association for Social Psychiatry (NCIASP), along with multiple other CME and international conferences. IASP promotes excellence in research in young scholars and honours the lifetime achievements of senior professionals by providing yearly national awards in the field of psychiatry and mental health during the annual national conference. The website of the association www.iasp.org.in was launched in 2008.

The Association came into being following certain fortuitous circumstances. During the transcultural psychiatry meet held in Madurai in August 1981 under the chairmanship of Professor A. Venkoba Rao, a group of behavioural scientists concerned with the relative neglect accorded to the study of social factors in mental illness in India decided to constitute an organization specifically devoted to further this cause. At that meeting it was generally felt by many professionals that there was a great need in the country to have a separate professional organization for social and/or transcultural psychiatry. Such an organization could also examine the interface between culture and personality and be conducive to the scientific study of the social issues relevant to the country and the society, in addition to examining the social and transcultural factors in the phenomenology, course, outcome and treatment of psychiatric disorders. The organization would primarily attempt academic and intellectual exercises and bring a multidisciplinary approach to bear on these issues. As a result in January 1982 in Madurai, an ad hoc committee was formed with Dr. V.K. Varma as the convener and Dr. Kirpal Singh as the chairman. This committee met at different places and discussed various aspects and organizational matters. Finally, The Indian Association for Social Psychiatry was formed on 14 January 1984 at Ranchi. Its constitution and by-laws were adopted, and the office-bearers were elected. Dr. A. Venkoba Rao was the first President and served in that capacity between 1984 and 1986. The Association is committed to studying the influence of culture in the causation, treatment and prevention of behavioural disorders; to promoting national and international collaborations among professionals related to social psychiatry, and making the knowledge and practice of social psychiatry available to other sciences and to advance the physical, social and psychological well-being of mankind.

The Association has been holding regular conferences, which have been held in various cities representing different parts of the country. Each conference was held with a socially relevant theme and included symposia, free papers and a number of guest lectures and popular lectures. The first annual conference was held in Kodaikanal in February 1985 under the chairmanship of Dr. A. Venkoba Rao and the second in Chandigarh. Prof. Shridhar Sharma was the founder member and President-Elect of IASP along with Prof. A. Venkoba Rao. Since then, the Indian Association has grown much stronger and is playing a bigger role in the growth of the World Association for Social Psychiatry (WASP) (https://iasp.org.in/about-iasp/). The Indian Association for Social Psychiatry (IASP) became formally affiliated to the WASP in October 1985 held the Regional Symposium of WASP in New Delhi in February 1989 and hosted the XIII WASP Congress in New Delhi in November 1992. The IASP hosted the Regional Symposium of the Transcultural Psychiatry Section of WPA in March 1995. It became a member society of the World Psychiatric Association (WPA) in June, 1993. IASP is one of the most active members of the WPA. Through its own activities and through the activities of its members, the IASP received greater recognition and visibility at the global level and at the level of the WPA and WASP. Professor S.D. Sharma, a past President of IASP has also served as the President of the World Association for Social Psychiatry. Prof Roy Abraham Kallivayalil, the past

President of IASP and Secretary General of WPA and President of WASP, contributed to a great extent to the development of social psychiatry in India.

The 20th World Congress of Social Psychiatry, in 2010, was organized under the leadership of Driss Moussaoui. The theme was "Promoting Integral of Health and Mental Health." The General Assembly elected Driss Moussaoui as President, Tom Craig as President-elect, and Roy Abraham Kallivayalil from India as secretary-general and resolved to revise the statutes. The event was a grand success with about 700 delegates participating.

The 21st Congress, Lisbon, was held in 2013. The theme was "The Biopsychosocial Model: The Future of Psychiatry." Organized by Maria Luisa Figueira. Tom Craig was elected as President, and Roy Abraham Kallivayalil as President-Elect.

The 22nd WASP Congress was held in New Delhi from November 30 to December 4, 2016, under the chairmanship of Prof R K Chadda, past President of IASP. More than 1100 delegates from 50 countries participated. The Congress theme was "Social Psychiatry in a Rapidly Changing World." With more than 1,000 delegates attending, it was one of the most successful WASP Congresses to date. The General Assembly elected Roy Kallivayalil as the President, Rachid Bennegadi as President-Elect, Fernando Lolas as secretary-general and Marianne Kastrup as treasurer.

The 23rd WASP Congress, Bucharest, was held from October 25 to 28, 2019. The theme was "Social Determinants of Health/Mental Health and Access to Care." Nearly 700 delegates from 66 countries participated. Roy Abraham Kallivayalil was the Congress President and it was organized under the dynamic leadership of Doina Cozman and Alexander Paziuc. The inauguration and release of the first issue of the World Journal of Social Psychiatry was one of the highlights of the Congress. Debasish Basu (Chandigarh, India) is the founding editor. The General Assembly elected Rachid Bennegadi as President, Vincenzo Di Nicola as President-Elect, Rakesh Chadda as secretary-general and Andrew Molodynski as treasurer. IASP has organized three World Congresses of Social Psychiatry and has given two Presidents to the WASP. India has also made an impressive contribution to the cause of the WASP (https://www.worldsocpsychiatry.org).

## 1.3 Indian Journal of Social Psychiatry

The first issue of the Indian Journal of Social Psychiatry was published in 1986 under the editorship of Dr B.B. Sethi. Indian Journal of Social Psychiatry, a peer-reviewed online journal with a quarterly print compilation of issues. The journal focuses on issues related to health, ethical and social factors in the field of social and community psychiatry and is highly acclaimed by the mental health academia. The journal is open-access and is indexed by Baidu Scholar, CNKI (China National Knowledge Infrastructure), EBSCO Publishing's Electronic Databases, Exlibris—Primo Central, Google Scholar, Hinari, Infotrieve, National Science Library, ProQuest, TdNet and Kudos.

## *1.4 World Association of Social Psychiatry Congresses in India*

XIII New Delhi, India 1992
XVII Agra, India 2001
XXII Delhi, India 2016

## *1.5 Presidents of the World Association of Social Psychiatry from India*

2001–2004: Shridhar Sharma, India
2016–2019: Roy Abraham Kallivayalil, India
2025–2028: Rakesh K Chadda, India

## *1.6 WASP Member Societies*

The organization of Member Societies within WASP is a relatively new development. Julio Arboleda-Flórez, President at the time, constituted the New Member Societies Committee in 2010, considering the importance of creating interest in new countries to develop their national Social Psychiatry Societies. Roy Abraham Kallivayalil, India, was the chair of this committee (Kallivayalil R. Notes from WASP President's desk, 2021).

A workshop on "National Social Psychiatric Societies: Best Practices & Lessons Learned" was held during the WASP Congress in Marrakech, October 2010, in which the following presentations were made:

1. Roy Abraham Kallivayalil (India): "Cultural Perspectives and Networking among National Social Psychiatry Societies."
2. J. K. Trivedi (India): "Indian Association for Social Psychiatry."

This was the beginning of the organization of WASP into Member Societies. The 2016–2019 WASP-EC, under the leadership of President Roy Kallivayalil, considered membership development as a priority item, and by the 2019 General Assembly, eight more Member Societies were added, taking the strength from 19 to 27. This was a significant leap forward in spreading the WASP movement to all parts of the globe (Kallivayalil, 2021).

## 1.7 Relevance of Social Psychiatry in India

The study of social factors in mental disorders has been at the forefront of psychiatric literature in the West. In India, though not totally absent, it has failed to be expressed in a coherent fashion. Epidemiological studies from India indicate the possible implications of factors like, social class, marital status, caste considerations, sibling position and family structure in relation to certain psychiatric disorders.

It has also been pointed out that the industrialization and modernization of India is changing the face of India from a predominantly rural and agrarian society to an urbanized one—the most telling impact of which is on the core of our society, i.e. the family which seems to be undergoing a transition from traditionally a joint pattern to a nuclear one. This phenomenon may be related to the increased frequency of mental disorders. At a clinical level, too, it has been emphasized that our patients express their mental problems in a pattern that is socio-culturally determined. Consequently, one hears of a need for therapies (e.g. psychotherapy) that are socially and culturally relevant. At this juncture however, it would be appropriate only to underline the fact that even though indirect evidence exists to link social factors to mental disorders in India, yet the attention paid has not been of a very high order. India is an excellent place for the study of the social and cultural processes as they relate to behaviour and more so now since the change from a conservative to a modern India is occurring at an unprecedented rate (Trivedi, & Kailash, 2012).

Much of the professional output of psychiatrists, psychologists and other mental health professionals in India can be subsumed under the rubric of social psychiatry. Previously, most Indian psychiatrists cut their psychiatric teeth either in the West or on the Western model. On returning to their home country, they often encountered significant difficulties in applying the Western model to the ground realities in India. "One major concern of the Indian psychiatrists was to translate modern psychiatry as it has evolved in the West to the Indian setting. This exercise has covered topics such as the epidemiology, types, manifestations, course and outcome of mental illness. Comparing the Indian situation to the Western textbooks has been a prime concern, particularly of the Indian psychiatrists trained in the West, and to a lesser extent all psychiatrists, as the Western frame of reference continues in their training and education."

Varma, in his write-ups of the souvenirs of the first (1985), the second (1986) and the fifth (1989) annual conferences of the IASP, has drawn attention to the social issues and problems of particular relevance to India. "The great diversity of the Indian culture both in temporal and spatial contexts" has been pointed out, particularly in view of the problem of national integration. In the national context, "problems of poverty and economic deprivation, technological backwardness, social and economic inequalities, urbanization, industrialization and social change, population control, cultural diversity and national integration and intra societal conflict and violence have been particularly identified as social problems. Increasingly, attention has also been drawn to crimes against women, including dowry death and rape and to the legal situation regarding attempted suicide and drug abuse" (Varma, 2012).

In India, the role of socio-cultural factors in mental health is indispensable. Rapid urbanization and growing technology have cut across national boundaries and are continuously testing the ability of people to adapt to this modernization. Disappearance of the joint family and the support system that comes along with it is resulting in the depletion of one of India's most valued resources. Stigma, problems of the deprived and socio-cultural issues specific to women are areas of interest in developing countries like India but also in developed countries. Family care and burden, disability, suicide including farmers suicide, religion, spirituality, help-seeking behaviour, pathway of care and preventive psychiatry are areas of specific interest in India and a great deal of work still needs to be done in these areas (Trivedi & Kailash, 2012).

## *1.8 Milestone Studies Related to Social Psychiatry in India*

In India, more than 90% of the severely and chronically mentally ill reside with their families (Thara et al., 1994). Family members are the key persons involved in the decision-making process regarding treatment and are primarily responsible for continued care and for ensuring adherence to treatment. In this area, one of the earliest studies was the measurement of expressed emotion (EE) in an Indian sample in comparison with the West as part of the WHO Determinants of Outcome project. It was found that in Indian families, EE was lower than in London families, and this may account for better outcomes for schizophrenia often observed in India (Wig et al., 1987).

Several scales on attitudes and burdens have been developed in India. Some of them are the Family Burden Scale by Pai and Kapur (Pai & Kapur, 1981) and the Burden Assessment Scale (BAS) developed by the Schizophrenia Research Foundation (SCARF) (Thara, Padmavati, et al., 1998). Attempts have been made to correlate the burden with the functioning of patients as well. Loganathan and Murthy, in 2008, assessed functioning in 100 patients with schizophrenia and the burden and methods of coping of their primary caregivers (Loganathan & Murthy, 2008). Fatalism and problem-solving were the two most preferred ways of coping. Problem-focused coping, i.e. problem-solving and expressive action, decreased the burden of caregivers, while emotion-focused coping, i.e. fatalism and passivity, increased it.

Rammohan et al. found that families of persons with schizophrenia used denial and problem-solving strategies (Rammohan et al., 2002). The strength of religious belief and perceived burden were significant predictors of the well-being of carers. The authors emphasized the need to reinforce religious coping methods as a component of family intervention programmes in India.

Murthy et al. showed reduction of burden on the family and better functioning of the patients with the onset of regular treatment in untreated or irregularly treated patients in a rural community (Murthy et al., 2005). In India, family burden is also reported by carers of persons with dysthymia, obsessive–compulsive disorder (OCD) and bipolar disorder (Chakrabarti et al., 1993). In the WHO Collaborative Study on

Strategies for Extending Mental Health Care in four developing countries (Colombia, India, Sudan and Philippines) for the social burden caused by mental illness in a family member, the social burden was found to be greatest in urban areas (Harding et al., 1983).

With the breaking up of joint families and the emergence of nuclear families and working women, families started seeking professional help to cope with mentally ill members of the family. Kulhara et al., in a randomized controlled trial of family psychoeducation, found that it was significantly better than routine outpatient care (Kulhara et al., 2008). The psychoeducational intervention package used was a simple, feasible and inexpensive viable facet of intervention for schizophrenia in India.

Family involvement in the process of care in India has led to the formation of family support groups in the last decade. They consider themselves as micro-organizations demonstrating the virtues of "small is powerful" and advocating family empowerment as the core of emotional strength and support to those with a disorder (Srinivasan, 2003).

## 2 Disability

Although the disability associated with mental illness was placed on a par with other disabilities in the Western world, and though we had an act for Persons with Disabilities since 1996, very little emphasis was given to India. Certification of disability of mental disorders was not regularly carried out, and as a result, many disabled persons did not get the benefits despite their eligibility.

The Indian Disability Evaluation and Assessment Scale (IDEAS) developed by the Indian Psychiatric Society was a significant leap in this regard (Thara, Rajkumar, & Valecha, 1988). Chaudhury et al. compared the disability of seven conditions using IDEAS in the north-Western state of Assam and found that while schizophrenia was most disabling, it was closely followed by alcohol abuse and OCD (Chaudhury et al., 2006). Disability in the occupational sphere was the most important concern since job not only provides self-respect and self-esteem but also a means of family income. Many rehabilitation programmes in India are therefore started towards increasing work-related skills and job placement efforts.

## 3 Stigma of Mental Disorders

The stigma of mental illness is as old as the disorder itself and its negative consequences seem to play a role in the outcome of many disorders. In India, caregivers and family members are subject to as much stigma as the patients. The nature and degree of stigma experienced by persons with schizophrenia was studied in Chennai (Srinivasan & Thara, 2001). Marriage, fear that neighbours would treat them differently and the extra efforts they had to make to hide the fact of mental illness from others were the predominant concerns. While 90% of marriages in India are "arranged" by the families, caregivers and family members are subject to greater stigma than the patients. If the fact of mental illness in a family is known to others, it could also jeopardize the chances of other members of the family getting married. In this study, stigma was higher if the patient was female and women carers perceived more stigma.

Another study on women with schizophrenia whose marriages had been broken revealed that families perceived this as a "dual tragedy" and felt very stigmatized (Thara et al., 2003a, b). Very few of these women received any support from their husbands after the onset of illness, and many were sent back to their parental families. Many women considered the break-in marriage more stigmatizing than schizophrenia since they felt socially ostracized because of the failure of their marriage. Many hoped that someday the husband would take them back.

### 3.1 Stigma in Urban/Rural Areas

Stigma is not confined to urban areas. An interesting ethnographic piece of work by Jadhav et al. showed significantly higher stigma among rural Indians, especially those with a manual occupation, and many appeared to deploy a punitive model towards the severely mentally ill (Jadhav et al., 2007). The urban group, in contrast, expressed a more liberal view of severe mental illness. Loganathan and Murthy also report the stigma of mental illness in rural areas (Loganathan & Murthy, 2008). While urban respondents of Karnataka (in southern India) felt the need to hide their illness and avoided illness histories in job applications, rural respondents experienced more ridicule, shame and discrimination.

### 3.2 Stigma Related to the Causation of Illness

Beliefs about the causation of mental illness can clearly influence the attitudes that families adopt towards patients and their help-seeking behaviour. Indian families have been typically described as often believing in causes like supernatural forces and therefore seeking help from magico-religious healers. In the changing mental health scenario in India, this impression was tested by Thara and Srinivasan by interviewing the key relatives of 254 chronic schizophrenia patients and asking them to name the causes they believed were responsible for the illness in their family members (Thara & Srinivasan, 2000). A supernatural cause was named by only 12% of families and as the only cause by 5%. Psychosocial stress was the most commonly cited cause, followed by personality defects and heredity. Urban families of patients rarely subscribe to the idea of supernatural causation of the illness. Rather, their causal attributions tend to be more biological and psychological.

Charles et al. in their study in Vellore in Tamil Nadu state observed that patients and families simultaneously held multiple and contradictory beliefs about the causation of illness and its treatment (Charles et al., 2007). A majority of respondents had approached at least two systems of healing, which included allopathic and traditional/magico-religious/religious modes. Stigma scores of patients were associated with a belief in disease models, as well as karma and evil spirits as a cause of illness. The authors argue that while planning mental health services, it should be kept in mind that beliefs regarding attributions, explanatory models and stigma play no small role in the help-seeking pattern of patients with mental disorders.

## 3.3 Suicide in India

Suicidal behaviour with consequent fatal outcomes has become an important public health problem in India. On average, 100,000 people per year commit suicide in India. Attempted and completed suicide was held to be a crime by an antiquated Indian law. India ranks 43rd in descending order of rates of suicide with a rate of 10.6/100,000 (Lee & Ortiz, 2015). A recent survey conducted by NIMHANS in 12 states of India on a random sample of 40,000 people shows that 1 million Indians are at high risk of suicide, and more women are found to be harbouring thoughts of suicide (NIMHANS: One crore Indians at high risk of suicide. The New Indian Express 10th September 2017).

## 3.4 Risk Factors for Suicide

Multiple factors impinge on the risk of suicide. In India, the causes that are reported for suicide differ in police records and in clinical experience. Maladjustment with significant family members, financial problems and domestic strife have been cited as the most important causes of suicide attempts in India· (Kumar et al., 1997).

Marital conflict is the most common cause of suicide among women, while interpersonal conflict is the most common cause among men (Banerjee et al., 1990). In Ponnudurai and Jayakar's study 12.5% females have committed suicide due to maladjustment with alcohol and drug abusing husbands (Ponnudurai & Jayakar, 1980).

An interesting finding, rarely seen in the West, is the high rate of suicide associated with sexual abuse (80 cases) and illegitimate pregnancy (49 cases) in India (Accidental Deaths & Suicides in India, 2019. New Delhi: Ministry of Home Affairs, Government of India; 2021. National Crime Records Bureau). This may be a reflection of cultural taboos related to sexuality in India. Chronic pain and illness are featured as a common reason in some studies (Srivastava et al., 2004).

A similar trend is seen for attempted suicide with interpersonal conflict, financial stressors, and educational burden being the most common triggers (Mohanty et al., 2007).

### 3.5 *Mental Disorders and Suicide*

In India, the relationship between suicidal behaviour and psychiatric diagnosis has always been a matter of debate. Western literature reports that about 90% of all those who commit suicide suffer from a psychiatric disorder (Bretolete & Fleischmann, 2002).

Studies in India show varying results with rates of psychiatric disorders ranging from 9.5 to 24.9% (Manoranjitham et al., 2010). Unfortunately, no reliable data are available from India on psychiatric diagnoses of suicide victims. In a series of studies on suicide attempters by the author, the predominant psychiatric problem was major depression closely followed by adjustment disorder and alcohol abuse/dependence. Several of these attempts were of impulsive type and were done within hours of some triggering factor (Kumar, 2013).

### 3.6 *Farmer Suicides*

Suicides in the farming industry continued to increase in 2022. According to the latest report of the National Crime Records Bureau (NCRB), 11,290 suicide cases were reported across the country last year. This is an increase of 3.7 per cent from 2021, when 10,281 deaths were reported. It is an increase of 5.7 per cent when compared with 2020 figures (National Crime Reports Bureau, ADSI Report Annual—2023, Government of India). The actual numbers may be larger, partly because the NCRB defines "farmers" as men (but not women) who work in agriculture.

In a study on farmer suicides in the Vidarbha region, Behere and Behere employed the psychological autopsy method to understand the phenomenon and identified the following reasons for farmer suicide (1) chronic indebtedness and inability to pay debts accumulated over the years, (2) economic decline that leads to complications, family disputes, depression, alcoholism, etc., (3) compensation following suicide helps the family repay debts, (4) grain drain and (5) rising costs of agricultural inputs and falling prices of agricultural produce (Behere & Behere, 2008).

In a psychological autopsy study conducted in Wayanad, an agrarian district of Kerala, factors contributing to the high rate of suicide in this vulnerable population were economic adversity, exclusive dependence on rainfall for agriculture, alcohol abuse, depression and possible monetary compensation to the family following suicide (Kumar, 2011).

## 3.7 Religion, Spirituality and Suicide

Religion seems to be a protective factor both at the individual and societal levels. The psychological autopsy study in Chennai by Vijaykumar and Rajkumar found that the lack of belief in God was over six times more common in completed suicides than in controls (Vijayakumar & Rajkumar, 1999). Victims had less belief in God, changed their religious affiliation and rarely visited places of worship. Eleven per cent had lost their faith in the three months prior to suicide (Vijayakumar, 2002). This finding was replicated by Gururaj et al. in their psychological autopsy study in Bangalore (Gururaj et al., 2004).

Altruistic suicide has a long history in India, even being noted in the Dharmashastras, an ancient religious text. In ancient India, two forms of altruistic suicide were practiced. One was Jauhar, a kind of mass suicide by women of a community when their menfolk suffered defeat in battle; the other was Sati, the suicide of a widow on the funeral pyre of her husband. The practice of Jauhar ended with the fall of the Muslim rule and the practice of Sati is against the law, although stray cases are still reported. The act of Sati is now seen as suicide, not as an altruistic act, and there are laws against abetment and glorification (Thara & Padmavati, 2010).

## 3.8 Mental Health, Religion and Help-Seeking

Religion and religious practices play a very important role in every aspect of life in India. Seeking help from a religious setting or faith healers is a common behaviour pattern among those suffering from mental illness (Campion & Brugha, 1997) (Sharma et al., 2007). The variety and diversity of traditional healthcare practices are an indication of the great influence that socio-cultural practices have on healing systems. The several sources of traditional and religious help available range from places of worship like temples, dargahs and churches to the ubiquitous roadside indigenous faith healer.

In a methodologically rigorous study in a rural population in south India, Thara et al. found that the explanations offered for psychoses, depression and hysteria were possessions by evil spirits, devils or a curse of God, warranting a religious or traditional mode of treatment (Thara et al., 1998). On the other hand, epilepsy and mental retardation were understood as having an organic basis. Another general population study, conducted in a rural area in northern India, found that magico-religious systems were utilized by a substantial number of persons who attributed the illness to supernatural causes (Sharma et al., 2007).

The coexistence of several kinds of healers treating mental illness has been well documented in India (Sharma et al., 2007) (Kapur, 1979). Healing methods included penance, visits to a shrine, astrology and spirit possession to negotiate with the evil spirit. The choice of a particular healer is often made because of the perceived effectiveness of the healers in dealing with mental illness. This choice may be independent of the level of education or the patient's belief in the cause of illness (Jiloha & Jugal, 1997).

The effectiveness of healing sites has been described in ethnographic studies. Raghuram et al. used standardized clinical assessments of psychopathology in a temple in south India (Raghuram et al., 2002). A near 20% reduction in observed psychopathology scores was noted. Family care givers also thought that most of the subjects had improved during their stay in the temple. The cultural power of residency in the temple, known for its healing potency, may have played a part in reducing the severe psychotic symptoms of the subjects. In another study, several ritualistic practices employed at various centres were documented (Padmavati, 2005). These included making offerings (money, in kind), engaging in physical acts like going around the place of worship, fasting, eating raw fruits like lime or letting oneself be chained. These rituals were viewed as necessary for recovery. These ritualistic practices appear to have a wide framework, incorporating social, religious and mythical domains, allowing the patients to express and resolve social and psychic suffering (Pfleiderer, 1988).

The pattern of utilization of traditional and indigenous systems has prompted the initiative of a formal collaboration between religious systems and the formal psychiatric care system. A rehabilitation centre was established in a place called Gunaseelam in south India, within the premises of a Hindu temple known for its religious healing of the mentally ill for over 200 years. A quasi-experimental integrated intervention programme was designed incorporating pharmacotherapy, rehabilitation strategies and spiritual (ritualistic) strategies (which have been followed as part of the temple's healing practices). Assessments of psychopathology, family burden and quality of life of caregivers indicated an improvement after the interventions. The authors hypothesized that the improvement may have been the result of a combination of psychiatric interventions with the existing spiritual and ritualistic strategies (Stanley & Shwetha, 2006).

## 3.9 *A Brief Overview of Epidemiology of Mental Illness in India*

Epidemiological studies report prevalence rates for psychiatric disorders varying from 9.5 to 370/1000 population in India. These varying prevalence rates of mental disorders are not only specific to Indian studies but are also seen in international studies (Math & Srinivasaraju, 2010). In National Mental Health Survey the overall weighted prevalence for any mental morbidity was 13.7% lifetime and 10.6% current (National Mental Health Survey (India)[56]

According the National Survey on Extent and Pattern of Substance Use in India, alcohol is the most common psychoactive substance used by Indians (14.6% of the population between 10 and 75 years of age uses alcohol). After Alcohol, Cannabis (2.8% of the population) and Opioids (2.1% of the country's population) are the next commonly used substances in India. About 1.08% of 10–75 year old Indians (approximately 1.18 crore people) are current users of sedatives (non-medical, non-prescription use). Other categories of drugs such as Cocaine (0.10%) Amphetamine Type Stimulants (0.18%) and Hallucinogens (0.12%) are used by a small proportion of country's population (National Survey on Extent and Pattern of Substance Use in India' 2019) (Magnitude of Substance Use in India, 2019).

The treatment gap for mental health in India is high, with 70–92% of people with mental disorders not receiving treatment. This is due to a lack of awareness, stigma and a shortage of mental health professionals (Singh, 2018).

**Indian contributions to social psychiatry**: There are many Indians who have made outstanding contributions to social psychiatry. Some of them are:

R L Kapur (1938–2006): He was a colossus in Indian Psychiatry, an original thinker and a great scientist. After his training in psychiatry in India, he went over to UK, had further training and research there, came back to India and worked in psychiatric settings in a medical school and a neuroscience hospital. Afterwards, he took keen interest in social science research apart from psychiatry. He is considered as one of the great beacons of social psychiatry in the world and especially from Asia (Kallivayalil et al., 2025). His contributions to psychiatric epidemiology, social and community psychiatry, postgraduate training and qualitative research on diverse social issues including violence and terrorism makes him an outstanding luminary in social psychiatry (Bibleau & Corin, 2010) (Bhide, 2006). His notable publications are: The Great Universe of Kota (1976) (Carstairs & Kapur, 1976), Indian Psychiatric Interview Schedule (1974), Indian Psychiatric Survey Schedule (1974), The role of traditional healers in mental healthcare in rural India (1979), Community involvement in mental healthcare (1994), Violence in India: A psychological perspective (1994), Qualitative methods in mental health research (1999) and Another Way to Live (2009).

Vidya Sagar (1909–1978) is a legendary figure in Indian Psychiatry who had dedicated his life to the service of the people first in the state of undivided Panjab and later in Haryana, India (Malhotra & Kallivayalil, 2025). Community psychiatry has come a long way in India and the building blocks were laid by Vidya Sagar, in 1950, by constructing tents and involving family members in the treatment of persons with mental illness in Amritsar. During the horrific times of partition of India, when a huge number of patients with mental illness were sent to Amritsar and kept in army barracks, he displayed phenomenal devotion to their care (Sethi & Batra, 2010). Vidya Sagar was the most renowned social psychiatrist of his times, a humanist, full of compassion for the mentally ill and their families, a self-less man, revered by his patients. He was ahead of his times in propagating family psychiatry, community psychiatry, psychoeducation and mass psychotherapy, in times when psychiatry was primarily practiced in mental hospitals.

A Venkoba Rao (1927–2005): A great teacher and an inspiring speaker, he was Chairman of the Institute of Psychiatry, Madurai Medical College for 23 years. He had many books authored or edited by him including *Psychiatry of Old Age in India*, *Depression and Suicide Behavior*, *Textbook of Psychiatry*, *Culture, Philosophy, Mental Health* and *Mind: Turbulent and Tranquil*. He was the founder President of the

Indian Association for Social Psychiatry and evolved a model of healthcare delivery to the rural aged in India. He also pioneered Geriatric Psychiatry research in India. He also interpreted and incorporated India's scriptures and ancient philosophies into contemporary mental health concepts. He was well known for his lectures and writings on the Bhagvad Gita and its implications for psychiatry (Kallivayalil, 2025).

N. N. Wig (1930–2018): had made seminal contributions to research in the area of nosology, culture-bound syndromes, course and outcome of psychoses, psychotherapy and social psychiatry. Apart from his role as a regional advisor for mental health of the EMRO—WHO, he had worked tirelessly to reduce stigma and discrimination due to mental illness (Avasthi & Chakrabarti, 2018).

J K Trivedi (1952–2013): was one of the most eminent social psychiatrists of India. He was an academician, researcher, teacher and leader of rare abilities. He was one of the foremost researchers in Psychiatry in India and conducted researches in collaboration with National Institute of Mental Health, USA; John Hopkins Institute, USA; Indian Council of Medical Research, etc., (Kallivayalil & Dalal, 2013).

**Culture-bound syndrome in India**: Among them, commonest are Possession Syndrome, Dhat Syndrome, Koro, Bhanmati, Gilhari syndrome, Compulsive spitting, Suchibai syndrome, culture-bound suicide (sati, santhra), Jhinjhinia, ascetic syndrome, etc., (Kapoor et al., 2018).

**Guru-Chela relationship**: meaning master-disciple or teacher-trainee, is a traditional Indian concept, particularly in Eastern traditions like Hinduism and Buddhism, where the guru guides the chela towards spiritual or practical knowledge and enlightenment through teachings and practice. As a therapeutic paradigm, the guru-chela relationship appears most suited to cultures valuing self-discipline rather than self-expression and creative harmony between individual and society (Neki, 1974).

**Hanuman complex**: in the context of Indian mythology and psychotherapy, refers to Hanuman's forgotten powers being restored by Jambavan during a crucial mission to rescue Queen Sita, illustrating a concept of regaining potential. Wig has often used this story in helping patients in psychotherapy as well as in teaching medical doctors and trainees in psychiatry. He had made a plea for wider use of stories from Indian mythology in psychiatric practice (Wig, 2004).

**Marriage and mental illness**: In India, marriage is regarded as an important and sacrosanct event in an individual's life, and everyone is supposed to get married and have a family so that he can continue his progeny. Marriage is essential not only for begetting a son to discharge his debt to the ancestors but also for the performance of other religious and spiritual duties, according to Hindu beliefs. Major mental disorders are listed both as preconditions of marriage and as grounds for divorce. Under the Hindu Marriage Act of 1955, conditions with respect to mental disorders have been included (Narayan et al., 2015).The Hindu Marriage Act (HMA) and the Special Marriage Act (SMA) address mental illness, with provisions for annulment or divorce based on "unsoundness of mind" or mental disorder, but these laws are often complicated by societal stigma and patriarchal attitudes.

**Stigma in India**: Stigma is an important issue here and needs to be addressed as a priority. It is one of the key reasons for people to shy away from seeking mental healthcare. Anti-stigma measures help to improve the quality of mental health services and even enhance the self-esteem of psychiatry and give mental health rich dividends (Kallivayalil & Enara, 2016).

**Social support systems in India**: It is heavily dependent on family and community networks. Families take up a dominant role and usually consider it their responsibility to care for the mentally ill. The problem occurs when the families themselves are poor and deprived. India needs a holistic approach in treatment which involves patients, their environment and other stakeholders. Non-governmental Organisations (NGOs) in India give a great opportunity to work collaboratively with all stakeholders, enabling the fight against stigma and discrimination (Kallivayalil, 2023a, b).

## 4 Conclusion

Social psychiatry is against biological reductionism and strongly advocates attention to the social paradigm in health and disease (Kallivayalil, 2020). The renewed interest in social psychiatry has led to the emergence of WASP as a powerful and influential organization. Social psychiatry's relevance to clinical practice is underlined in the recently published WASP Textbook on social psychiatry, a comprehensive book with editorial contributions from India (Kallivayalil, 2023a, b). Social psychiatry is inclusive, as in ancient India, and also uses the concepts of social sciences like psychology, sociology and anthropology (Kallivayalil, 2023a, b). Psychosocial issues and social approaches to care are paramount in India (Chadda & Kallivayalil, 2023) and many other countries.

We have provided a brief overview of the roots of social psychiatry in India, the formation of IASP and significant contributions by stalwarts from the country. We have also outlined key studies related to social psychiatry in India, focusing on the role of families, disabilities, stigma, the specific problem of suicide and farmer's suicide, spirituality and the plurality of help-seeking responses and resources. The findings of these studies pose specific challenges in the Indian context. Understanding and meeting these challenges requires a social psychiatry perspective, both in research and in the delivery of care to those with a mental illness and their families—a paradigm shift in our thinking. This should happen now!

## References

Accidental Deaths and Suicides in India. (2019). New Delhi: Ministry of Home Affairs, Government of India; 2021. National Crime Records Bureau.

Avasthi, A., & Chakrabarti, S. (2018). Prof. NN Wig… The living legend of Indian Psychiatry. *Journal of Postgraduate Medicine, Education and Research, 52*(3), 164–165. https://doi.org/10.5005/jp-journals-10028-1294

Banerjee, G., Nandi, D. N., & Nandi, S. (1990). The vulnerability of Indian women to commit suicide-a field study. *Indian Journal of Psychiatry, 32,* 305–308.

Behere, P. B., & Behere, A. P. (2008). Farmers' suicide in Vidarbha region in Maharashtra State: A myth or reality? *Indian Journal of Psychiatry, 50,* 124–7. https://doi.org/10.4103/0019-5545.42401

Bhide, A. (2006). Remembering a Giant. *Indian Journal of Psychological Medicine, 28,* 6–7.

Bibleau, G., & Corin, E. (2010). Dr Ravi L Kapur (1938–2006): A psychiatrist at the crossroads of multiple worlds. *Transcultural Psychiatry, 47,* 159–180. https://doi.org/10.1177/1363461510364688

Bretolete, J. M., & Fleischmann, A. (2002). Suicide and psychiatric diagnosis: A worldwide perspective. *World Psychiatry, 1*(3), 181–185.

Campion, J., & Brugha, D. (1997). Experiences of religious healing in psychiatric patients in south India. *Social Psychiatry and Psychiatric Epidemiology, 32,* 215–221. https://doi.org/10.1007/BF00788241

Carstairs, G. M., & Kapur, R. L. (1976). *The great universe of Kota: Stress, change and mental disorder in an Indian village.* Hogarth Press.

Chadda, R. K., & Kallivayalil, R. A. (2023). Substance use and addictive disorders. *The wasp textbook on social psychiatry: Historical, developmental, cultural, and clinical perspectives* (p. 360).

Chakrabarti, S., Kulhara, P., & Verma, S. K. (1993) The pattern of burden in families of neurotic patients. *Social Psychiatry and Psychiatric Epidemiology, 28*(4), 172–177. https://doi.org/10.1007/BF00797319

Charles, H., Manoranjitham, S. D., & Jacob, K. S. (2007). Stigma and explanatory models among people with schizophrenia and their relatives in Vellore, South India. *International Journal of Social Psychiatry, 53*(4), 325–332. https://doi.org/10.1177/0020764006074538

Chaudhury, P. K., Deka, K., & Chetia, D. (2006). Indian disability evaluation and assessment scale. *Indian Psychiatric Society, 48*(2), 95–101. https://doi.org/10.4103/0019-5545.31597

Gururaj, G., Isaac, M., Subhakrishna, D. K., & Ranjani, R. (2004). Risk factors for completed suicides: A case-control study from Bangalore, India. *International Journal of Injury Control and Safety Promotion, 11,* 183–191. https://doi.org/10.1080/156609704/233/289706

Harding, T. W., Climent, C. E., Diop, M., Giel, R., Ibrahim, H. H., Murthy, R. S., Suleiman, M. A., & Wig, N. N. (1983). The WHO collaborative study on strategies for extending mental health care, II: The development of new research methods. *American Journal of Psychiatry, 140*(11), 1474–1480. https://doi.org/10.1176/ajp.140.11.1474

Jadhav, S., Littlewood, R., Ryder, A. G., Chakraborty, A., Jain, S., & Barua, M. (2007). Stigmatization of severe mental illness in India: Against the simple industrialization hypothesis. *Indian Journal of Psychiatry, 49*(3), 189–194. https://doi.org/10.4103/0019-5545.37320

Jiloha, R. C., & Jugal, K. (1997). Supernatural beliefs, mental illness and treatment out come in Indian patients. *Indian Journal of Social Psychiatry, 13*(3/4), 106–113.

Kallivayalil, R. (2021). Notes from WASP president's desk.

Kallivayalil, R. A. (2020). Psychiatry—From biological reductionism to a biopsycho-social perspective. *World Social Psychiatry, 2,* 3–6. https://doi.org/10.4103/WSP.WSP_4_20

Kallivayalil, R. A. (2023a). The relevance and need for a comprehensive textbook on social psychiatry. *The WASP Textbook On Social Psychiatry: Historical, Developmental, Cultural, and Clinical Perspectives.* https://doi.org/10.1093/med/9780197521359.001.0001

Kallivayalil, R. A. (2023b). Public mental health: Collaborating with nongovernment organizations. *World Social Psychiatry, 5*(2), 127-128. https://doi.org/10.4103/wsp.wsp_40_23

Kallivayalil, R. A. (2025). A Venkoba Rao (1927–2005). The Glow of Synthesis: Twelve Beacons of Light in Social Psychiatry: Jaypee Publications, New Delhi (under print).

Kallivayalil, R. A., & Enara, A. (2016). Stigma toward psychiatric disorders—National and International perspectives. *Indian Journal of Social Psychiatry, 32,* 115–119. https://doi.org/10.4103/0971-9962.181096

Kallivayalil, R. A., & Dalal, P. K. (2013). Prof. J. K. Trivedi. *Indian Journal of Psychiatry, 55*(4):311–312. https://doi.org/10.4103/0019-5545.120527.

Kallivayalil, R. A., Gogineni, R. R., Salman, & Akhtaret. (2025). Ravi L Kapur (1938–2006). The Glow of Synthesis: Twelve Beacons of Light in Social Psychiatry: Jaypee Publications, New Delhi (under print).

Kapoor, A., Juneja, R., & Chand Singh, D. (2018). Cultural Specific Syndromes in India—An Overview. *International Journal of Current Research and Review, 10*(11), 2–6. https://doi.org/10.31782/IJCRR.2018.10111

Kapur, R. (1979). The role of traditional healers in mental health care in rural India. *Social Science and Medicine, 13B,* 27–31. https://doi.org/10.1016/0160-7987(79)90015-2

Kulhara, P., Chakrabarti, S., Avasthi, A., Sharma, A., & Sharma, S. (2008). Psychoeducational intervention for care givers of Indian patients with schizophrenia: A randomised-controlled trial. *Acta Psychiatrica Scandinavica, 119*(6), 472–483. https://doi.org/10.1111/j.1600-0447.2008.01304.x

Kumar, P. N. S. (2011). A case—controlled Study of Suicides in an agrarian district in Kerala. *Indian Journal of Social Psychiatry, 27*(1–2), 9–15. https://doi.org/10.4103/ipj.ipj_136_24

Kumar, P. N. S. (2013). Life events, social support, coping strategies and quality of life in attempted suicide: A case control study. *Indian Journal of Psychiatry, 55*(1), 46–51. https://doi.org/10.4103/0019-5545.105504

Kumar, P. N. S., Kuruvilla, K., Dutta, S., John, G., & Nair, S. M. (1997). Hundred cases of suicide attempters admitted in a medical intensive care unit: Study of psychosocial factors in relation to age and sex. *Annals of National Academy of Medical Sciences, 33,* 223–233. https://doi.org/10.30834/KJP.32.1.2019.177

Lee, L., Roser, M., & Ortiz-Ospina, E. (2015). Suicide- Our world data.

Loganathan, S., & Murthy, S. R. (2008). Experience of stigma and discrimination endured by people suffering from schizophrenia. *Indian Journal of Psychiatry, 50*(1), 39–46. https://doi.org/10.4103/0019-5545.39758

Magnitude of Substance Use in India. (2019). https://www.lgbrimh.gov.in/resources/Addiction_Medicine/elibrary/magnitude_substance_abuse_india.pdf

Malhotra, S., & Kallivayalil, R. A. (2025). Vidya Sagar (1909–1978). The Glow of Synthesis: Twelve Beacons of Light in Social Psychiatry: Jaypee Publications, New Delhi (under print).

Manoranjitham, S. D., Rajkumar, A. P., Thangadurai, P., Prasad, J., Jayakaran, R., & Jacob, K. S. (2010). Risk factors for suicide in rural south India. *British Journal of Psychiatry, 196,* 26–30. https://doi.org/10.1192/bjp.bp.108.063347

Math, S. B., & Srinivasaraju, R. (2010). Indian Psychiatric epidemiological studies: Learning from the past. *Indian Journal of Psychiatry, 52*(Suppl 1):S95-S103. https://doi.org/10.4103/0019-5545.69220. PMID: 21836725; PMCID: PMC3146182.

Mezzich, J. E. (2007). Psychiatry for the person: Articulating medicine's science and humanism. *World Journal of Psychiatry, 6*(2), 65.

Mohanty, S., Sahu, G., Mohanty, M. K., & Patnaik, M. (2007). Suicide in India: A four-year retrospective study. *Journal of Forensic and Legal Medicine, 14,* 185–189. https://doi.org/10.1016/j.jcfm.2006.05.007

Murthy, R. S., Kishore Kumar, K. V., Chisholm, D., Thomas, T., Sekar, K., & Chandrashekari, C. R. (2005). Community outreach for untreated schizophrenia in rural India: A follow-up study of symptoms, disability, family burden and costs. *Psychological Medicine, 35*(3), 341–351. https://doi.org/10.1017/s0033291704003551

Narayan, C. L, Narayan, M., Shikha, D., & Shekhar, S. (2015). Indian marriage laws and mental disorders: Is it necessary to amend the legal provisions? *Indian Journal of Psychiatry, 57*(4), 341-344. https://doi.org/10.4103/0019-5545.171836. PMID: 26816420; PMCID: PMC4711231.

National Crime Reports Bureau, ADSI Report Annual—2023, Government of India.

National Mental Health Survey India. (2015–16). https://indianmhs.nimhans.ac.in/phase1/Docs/Summary.pdf

Neki, J. S. (1974). A reappraisal of the guru-chela relationship as a therapeutic paradigm. *International Mental Health Research Newsletter, 16*(2), 2–7.

NIMHANS: One crore Indians at high risk of suicide. The New Indian Express10th September 2017.

Padmavati, R. (2005). Community mental health care in India. *International Review of Psychiatry, 17*(2), 103–107. https://doi.org/10.1080/09540260500073562

Pai, S., & Kapur, R. L. (1981). The burden on the family of a psychiatric patient: Development of an interview schedule. *British Journal of Psychiatry, 138,* 332–335.

Pfleiderer, B. (1988). The semiotics of a ritual healing in a north Indian Muslim shrine. *Social Science and Medicine, 27,* 417–424. https://doi.org/10.1016/0277-9536(88)90364-4

Ponnudurai, R., & Jayakar, J. (1980). Suicide in Madras. *Indian Journal of Psychiatry, 22,* 203–205.

Raghuram, R., Venkateshwaran, A., Ramakrishna, J., & Weiss, M. G. (2002). Traditional community resources for mental health: A report of temple healing from India. *British Medical Journal, 325,* 38–40. https://doi.org/10.1136/bmj.325.7354.38

Rammohan, A., Rao, K., & Subbakrishna, D. K. (2002). Religious coping and psychological wellbeing in carers of relatives with schizophrenia. *Acta Psychiatrica Scandinavica, 105*(5), 356–362. https://doi.org/10.1034/j.1600-0447.2002.1o149.x

Sethi, S., & Batra, R. (2010). Dr. Vidya Sagar in Icons of Indian Psychiatry. *Indian Journal of Psychiatry,* 197–200.

Sharma, P., Vohra, A. K., & Khurana, H. (2007). Treatment seeking behavior of mentally ill patients in a rural area: A cross-sectional study. *Indian Journal of Community Medicine, 32*(4), 290–291. https://doi.org/10.4103/0970-0218.37699

Singh O. P. (2018). Closing treatment gap of mental disorders in India: Opportunity in new competency-based Medical Council of India curriculum. *Indian Journal of Psychiatry, 60*(4), 375–376. https://doi.org/10.4103/psychiatry.IndianJPsychiatry_458_18. PMID: 30581200; PMCID: PMC6278227.

Srinivasan, N. (2003). *The story of AMEND–The Association for the Mentally Disabled, in Meeting the Mental Health Needs of Developing Countries.* In V. Patel & R. Thara (Eds.), (vol. 17, pp. 329–349). SAGE Publications. https://doi.org/10.1177/004908570403400210

Srinivasan, T. N., & Thara, R. (2001). Beliefs about causation of schizophrenia: Do Indian families believe in supernatural causes? *Social Psychiatry and Psychiatric Epidemiology, 36*(3), 134–140. https://doi.org/10.1007/s001270050302

Srivastava, M. K., Sahoo, R. N., Ghotekar, L. H., Dutta, S., Danabalan, M., Dutta, T. K., & Das, A. K. (2004). Risk factors associated with attempted suicide: A case control study. Indian *Journal of Psychiatry, 46,* 33–38.

Stanley, S., & Shwetha, S. (2006). Integrated psycho social intervention in schizophrenia: Implications for patients and caregivers. *International Journal of Psychosocial Rehabilitation, 10*(2), 113–128.

Thara, R., Henrietta, M., Joseph, A., Rajkumar, S., & Eaton, W. W. (1994). Ten-year course of schizophrenia—the Madras longitudinal study. *Acta Psychiatrica Scandinavica, 90,* 329–336.

Thara, R., & Srinivasan, T. N. (2000). How stigmatizing is schizophrenia in India? *International Journal of Social Psychiatry, 46*(2), 135–141. https://doi.org/10.1177/002076400004600206

Thara, R., Islam, A., & Padmavati, R. (1998). Beliefs about mental illness: A study of a rural South Indian community. *International Journal of Mental Health, 27*(3), 70–85.

Thara, R., Kamath, S., & Kumar, S. (2003a). Women with schizophrenia and broken marriages doubly disadvantaged? Part I: Patient perspective. *International Journal of Social Psychiatry, 49*(3), 225–232.

Thara, R., Kamath, S., & Kumar, S. (2003b). Women with schizophrenia and broken marriages–doubly disadvantaged? Part II: Family perspective. *International Journal of Social Psychiatry, 49*(3), 233–240. https://doi.org/10.1177/00207640030493008

Thara, R., & Padmavati, R. (2010). Social psychiatry in India. In C. Morgan, & D. Bhugra (Eds.), *Principles of Social Psychiatry* (2nd ed., pp. 531–540). John Wiley & Sons Ltd. https://doi.org/10.1002/9780470684214.ch40

Thara, R., Padmavati, R., Kumar, S., & Srinivasan, L. (1998). Burden assessment schedule. *Indian Journal of Psychiatry, 40,* 21–29. https://pmc.ncbi.nlm.nih.gov/articles/PMC2964812/

Thara, R., Rajkumar, S., & Valecha, V. (1988). Schedule for the assessment of psychiatric disability—A modification of DAS. *Indian Journal of Psychiatry, 30*(1), 47–53.

Trivedi, J. K., Kaialsh, S. (2012). Relevance of social psychiatry in india—a reappraisal. *Indian Journal of Social Psychiatry, 28* (1–2), 8–9.

Varma, V. K. (2012). Whither social psychiatry? *Indian Journal of Social Psychiatry, 28*(1–2), 4–7.

Vijayakumar, L. (2002). Religion: A protective factor in suicide. *Suicidology, 2,* 9–12.

Vijayakumar, L., & Rajkumar, S. (1999). Are risk factors for suicide universal? A case-control study in India. *Acta Psychiatrica Scandinavica, 99,* 407–411. https://doi.org/10.1111/j.1600-0447.1999.tb00985.x

Wig, N. N. Menon, D. K., Bedi, H., Leff, J., Kuipers, L, Ghosh, A., Day, R., Korten, A., & Ernberg, G. (1987). Expressed emotion and schizophrenia in north India. II. Distribution of expressed emotion components among relatives of schizophrenic patients in Aarhus and Chandigarh. *British Journal of Psychiatry, 151,* 870.

Wig, N. N. (2004). Hanuman Complex and its Resolution: An illustration of psychotherapy from Indian mythology. *Indian Journal of Psychiatry, 46*(1):25–28.

# Chapter 5
# Social Psychiatry in Nepal

**Pawan Sharma, Anoop Krishna Gupta, and Kamal Gautam**

**Abstract** Nepal is a diverse nation with rich cultural and social traditions. It has faced unique challenges in mental health due to factors like poverty, natural disasters, political instability, and deep-rooted stigma throughout the history. Though mental health services in Nepal have been limited and largely centered in urban areas in the past, there has been an upliftment of services in the last decade. Efforts have been made to decentralize mental health services and integrate them into primary healthcare and community settings. The disasters at regular intervals and the COVID-19 pandemic exposed vulnerabilities in Nepal's mental health system. Traditional faith healing practices continue to coexist with modern psychiatric care, necessitating collaboration between mental health professionals and local healers to ensure proper pathways of care. There is a need for policy reform, capacity building, and research to generate evidence-based interventions to suit the social context of Nepal. In this chapter, we discuss the social aspects of psychiatric disorders and their management in the Nepalese context.

**Keywords** Social psychiatry · Social determinants · Mental Health · Stigma · Nepal

## 1 Introduction

Nepal is a landlocked country in South Asia with China in the North and India in the east, west, and south. The population of Nepal is approximately 30 million, and there are more than 142 caste/ethnic groups and 124 languages spoken (National Statistics

P. Sharma (✉)
Department of Psychiatry, Patan Academy of Health Sciences, Lalitpur, Nepal
e-mail: pawansharma@pahs.edu.np

A. K. Gupta
Department of Psychiatry, National Medical College, Birgunj, Nepal

K. Gautam
Transcultural Psychosocial Organization Nepal (TPO), Kathmandu, Nepal



S. M. Y. Arafat et al. (eds.), *Social Psychiatry in South Asia*, South Asian Perspectives in Mental Health and Psychology , https://doi.org/10.1007/978-981-96-8078-8_5

Office, 2021; Regmi, 2024). There is a federal democratic system with governance through a three-tier federal structure, including federal, provincial, and local levels. The constitution of Nepal 2015 ensures social inclusion and equal rights for all citizens of Nepal. Nepal is known for its geographical diversity, rich cultural heritage, and multi-ethnic society. The social structure is influenced by historical caste divisions, economic disparities, and cultural traditions. Even today, there is a communal lifestyle with a joint family system and social bonds which play a significant role in everyday life (Yadav, 2023). Hinduism and Buddhism are the major religions in the country with minority of Christian and Muslim communities (National Statistics Office, 2021). There is a disparity in access to education, healthcare, and employment opportunities between urban and rural areas. Though urban areas have undergone rapid modernization, there are many rural regions which lack basic healthcare infrastructure, including mental health services (Luitel et al., 2015). Nepal has undergone a rapid shift in its migration pattern in the last three decade and this has also created an impact in the social structure of Nepal (Adhikari et al., 2023).

Nepal underwent decades of political turmoil, mainly a decade-long civil war from 1996 to 2006. There was an abolition of monarchy in 2008. Nepal faced a mega earthquake in 2015 followed by COVID-19 Pandemic. These events have created an impact in the mental health status of people living in Nepal (Poudel & Subedi, 2020; Sherchan et al., 2017). In this chapter we aim to discuss the social determinants of mental health in the Nepalese population, the social epidemiology of mental health, the unique issues of social psychiatry pertinent to Nepal, and the challenges and ways out in this field.

## 2 Social Epidemiology of Psychiatric Disorders in Nepal

### *2.1 Prevalence and Social Determinants of Mental Health in Nepal*

A study using global burden of disease 2019 data reported an estimate that around 13.5% of the population suffers from mental illness in Nepal while the prevalence in 1990 was around 12.9% (Dhungana et al., 2023). Similarly, the National Mental Health Survey of Nepal 2019–2020 showed a lifetime prevalence of mental illness of 10% among the adult population and 5.2% among adolescents (Dhimal et al., 2022). Earthquake, old age, divorce, poverty, low social class, civil conflicts, and exposure to violence have been shown to contribute to mental illness in adults and children (Chaulagain et al., 2019; Jha et al., 2019). Children and adolescents have been affected by the post-earthquake and civil conflict. PTSD was on the rise post-conflict and post-2015 earthquake (Luitel et al., 2013). Lack of educational opportunities have pushed adolescents into substance use disorders. As per the National mental health Survey, 2020 the prevalence of alcohol use disorder (past 12 months) was 4.2% and other substance use disorder (past 12 months) was 0.2% excluding nicotine use (Dhimal et al., 2022). As per the WHO STEPwise approach to NCD risk factor surveillance (STEPS) survey of Nepal 28.9% (48.3% male and 11.6% females) were current users of tobacco, in any form. 17.1% of adults smoked tobacco and 18.3% used smokeless tobacco (Mandal, 2022). Recent trends in migration are on the rise, and migrant workers show poorer mental health than the general population (Devkota et al., 2021a, 2021b). The left-behind wives and children of the migrant population have poorer mental health as well (Aryal et al., 2019, 2020). Women are affected after being burdened by the family responsibilities of the migrant workers. Females have also suffered from domestic violence and substance use of spouse. Men and women of marginalized communities like Dalits and indigenous groups have suffered. Poverty, unemployment, lack of education, belonging to low casts, male dominance, and poor living conditions contribute to mental health issues in Nepal (Chase et al., 2018). Unemployment, especially among youth, contributes to a sense of hopelessness and social isolation, which are the major risk factors for mental illness (Regmi et al., 2020). Gender norms and masculinity in Nepal are deeply entrenched in cultural traditions, reinforcing social expectations for men to exhibit strength, resilience, and emotional stoicism. These ideals, while seemingly empowering, often create mental health challenges, including stress, anxiety, depression, and reluctance to seek psychological support (Uprety & Lamichanne, 2016).

## *2.2 Suicide and Its Correlates in Nepal*

The prevalence of suicidality in Nepal is 7.2% among adults and 4.1% of adolescents as per the National Mental Health Survey. The current prevalence of suicidal thoughts and lifetime suicidal attempts were among 6.5% and 1.1% of adults, respectively (Dhimal et al., 2022). A scoping review of studies on suicide in Nepal has found that the rates of suicide and self-harm behaviors were higher among women and younger age groups, migrant workers, and marginalized and disaster-affected populations. The role of psycho-social factors was more prominent than mental illness alone (Thapaliya et al., 2018). The most consistent risk factors of suicide in Nepal are younger age and the presence of a mental disorder, especially depression. Apart from marriage and relationship issues, interpersonal and family conflicts, family history of attempted suicide, and substance-use disorders have also been identified as risk factors for suicide in the Nepalese population (Marahatta et al., 2017). A mixed-method psychological autopsy study suggested a social pattern across cases like lack of education, life stressors such as poverty, violence, migrant labor, family disputes, and family histories of suicidal behavior. Among females, attributed factors were hopeless situations like spousal abuse and social stigma, whereas, among males, suicides were most commonly associated with alcohol abuse and internalized stigma, such as financial failure or an inability to provide for their family (Hagaman et al., 2018).

### 2.3 *Mental Health During Disasters and Political Conflict in Nepal*

In Nepal, floods, landslides, and earthquakes are the most regularly occurring disasters. There have been negative impacts of these disasters in the context of Nepal. Apart from this, political conflict and civil war also have also contributed to mental health problems (Tol et al., 2010). A prospective study that compared mental health before and after exposure to direct political violence during the People's War in Nepal showed that there was an increase of depression from 30.9% to 40.6%, and anxiety from 26.2% to 47.7%. The prevalence of post-traumatic stress disorder (PTSD) was 14.1% (Kohrt et al., 2012). A cross-sectional study conducted among 750 earthquake-affected individuals in six districts in central Nepal 15 months post-earthquake showed that the symptoms of depression and anxiety symptoms were significantly higher in females and individuals between 40 and 50 years old (Powell et al., 2019). The recent COVID-19 pandemic and the measure to contain like lockdown curfews, self-isolation, social distancing, and quarantine have affected the overall mental, spiritual, and social well-being of the Nepalese population (Poudel & Subedi, 2020). A community-level survey showed that during the COVID-19 pandemic, the psychological distress was higher among age group > 45 years, female gender, and post-secondary education group and health professionals (Shrestha et al., 2020).

### 2.4 *Culture Bound Syndrome in Nepal*

There are many culture-bound syndromes identified in Nepal. Table 1 presents the common syndromes with the cultural context and its impact in Nepalese context.

## 3 Help-Seeking Behavior for Mental Illness in Nepal

The help-seeking behavior for mental health problems in Nepal ranges from traditional faith healers, supernatural role practitioners, general practitioners, and community health workers to mental health professionals. In Nepal, traditional faith healers are often the first contact while compared to the psychiatrist as they are easily approachable and people have belief in supernatural cause for mental disorders (Pradhan et al., 2013). A 14-center nationwide study found out most of the patients with severe mental illnesses (SMIs) had their first contact with faith healers (49%). 29.8% of patients with common mental disorders (CMDs) had first contact with faith healers and 26% of the patients had first contact with psychiatrists (Gupta et al., 2021). As per the National Mental Health Survey, 2020, among the treatment-seeking patients, 8.8% visited non-specialist doctors, 6.7% visited faith healers (6.7%), and 6.5% visited psychiatrists for treatment (National Mental Health Survey, 2020).

**Table 1** Culture bound syndrome (CBS), their cultural context and impact in Nepal

| CBS | Cultural context | Impact |
|---|---|---|
| **Dhat syndrome**: It is the most commonly reported culture-bound syndrome in Nepal. It involves the fear of losing semen in urine (often linked to excessive physical or mental exertion), which is believed to cause weakness, fatigue, anxiety, and depression | It is often associated with feelings of shame and guilt, particularly in the context of societal views on masculinity and sexual performance. A range of psychological and somatic symptoms associated with Dhat syndrome were revealed from a study among 50 patients of Dhat syndrome like excessive worries, tingling sensation of body, weakness, decreased interest, fatigue, depressed mood, and generalized body ache (Dhungana et al., 2017) | Those suffering from Dhat syndrome may avoid social situations, express significant distress, and avoid seeking professional psychiatric help, fearing social stigma or embarrassment<br>A study among 50 patients revealed that 2/3rd had other co-morbid ICD 10 diagnosis (Shakya, 2019) |
| **Koro syndrome**: It is marked by the fear that one's genitals (usually male) are retracting into the body and that they will disappear or cause death. This syndrome is primarily reported in Southeast Asia but has also been observed in Nepal (Shakya et al., 2021) | In Nepalese culture, a few cases have been reported, but the studies on detailed cultural context and impact are not available (Shakya et al., 2021) | NA |
| **Mass Hysteria**: Mass hysteria often occurs in communities where there is a significant amount of stress or anxiety. It manifests as uncontrollable laughter, crying, shouting, brief writhing movement or fainting | In Nepal, it often occurs among young women and girls, particularly in rural areas, and is linked to social and economic stressors, such as pressure to marry or cope with familial responsibilities (R. Shakya, 2005). The condition is often seen as a response to unexpressed emotions or repressed desires. A case control study identified physical abuse, peritraumatic dissociation, and hypnotizability as contributing factors for mass dissociation in Nepal (Sapkota et al., 2020) | It is typically viewed as a transient condition that can be resolved through rest and family support. However, when episodes persist or become chronic, individuals may be referred to local healers or religious leaders for spiritual intervention |

(continued)

**Table 1** (continued)

| CBS | Cultural context | Impact |
|---|---|---|
| ***Mata aaune or Devi chadhne* (Trance and possession)**: Such episodic illness is characterized by rolling head and upper trunk in a circular motion with loose hairs mostly seen in females. They may speak their repressed wishes or command authoritative figures like husbands and parents, often followed by voicing threats of misfortune if their commands are not followed. The memory of the episode may or may not be remembered | This syndrome is often associated with domestic violence in past, unresolved grief, or perceived abuse in assumed protective environment (e.g., sexual abuse, marital rape, alcoholic husband or family conflict). In rural Nepal, this phenomenon may be interpreted as a sign of spiritual possession or a deep need for social respect | While individuals in rural region may receive traditional offerings and respect due to fear, those in urban areas may eventually be referred to psychiatric care. However, the reluctance to seek professional help due to stigma or lack of access remains a significant barrier. Such illness acts like a neurotic defense to psychosocial stressors and may continue if not resolved (Gupta et al., 2021) |
| **Jhum-Jhum**: It is characterized by a tingling sensation in limbs and body where individuals may lose consciousness, often followed by physical symptoms such as trembling, falling into trance-like states, or exhibiting a loss of coordination | This phenomenon has been both described as a syndrome (Kohrt & Schreiber, 1999) and also as a symptom suggestive of paresthesia (Basnyat et al., 1999) | This phenomenon may be a somatic symptom of depression. It can also be a symptom of medical disorder or a symptom of somatization (Kohrt, 2005) |

Evidence demonstrates that people trust traditional faith healers, and those who do so are more likely to seek help from healthcare providers recommended by them (Thapa et al., 2018). Seeking traditional faith healing care has both positive and negative outcomes. While negative outcomes pertain to the infliction of physical injuries, providing false hope and assurance to delay in seeking appropriate care, there are several positive outcomes like building self-esteem, psychological care, and opportunities for early detection and initiation of treatment. A study among 1983 adults in a community where screening for depression and alcohol use disorder was done showed that more than 90% didn't seek treatment for their condition. The barriers to treatment were lacking financial means to afford care, fear of being perceived as "weak" for having mental health problems, fear of being perceived as "crazy," and being too unwell to ask for help (Luitel et al., 2017). A qualitative study has shown mental health stigma and inadequate awareness as major factors that cause barriers to mental health service utilization at the community level (Devkota et al., 2021a, 2021b). Financial barriers often lead individuals to seek alternative healing practices rather than evidence-based psychiatric treatments, which contributes to delaying appropriate care and worsens the outcomes (Pham et al., 2021).

## 4 Community Understanding and Attitude toward Mental Health in Nepal

Nepalese communities view individuals with mental illnesses with stigma and consider them as either cursed or sufferers of past sins. Despite that, suffering families often serve as the first line of support for individuals with mental health conditions. Caregivers' attitudes toward the mentally ill differ by the gender of the caregiver, the education and gender of the patient, and the type of mental illness. Similarly, the perceived stigma is different between genders of caregiver, education, occupation, and relation with patient. Not much difference in perceived stigma was seen between urban and rural communities (Neupane et al., 2016). There has been an improvement in knowledge about mental illness in communities of Nepal, however, negative attitudes still persists (Jha & Mandal, 2021) (Das & Adhikari, 2013). The knowledge of issues like the human rights of mentally ill patients is still inadequate in the community setting (Koirala et al., 2019).

## 5 Resilience among the Nepalese Population

A study among adolescents of Nepal showed that 17.5% of adolescents were classified as having low resilience. The socio-demographic factors associated with having low resilience were female gender, attending a private school, higher birth order compared to firstborn, living in an urban area, and being physically inactive (Singh et al., 2019). The lower incidence of 12-month prevalence of mental disorders as compared to Western setting have provided an indirect evidence of good resilience among Nepalese people (Scott et al., 2021). A study among 100 clinical population from tertiary center of Nepal showed that resilience had negative correlations with PTSD, anxiety, and depression symptoms with a history of trauma after adjusting for social variables (S. Dhungana et al., 2022). The resilience of the Nepalese population has been tested time and again by different disasters and political unrest, and factors like self-efficacy, perceived stress, spirituality, self-esteem, and social support have played a major role in this context (Timalsina et al., 2022).

## 6 Social Security and Health Economics in Psychiatry in Nepal

A 24-year family panel study among 10,516 Nepalese has shown that transition to marriage was associated with increased odds of first onset depression. The factors like divorce and early widowed increased odd of having depression among females and becoming widowed increased the odds of depression in males (Axinn et al., 2020). In the social context of Nepal, the family plays an important role not only in the identification of symptoms but also in the management and rehabilitation of people with mental disorders. The family plays an important role not only in the identification of symptoms but also in the management and rehabilitation of people with mental disorders. The caregiving burden for family members among admitted patients was moderate to severe, indicating the involvement in treatment (Bhandari et al., 2015). The subjective burden by the family members have been reported up to 95% (Kunwar et al, 2020). Mental illness in the family disrupts normal functioning, and as per a qualitative study, family members in Nepal are responsible for improving the detection and identification of mental health problems, and they sometimes are recognized as key barriers to this process (Brenman et al., 2014).

Though the constitution of Nepal states basic healthcare is a fundamental right, individuals with mental disorders rely on out-of-pocket expenses for treatment (Sharma et al., 2024). The Government of Nepal launched the national health insurance policy in 2014 and currently, this scheme provides insured individuals with treatment of one lakh for out-patients or in-patients set up where this program is ongoing. This is a co-pay system (10% to be paid by the insured individual) and not all psychotropics are available in this system, indicating the inadequacy and inaccessibility for all citizens (Paneru et al., 2022). Nepal's social security system does not provide adequate financial support for elderly individuals suffering from dementia and other psychiatric illnesses (Thapa et al., 2024).

## 7 Media Representation of Mental Illness in Nepal

In Nepal, having a mental health condition is often synonymous with having a psychotic illness and is often associated with stigma and discrimination. Dissociative (Conversion) disorders are the most commonly reported mental illness in social and mass media in the country. Media and news often cover episodes of mass conversion disorders in schools in rural settings of Nepal. Information is often misleading and often reported as "Hysteria"(Seale-Feldman, 2019). Similarly, several media report incidents of suicide. Responsible media reporting on suicide is very much lacking, and media often portray incidents verbatim to the witness and often publish pictures of the deceased, details of the incident, means of suicide and family members in grief (Sharma et al., 2022). The depictions of suicidality in Nepali motion pictures minimally adhere to the WHO media guidelines indicating poor awareness (Singh et al., 2024). Though a guideline for responsible media reporting of suicide has been endorsed by the National Health Education Information and Communication Centre (NHEICC), MoHP, the rollout of this guideline and its impact on the reporting of suicide is yet to be analyzed (WHO, 2023).

## 8 Mental Health Literacy and Stigma

The awareness about mental health issues is low in the community, especially in the rural areas (Luitel et al., 2015). Nepal's mental health and suicide literacy are also low as studied by medical students (Gupta et al., 2023; Mishra et al., 2023). Additionally, it is believed that mental illness is incurable and requires life-long medications. Suicide is considered not only a sin but stigmatizing terms are used for patients with mental disorders and suicide attempters (Gupta et al., 2023). The stigma has led to disease concealment, low help-seeking, and poor treatment compliance (Gurung et al., 2022). Among psychotic patients, those with supernatural beliefs had a longer duration of untreated psychosis (Gupta et al., 2021). This is one of the challenges.

Measuring stigma with standardized tools along with implementation and evaluation of interventions need to be done. Policies and campaigns to reduce stigma and promotion of mental health awareness by government bodies, NGOs, and community programs are needed. The initiatives that train family members to help recognize early symptoms, provide emotional support, and help in reintegration after hospitalization would be helpful (Jordans et al., 2015). Additionally, peer-support programs within families help reduce stigma and encourage open discussions about mental health, which helps contribute to more sustainable recovery pathways. The involvement of family members and community health workers in psychiatric treatment would enhance medication adherence and overall patient well-being in Nepalese communities.

## 9 Mental Health of Migrant Workers

A study done among 502 Nepalese migrant workers suggested that 14.4% had mild to severe depression, while 4.4% had moderate anxiety. Also, 14.1% of the respondents had WHO 5 well-being scores suggestive of poor psychological well-being (Sharma et al., 2023). Similarly, a qualitative study conducted with Nepalese migrating and returnee migrant workers identified several risk factors such as high expectations from families back home, unfair treatment at work, poor working and living arrangements, discrimination at work and social isolation abroad which may trigger poor mental health among the Nepali migrants (Regmi et al., 2020). Migration not only impacts the health and well-being of migrants themselves, but it also has a significant effect on those people left behind. A study conducted with wives of Nepalese migrants reported three times higher depression rates in left-behind wives than those living with their husbands (Bhirtyal & Wasti, 2021). A study reported that separated family members were feeling lonely and experiencing marital conflict (Thapa et al., 2019).

To counter the problem, comprehensive pre-immigration sessions and screenings would be needed. Further mental health services need to be strengthened by collaborative effort from government and embassies. Strengthening of tele-mental health services may be one option for early detection and treatment.

## 10 Opportunities

There are several challenges in Nepal, like lack of regular supply of psychotropic medications enlisted in the essential free drug list, lack of supervision and mentoring after the training of health workers, frequent transfer of trained health workers, prevailing stigma and discrimination among health workers toward patients with mental health conditions, inadequate recording and reporting of diagnosed cases and inadequate resource allocation on mental health by the government, etc., (Sharma et al, 2024). On the positive side, mental health services have developed tremendously over the past decade in Nepal especially in terms of the increased number of mental health professionals, scaling up of community mental health programs, the establishment of the country's first child and adolescent psychiatry unit, designation of a focal mental health unit at the Ministry of Health and Population, initiation of the National Mental Health Survey, formulation and implementation of National Mental Health Strategy and Action Plan (Rai et al., 2021). A task-sharing approach as envisioned by WHO was initiated in Nepal in 2011, and the WHO mhGAP training manual has been translated, adapted, endorsed, and rolled out across several regions of the country by the Ministry of Health & Population (Sharma et al., 2024). However, a shortcoming of these in-service training programs has been the lack of accurate detection of patients with mental health conditions who need mental health services (Kohrt et al., 2025). Similarly, there are post-graduate trainings, incorporation of psychiatry in undergraduate training, psychology courses, and psychiatric nursing courses ongoing in Nepal. A tele-health guideline has been developed by the Curative Service Division, Ministry of Health and Population, tailored to mental health service delivery including prescription of psychotropics. However, there is still a need of policy reform, capacity building, and research to generate evidence-based interventions to suit the social context of Nepal.

## 11 Conclusion

Mental health in Nepal is shaped by diverse factors, including socio-economic conditions, rapid urbanization, and the challenges faced by vulnerable populations. The mental health services have developed tremendously over the past decade but more needs to be done considering the problem statement. There needs to be a comprehensive approach that includes both preventive measures and robust support systems in the social context of Nepal in order to provide collaborative mental healthcare to all.

Mental health services should be expanded, particularly for vulnerable groups, and efforts to reduce stigma and increase awareness should be prioritized. Strengthening resilience at the community level and integrating mental health support into everyday social practices will be key to improving mental health outcomes along with policy reform, capacity building, and research to generate evidence-based interventions to suit the social context of Nepal.

## References

Adhikari, J., Rai, M. K., Baral, C., & Subedi, M. (2023). Labour migration from Nepal: Trends and explanations. In S. I. Rajan (Ed.), *Migration in South Asia: IMISCOE regional reader* (pp. 67–81). Springer International Publishing. https://doi.org/10.1007/978-3-031-34194-6_5

Aryal, N., Regmi, P. R., Van Teijlingen, E., Simkhada, P., & Mahat, P. (2019). Perspective adolescents left behind by migrant workers: A call for community-based mental health interventions in Nepal. WHO South-East Asia. *Journal of Public Health, 8*(1). https://doi.org/10.4103/2224

Aryal, N., Regmi, P. R., van Teijlingen, E., Trenoweth, S., Adhikary, P., & Simkhada, P. (2020). The impact of spousal migration on the mental health of Nepali women: A cross-sectional study. *International Journal of Environmental Research and Public Health, 17*(4). https://doi.org/10.3390/ijerph17041292

Axinn, W. G., Zhang, Y., Ghimire, D. J., Chardoul, S. A., Scott, K. M., & Bruffaerts, R. (2020). The association between marital transitions and the onset of major depressive disorder in a South Asian general population. *Journal of Affective Disorders, 266,* 165–172.

Basnyat, B., Zimmerman, M., Sleggs, J., & Vaidhya, H. (1999). Jhum-jhum is a symptom. *The Lancet, 353*(9169), 2074. https://doi.org/10.1016/S0140-6736(05)77894-6

Bhandari, A. R., Marahatta, K., Rana, M., Ojha, S. P., & Regmi, M. P. (2015). Caregiving burden among family members of people with mental illness. *Journal of Psychiatrists' Association of Nepal, 4*(1), 36–42.

Bhirtyal, Y. M., & Wasti, S. P. (2021). Effects of male international migration on mental health of wives left behind in Nepal. *Journal of Manmohan Memorial Institute of Health Sciences, 7*(1). https://doi.org/10.3126/jmmihs.v7i1.43151

Brenman, N. F., Luitel, N. P., Mall, S., & Jordans, M. J. (2014). Demand and access to mental health services: A qualitative formative study in Nepal. *BMC International Health and Human Rights, 14,* 1–12.

Chase, L. E., Sapkota, R. P., Crafa, D., & Kirmayer, L. J. (2018). Culture and mental health in Nepal: An interdisciplinary scoping review. *Global Mental Health, 5.* https://doi.org/10.1017/gmh.2018.27

Chaulagain, A., Kunwar, A., Watts, S., Guerrero, A. P. S., & Skokauskas, N. (2019). Child and adolescent mental health problems in Nepal: A scoping review. *International Journal of Mental Health Systems, 13,* 1–8.

Das, R., & Adhikari, P. (2013). Knowledge, attitude and practice survey of community people regarding mental illness: Evidence from Dang District of Nepal. *Journal of Young Medical Researchers.*

Devkota, G., Basnet, P., Thapa, B., & Subedi, M. (2021a). Factors affecting utilization of mental health services from Primary Health Care (PHC) facilities of western hilly district of Nepal. *PLOS ONE, 16*(4), e0250694. https://doi.org/10.1371/journal.pone.0250694

Devkota, H. R., Bhandari, B., & Adhikary, P. (2021b). Perceived mental health, wellbeing and associated factors among Nepali male migrant and non-migrant workers: A qualitative study. *Journal of Migration and Health, 3,* 100013. https://doi.org/10.1016/j.jmh.2020.100013

Dhimal, M., Dahal, S., Adhikari, K., Koirala, P., Bista, B., Luitel, N., Pant, S., Marahatta, K., Shakya, S., Sharma, P., Ghimire, S., Gyanwali, P., Ojha, S. P., & Jha, A. K. (2022). A Nationwide prevalence of common mental disorders and suicidality in Nepal: Evidence from national mental health survey, 2019–2020. *Journal of Nepal Health Research Council, 19*(4), 740–747. https://doi.org/10.33314/jnhrc.v19i04.4017

Dhungana, M., Ghimire, S. R., & Thapa, M. (2017). A study of Dhat syndrome—a culture bound syndrome in Nepalese context. *Journal of Psychiatrists' Association of Nepal, 6*(1), Article 1. https://doi.org/10.3126/jpan.v6i1.21770

Dhungana, R. R., Pandey, A. R., Joshi, S., Luitel, N. P., Marahatta, K., Aryal, K. K., & Dhimal, M. (2023). The burden of mental disorders in Nepal between 1990 and 2019: Findings from the global burden of disease study 2019. *Cambridge Prisms: Global Mental Health, 10*. https://doi.org/10.1017/gmh.2023.55

Dhungana, S., Koirala, R., Ojha, S. P., & Thapa, S. B. (2022). Resilience and its association with post-traumatic stress disorder, anxiety, and depression symptoms in the aftermath of trauma: A cross-sectional study from Nepal. *SSM—Mental Health,2,* 100135. https://doi.org/10.1016/j.ssmmh.2022.100135

Gupta, A. K., Joshi, S., Kafle, B., Thapa, R., Chapagai, M., Nepal, S., Niraula, A., Paudyal, S., Sapkota, P., Poudel, R., Gurung, B. S., Pokhrel, P., Jha, R., Pandit, S., Thapaliya, S., Shrestha, S., Volpe, U., & Sartorius, N. (2021). Pathways to mental health care in Nepal: A 14-center nationwide study. *International Journal of Mental Health Systems, 15*(1). https://doi.org/10.1186/s13033-021-00509-4

Gupta, A. K., Sharma, R., Sah, R. P., Sharma, S., Jha, A., Chapagai, M., Saeed, F., & Shoib, S. (2023). Cross-cultural adaptation of Nepalese literacy and stigma of suicide scales (LOSS-SF-Nep and SOSS-SF-Nep) among Nepalese medical and nursing students. *Brain and Behavior,13*(12). https://doi.org/10.1002/brb3.3344

Gurung, D., Poudyal, A., Wang, Y. L., Neupane, M., Bhattarai, K., Wahid, S. S., Aryal, S., Heim, E., Gronholm, P., Thornicroft, G., & Kohrt, B. (2022). Stigma against mental health disorders in Nepal conceptualised with a 'what matters most' framework: A scoping review. *Epidemiology and Psychiatric Sciences, 31,* e11. https://doi.org/10.1017/S2045796021000809

Hagaman, A. K., Khadka, S., Wutich, A., Lohani, S., & Kohrt, B. A. (2018). Suicide in Nepal: Qualitative findings from a modified case-series psychological autopsy investigation of suicide deaths. *Culture, Medicine, and Psychiatry, 42*(3), 704–734. https://doi.org/10.1007/s11013-018-9585-8

Jha, A. K., Ojha, S. P., Dahal, S., Sharma, P., Pant, S. B., Labh, S., Marahatta, K., Shakya, S., Adhikari, R. P., Joshi, D., Luitel, N. P., & Dhimal, M. (2019). Prevalence of mental disorders in Nepal: Findings from the pilot study. *Journal of Nepal Health Research Council, 17*(2), 141–147. https://doi.org/10.33314/jnhrc.v0i0.1960

Jha, P., & Mandal, P. K. (2021). Knowledge and attitude on mental illness among people of a selected community of Biratnagar. *Journal of Psychiatrists' Association of Nepal, 10*(1), https://doi.org/10.3126/jpan.v10i1.40347

Jordans, M. J. D., Kohrt, B. A., Luitel, N. P., Komproe, I. H., & Lund, C. (2015). Accuracy of proactive case finding for mental disorders by community informants in Nepal. *The British Journal of Psychiatry: THe Journal of Mental Science, 207*(6), 501–506. https://doi.org/10.1192/bjp.bp.113.141077

Kohrt, B. A. (2005). "Somatization" and "Comorbidity": A Study of Jhum-Jhum and Depression in Rural Nepal. *Ethos, 33*(1), 125–147. https://doi.org/10.1525/eth.2005.33.1.125

Kohrt, B. A., Gurung, D., Singh, R., Rai, S., Neupane, M., Turner, E. L., Platt, A., Sun, S., Gautam, K., Luitel, N. P., & Jordans, M. J. D. (2025). Is there a mental health diagnostic crisis in primary care? Current research practices in global mental health cannot answer that question. *Epidemiology and Psychiatric Sciences, 34,* e7. https://doi.org/10.1017/S2045796025000010

Kohrt, B. A., Hruschka, D. J., Worthman, C. M., Kunz, R. D., Baldwin, J. L., Upadhaya, N., Acharya, N. R., Koirala, S., Thapa, S. B., Tol, W. A., Jordans, M. J. D., Robkin, N., Sharma,

V. D., & Nepal, M. K. (2012). Political violence and mental health in Nepal: Prospective study. *The British Journal of Psychiatry, 201*(4), 268–275. https://doi.org/10.1192/bjp.bp.111.096222

Kohrt, B. A., & Schreiber, S. S. (1999). Jhum-jhum: Neuropsychiatric symptoms in a Nepali village. *The Lancet, 353*(9158), 1070. https://doi.org/10.1016/S0140-6736(98)05782-1

Koirala, D., Silwal, M., Gurung, A., Gurung, R., & Paudel, S. (2019). A study to assess the knowledge regarding human right of mentally ill patient among community people in Kaski, Pokhara, Nepal. *Journal of Gandaki Medical College-Nepal, 12*(2), Article 2. https://doi.org/10.3126/jgmcn.v12i2.27171

Kunwar, D., Lamichhane, S., Pradhan, N., Shrestha, B., Khadka, S., Gautam, K., & Risal, A. (2020). The study of burden of family caregivers of patients living with psychiatric disorders in remote area of Nepal. *Kathmandu University Medical Journal, 18*(2), 41–45.

Luitel, N. P., Jordans, M. J., Adhikari, A., Upadhaya, N., Hanlon, C., Lund, C., & Komproe, I. H. (2015). Mental health care in Nepal: Current situation and challenges for development of a district mental health care plan. *Conflict and Health, 9*(1), 3. https://doi.org/10.1186/s13031-014-0030-5

Luitel, N. P., Jordans, M. J. D., Kohrt, B. A., Rathod, S. D., & Komproe, I. H. (2017). Treatment gap and barriers for mental health care: A cross-sectional community survey in Nepal. *PLOS ONE, 12*(8), e0183223. https://doi.org/10.1371/journal.pone.0183223

Luitel, N. P., Jordans, M. J. D., Sapkota, R. P., Tol, W. A., Kohrt, B. A., Thapa, S. B., Komproe, I. H., & Sharma, B. (2013). Conflict and mental health: A cross-sectional epidemiological study in Nepal. *Social Psychiatry and Psychiatric Epidemiology, 48*(2), 183–193. https://doi.org/10.1007/s00127-012-0539-0

Mandal, A. K. (2022). Trend of tobacco use: Reviewing the STEPS surveys conducted in Nepal. *Journal of Health Promotion, 10*(1), 89–100.

Marahatta, K., Samuel, R., Sharma, P., Dixit, L., & Shrestha, B. R. (2017). Suicide burden and prevention in Nepal: The need for a national strategy. *WHO South-East Asia Journal of Public Health, 6*(1), 45. https://doi.org/10.4103/2224-3151.206164

Mishra, A., Bhattarai, K., KC, H., Shah, R., & Parajuli, S. B. (2023). Mental health literacy among undergraduate medical students in Eastern Nepal. *Journal of Chitwan Medical College, 13*(2), 14–19. https://doi.org/10.54530/jcmc.1312

National Mental Health Survey. (2020). Reports, Nepal health research council. Retrieved August 6, 2023, from https://nhrc.gov.np/wp-content/uploads/2022/10/National-Mental-Health-Survey-Report2020.pdf

National Statistics Office. (2021). National population and housing census 2021 Results. Retrieved February 7, 2025, from https://nsonepal.gov.np/

Neupane, D., Dhakal, S., Thapa, S., Bhandari, P. M., & Mishra, S. R. (2016). Caregivers' attitude towards people with mental illness and perceived stigma: A cross- sectional study in a tertiary hospital in Nepal. *PLOS ONE, 11*(6). https://doi.org/10.1371/journal.pone.0158113

Paneru, D. P., Adhikari, C., Poudel, S., Adhikari, L. M., Neupane, D., Bajracharya, J., Jnawali, K., Chapain, K. P., Paudel, N., Baidhya, N., & Rawal, A. (2022). Adopting social health insurance in Nepal: A mixed study. *Frontiers in Public Health, 10*. https://doi.org/10.3389/fpubh.2022.978732

Pham, T. V., Kaiser, B. N., Koirala, R., Maharjan, S. M., Upadhaya, N., Franz, L., & Kohrt, B. A. (2021). Traditional Healers and Mental Health in Nepal: A Scoping Review. *Culture, Medicine, and Psychiatry, 45*(1), 97–140. https://doi.org/10.1007/s11013-020-09676-4

Poudel, K., & Subedi, P. (2020). Impact of COVID-19 pandemic on socioeconomic and mental health aspects in Nepal. *International Journal of Social Psychiatry, 66*(8), 748–755. https://doi.org/10.1177/0020764020942247

Powell, T., Li, S.-J., Hsiao, Y., Ettari, C., Bhandari, A., Peterson, A., & Shakya, N. (2019). Investigating the aftershock of a disaster: A study of health service utilization and mental health symptoms in post-earthquake Nepal. *International Journal of Environmental Research and Public Health, 16*(8), Article 8. https://doi.org/10.3390/ijerph16081369

Pradhan, S. N., Sharma, S. C., Malla, D. P., & Sharma, R. (2013). A study of help seeking behavior of psychiatric patients. *Journal of Kathmandu Medical College, 2*(1), Article 1. https://doi.org/10.3126/jkmc.v2i1.10538

Rai, Y., Gurung, D., & Gautam, K. (2021). Insight and challenges: Mental health services in Nepal. *Bjpsych International, 18*(2), E5. https://doi.org/10.1192/bji.2020.58

Regmi, D. R. (2024). Status of the mother tongues in the 2021 census of Nepal. *Journal of Nepalese Studies, 16*(1), Article 1. https://doi.org/10.3126/jns.v16i1.71780

Regmi, P. R., Aryal, N., van Teijlingen, E., Simkhada, P., & Adhikary, P. (2020). Nepali migrant workers and the need for pre-departure training on mental health: A qualitative study. *Journal of Immigrant and Minority Health, 22*(5), 973–981. https://doi.org/10.1007/s10903-019-00960-z

Sapkota, R. P., Brunet, A., & Kirmayer, L. J. (2020). Characteristics of adolescents affected by mass psychogenic illness outbreaks in schools in Nepal: A case-control study. *Frontiers in Psychiatry, 11*. https://doi.org/10.3389/fpsyt.2020.493094

Scott, K. M., Zhang, Y., Chardoul, S., Ghimire, D. J., Smoller, J. W., & Axinn, W. G. (2021). Resilience to mental disorders in a low-income, non-Westernized setting. *Psychological Medicine, 51*(16), 2825–2834. https://doi.org/10.1017/S0033291720001464

Seale-Feldman, A. (2019). Ethos | AAA Sociocultural Anthropology Journal | Wiley Online Library. https://doi.org/10.1111/etho.12245

Shakya, D. R. (2019). Dhat syndrome: Study of clinical presentations in a teaching institute of eastern Nepal. *Journal of Psychosexual Health, 1*(2), 143–148. https://doi.org/10.1177/2631831819853742

Shakya, R. (2005). Epidemic of hysteria in a school of rural eastern Nepal: A case report. *Journal of Indian Association for Child and Adolescent Mental Health, 1*(4), 20–24. https://doi.org/10.1177/0973134220050404

Shakya, Y., Nazim, A., & Joshi, D. (2021). Koro like syndrome with genital retraction fear in two Nepalese men: A case series. *Journal of Psychiatrists' Association of Nepal, 10*(2), Article 2. https://doi.org/10.3126/jpan.v10i2.49010

Sharma, A., Adhikari, R., Parajuli, E., Buda, M., Raut, J., Gautam, E., & Adhikari, B. (2023). Psychological morbidities among Nepalese migrant workers to Gulf and Malaysia. *PLOS ONE, 18*(11), e0267784. https://doi.org/10.1371/journal.pone.0267784

Sharma, P., Gautam, K., & Marahatta, K. (2024). Access to mental health care in Nepal: Current status, potential challenges, and ways out. In S. M. Y. Arafat & S. K. Kar (Eds.), *Access to mental health care in south Asia: Current status, potential challenges, and ways out* (pp. 91–111). Springer Nature. https://doi.org/10.1007/978-981-99-9153-2_6

Sharma, P., Timasina, R. R., Singh, S., Gyawali, S., Marahatta, K., & Arafat, S. M. Y. (2022). Quality of media reporting of suicide in Nepal. *Psychiatry Journal, 2022*(1), 5708092. https://doi.org/10.1155/2022/5708092

Sherchan, S., Samuel, R., Marahatta, K., Anwar, N., Van Ommeren, M. H., & Ofrin, R. (2017). Post-disaster mental health and psychosocial support: Experience from the 2015 Nepal earthquake. *WHO South-East Asia Journal of Public Health, 6*(1), 22. https://doi.org/10.4103/2224-3151.206160

Shrestha, D. B., Thapa, B. B., Katuwal, N., Shrestha, B., Pant, C., Basnet, B., Mandal, P., Gurung, A., Agrawal, A., & Rouniyar, R. (2020). Psychological distress in Nepalese residents during COVID-19 pandemic: A community level survey. *BMC Psychiatry, 20*(1), 491. https://doi.org/10.1186/s12888-020-02904-6

Singh, R., Mahato, S., Singh, B., Thapa, J., & Gartland, D. (2019). Resilience In Nepalese adolescents: Socio-demographic factors associated with low resilience. *Journal of Multidisciplinary Healthcare, 12,* 893–902. https://doi.org/10.2147/JMDH.S226011

Singh, R., Mahato, S., Singh, K., Puri, N. R., Baniya, S., & Arafat, S. Y. (2024). Suicidal behavior in Nepali motion pictures of three decades (1990–2020): A content analysis. *Brain and Behavior, 14*(1), e3366. https://doi.org/10.1002/brb3.3366

Thapa, D. K., Lamichhane, N., & Subedi, S. (2018). Traditional faith healers as referral sources: A hospital-based descriptive study. *Journal of Psychiatrists' Association of Nepal, 7*(2), Article 2. https://doi.org/10.3126/jpan.v7i2.24614

Thapa, N., Paudel, M., Guragain, A. M., Thapa, P., Puri, R., Thapa, P., Aryal, K. K., Paudel, B. K., Thapa, R., & Stray-Pedersen, B. (2019). Status of migration and socio-reproductive impacts on migrants and their families left behind in Nepal. *Migration and Development, 8*(3), 394–417. https://doi.org/10.1080/21632324.2019.1567097

Thapa, P., Marahatta, K., Upadhyay Raj, S., Sapkota, N., Baral, P., Lama, S., Kamholz, B., Paudel, S., & Basnet, M. (2024). Dementia care landscape in Nepal: Understanding the context, barriers, and opportunities for the development of a national dementia care plan. *International Journal of Geriatric Psychiatry, 39*(6), e6111. https://doi.org/10.1002/gps.6111

Thapaliya, S., Sharma, P., & Upadhyaya, K. (2018). Suicide and self harm in Nepal: A scoping review. *Asian Journal of Psychiatry, 32,* 20–26. https://doi.org/10.1016/j.ajp.2017.11.018

Timalsina, R., Songwathana, P., & Sae-Sia, W. (2022). Factors explaining resilience among Nepalese older adults experiencing disasters: A cross-sectional study. *International Journal of Disaster Risk Reduction, 69,* 102756. https://doi.org/10.1016/j.ijdrr.2021.102756

Tol, W. A., Kohrt, B. A., Jordans, M. J. D., Thapa, S. B., Pettigrew, J., Upadhaya, N., & de Jong, J. T. V. M. (2010). Political violence and mental health: A multi-disciplinary review of the literature on Nepal. *Social Science & Medicine, 70*(1), 35–44. https://doi.org/10.1016/j.socscimed.2009.09.037

Uprety, S., & Lamichanne, B. (2016). Mental Health in Nepal: A Backgrounder. https://doi.org/10.13140/RG.2.2.16817.45923

WHO. (2023). Responsible media reporting for suicide prevention. Retrieved March 3, 2025, from https://www.who.int/nepal/news/detail/27-09-2023-responsible-media-reporting-for-suicide-prevention

Yadav, S. K. (2023). Socio-cultural aspects of federal structure in Nepal. *Academic View, Journal of TUTA Tri-Chandra Campus Unit,* 127–135. https://doi.org/10.3126/acadview.v9i1.71251

# Chapter 6
# Social Psychiatry in Pakistan

**Widad Malik, Samiya Iqbal, Aimen Iqbal, and Salahudeen Mirza**

**Abstract** The Islamic Republic of Pakistan is the fifth-largest country in the world. A lower- and middle-income country (LMIC), Pakistan was founded in 1947 on partition from India. Pakistan is a regional and global powerhouse, but its tumultuous history and its young age have conferred serious vulnerabilities. Social determinants are key in the etiology of Pakistan's present mental health burden. With the most recent psychiatric epidemiological survey establishing a high rate of psychiatric problems, new scalable strategies are needed to address the struggles of the Pakistani population. In this Chapter, we describe the nature of the mental health landscape in Pakistan, with a focus on the epidemiology of mental health problems and their social components, as well as the infrastructures—both available and absent—which could be leveraged to support well-being.

**Keywords** Pakistan · South Asia · Mental health · Public mental health · Social psychiatry · Psychiatric epidemiology · Mental health legislation

## 1 Introduction

The Islamic Republic of Pakistan is situated in South Asia with India to its East, Iran-Afghanistan to its West, China to its North and Arabian Sea to its South. It is classified as a lower- and middle-income country (LMIC) with a geographical area of approximately 803,940 square kilometers (Dayani et al., 2024). Pakistan is a federation of four provinces (Punjab, Sindh, Balochistan, and Khyber Pakhtunkhwa)

---

Widad Malik and Samiya Iqbal are Co-first authors

W. Malik · A. Iqbal
Department of Psychiatry, Watim Medical & Dental College, Rawat, Islamabad, Pakistan

S. Iqbal
Department of Psychiatry, Aga Khan University, Karachi, Sindh, Pakistan

S. Mirza (✉)
Child Study Centre, Yale School of Medicine, New Haven, CT, USA
e-mail: salahudeen.mirza@yale.edu



S. M. Y. Arafat et al. (eds.), *Social Psychiatry in South Asia*, South Asian Perspectives in Mental Health and Psychology , https://doi.org/10.1007/978-981-96-8078-8_6

and three regions (Islamabad Capital Territory, Azad Jammu & Kashmir, and Gilgit Baltistan). According to the seventh national population and housing census (2023), Pakistan had a population of 241.49 million people, making it the fifth most populated country in the world and the fourth largest in South and East Asia (*7th Population and Housing Census—Detailed Results*, n.d.).

In terms of the financial budget, in 2021–2022, a total of 1,962 billion was earmarked for the health budget, indicating a major increase of 34% from 2019 to 2020. This allocated amount accounted for 2.91% of Pakistan's total GDP. Currently, Pakistan's yearly per capita healthcare expenditure is $48.05 USD, the lowest compared to its neighboring countries, which includes India with $56.63 USD, Bangladesh $50.66 USD, Afghanistan $80.29 USD, and China $583.00 USD (*National Health Accounts*, n.d.). Even though Pakistan still has the lowest per capita health care expenditure compared to its neighbors, the social markers indicative of physical health have improved dramatically in recent years. The average life expectancy has gone up from 65.7 years in 2015 to 67.3 years in 2020, compared to the global average of 71.4 years, and is anticipated to further improve to 68.08 years by 2025. Additionally, health-adjusted life expectancy increased by 3.7 years, from 53.2 years in 2000 to 56.9 years in 2019 (*GHO | By category | Life expectancy and Healthy life expectancy—Data by country*, n.d.).

The governance of the health sector in Pakistan has seen some major shifts in the past. Before 2011, the Federal Ministry of Health was in charge of health planning, service delivery, policymaking and program implementation. However, in 2011, the 18th amendment to the 1973 constitution transferred all of these services to the provinces. This transfer posed various issues for the provincial governments such as lack of experience in policymaking and difficulty in program implementation. To overcome this challenge, the Federal Ministry of Health was reconstituted as the Ministry of National Health Services, Regulations and Coordination (NHSRC) (MINISTRY OF NATIONAL HEALTH SERVICES REGULATIONS AND COORDINATION, n.d.). This ministry bears the responsibility of guiding and supervising the healthcare system. Pakistan's health policy, with support from the World Health Organization (WHO), is the "National Health Vision Plan 2016–2025" launched in 2016 (*National Vision 2016–2025*, n.d.). Its goal is to improve the health of all Pakistanis, particularly women and children, by providing universal access to affordable, quality, essential health services delivered through a resilient and responsive health system capable of attaining the Sustainable Development Goals (SDGs). It should be noted that mental health was not a part of the specific objectives of the National Health Vision Plan.

## 2 Healthcare System in Pakistan

Healthcare delivery in Pakistan is provided by the public and private sectors. The federal and provincial governments are both considered to be part of the public sector. Federal hospitals, cantonment boards of Pakistan, and the military healthcare system all come under the domain of the Federal Government. The military healthcare system serves soldiers, their families, parents, retired soldiers, civilians funded by defense estimates, and non-entitled civilians. The provincial government operates under the framework of the district health system and is divided into three main sectors, viz. primary, secondary, and tertiary health sectors. Primary healthcare is provided by Basic Health Units (BHUs), Rural Health Centers (RHCs), Maternal and Child Health Centers (MCHCs), and Dispensaries where the main facilities are preventive and outpatient care, outreach and community-based activities, which focus on immunization, sanitation, malaria control, maternal and child health, and family planning. Secondary healthcare facilities offer acute, ambulatory, and inpatient care through Tehsil Headquarter Hospitals (THQs) and District Headquarter Hospitals (DHQs). Hospitals with more specialized care located mostly in big cities offer tertiary healthcare. Private healthcare facilities are highly diverse and are mostly ungoverned. These include major hospitals with specialized medical facilities, independently operated clinics, homeopaths, hakims, and other traditional healthcare providers, as well as medical facilities provided by non-governmental organizations. Figures from National Health Accounts (NHA) 2021–2022 show that 83% of the Pakistani population access healthcare from the private sector while only 17% prefer the public sector.

## 3 Social Epidemiology of Mental Illness in Pakistan

It is a widely acknowledged fact that the burden of psychiatric morbidity is more significant in LMICs. This fact is corroborated by the findings of the National Psychiatric Morbidity Survey of Pakistan (NPMS) 2022 conducted by the Pakistan Psychiatric Society. According to this survey, one in every three adults is believed to have a mental health condition at any given moment. The NPMS statistics suggest that the lifetime prevalence of any psychiatric illness in Pakistan is 37.1%, which is higher than the rates recorded in other middle- and low-income nations such as Malaysia, Nigeria, and Iran, where estimates range from 5.2% to 23.2%. The prevalence of depressive disorder was 17.8%, which is lower than reported in several earlier Pakistani studies. Schizophrenia and other psychotic illnesses accounted for the bulk of serious psychiatric diseases (4.52%) (Rahman et al., 2024). In a country like Pakistan, this high frequency of psychiatric diseases can be linked to a multitude of factors like poor socio-economic conditions, the stigma surrounding mental illness, lack of awareness of mental health issues, inadequate resources for treatment and management of mental illnesses, and limited access to mental healthcare. The staggering fact that one in every three people has a psychiatric disorder begs for more extensive and detailed epidemiological studies.

## 4 Mental Disorders and Their Treatment

The spectrum of mental disorders in Pakistan reflects both universal psychiatric conditions and culturally specific manifestations. The most common mental health disorders include depression, anxiety, post-traumatic stress disorder (PTSD), schizophrenia, and substance use disorders. Hussain et al. describe a high prevalence of common mental disorders in Pakistan, ranging from 25% in urban areas to 72% in rural areas for women and from 10% (urban) to 44% (rural) for men (*Integration of mental health into primary healthcare: perceptions of stakeholders in Pakistan*, n.d.). Depression and anxiety are particularly widespread (Mirza & Jenkins, 2004). Socio-economic stressors, political instability, and domestic violence often trigger them. PTSD is prevalent among survivors of terrorism, natural disasters, and war (Minas & Lewis, 2017). Despite the high prevalence of these conditions, a significant number of cases remain undiagnosed due to stigma and limited access to professional care (Hussain et al., 2018).

Treatment modalities range from pharmacological interventions to psychotherapy. Access to treatment remains a significant challenge, exacerbated by a severe shortage of mental health professionals. Pakistan has only a few hundred psychiatrists for a population exceeding 240 million. Psychologists and psychotherapists, while growing in numbers, do not have any accreditation or licensing body in Pakistan, which may compromise the quality of the treatment delivered (Javed et al., 2020). Psychiatric hospitals are limited and mostly concentrated in major cities, making them largely inaccessible to rural populations. Furthermore, psychiatric medication is expensive and not readily available in public hospitals (Karim et al., 2004). The same is true for psychotherapeutic treatment modalities.

There is a growing movement among mental health professionals to modernize and expand psychiatric care. Innovations in community-based mental health programs and telepsychiatry offer a glimmer of hope in bridging the gap between need and service (Ahmad & Koncsol, 2022). Additionally, online psychotherapy and private counseling services are gaining popularity, particularly among younger generations. However, affordability for most people remains a concern (Choudhry et al., 2023).

## 5 Community Mental Health

The global burden of mental health is immense, under-appreciated, and under-resourced, particularly in developing nations, with Pakistan being no exception. With only a small portion of the overall health budget being allocated to mental health, the financial strain of mental illness in Pakistan is increasing at an alarming rate, from 250.5 billion Pakistani rupees (PKR) in 2006 to 616.9 billion PKR in 2020 (Alvi et al., 2023). In Pakistan, mental health policy is a neglected topic, as evidenced by Pakistan's placement of 164th out of 193 nations in the United Nations Development Program's (UNDP) human development index (HDI) (*UNDP's 2023–2024 Human Development Report points to a global 'gridlock' of increased inequality and political polarization*, n.d.).

Existing mental healthcare services are inefficacious in terms of accessibility, quality, and affordability. There are primarily three formal and informal sources for mental health services in Pakistan. Formal sources include those provided by public and private psychiatric units and non-governmental organizations (NGOs), as well as community-based programs. Spiritual and faith healers are part of informal mental health treatments. A 2023 WHO press release estimates that 24 million people in Pakistan need mental healthcare. A population of 24 million is served by less than 500 certified psychiatrists and approximately 500 psychologists to meet these demands. It is indeed concerning that there are 0.19 psychiatrists for every 100,000 individuals (Main Thompson & Saleem, 2025).

Public mental health services include government-run hospitals and clinics, inpatient outpatient psychiatric units, and community-based mental health facilities. According to the Mental Health Atlas 2020, the nation has 11 mental health hospitals, 800 psychiatric units in general hospitals, and 578 community residential institutions. There are 624 community-based mental health outpatient facilities and 3729 hospital-affiliated mental health outpatient facilities accessible for outpatient care. This brings the number of community-based mental health facilities per 100,000 population to 0.56 (*Mental Health Atlas 2020 Country Profile: Pakistan*, n.d.).

The Pakistani government has been making strides in the health sector and has introduced a number of health insurance schemes for its people. Universal Health Coverage (UHC) is one, which aims to enhance health outcomes by providing everyone with comprehensive care (World Health Organization, n.d.). The essential package of health services under the UHC covers the treatment of anxiety, depression, and certain childhood disorders, but it excludes more severe mental illnesses that require inpatient care. Although the support for the integration of mental health within UHC has gained momentum in the past couple of years, there are still no apparent routes for doing so. A few other insurance programs, such as the Sehat Sahulat Program and Qaumi Sehat Card, were also introduced, including mental healthcare, but they only cover hospital stays, and the burden of the cost of medications still falls on the patients and their family members.

Due to Pakistan's particular issue with sustainable delivery, the country has a notably large treatment gap for mental disorders. In 2009, WHO took the initiative of starting the Mental Health Global Action Program (mhGAP) to offer evidence-based treatments at the primary and secondary levels for the prevention and treatment of neurological and psychiatric illnesses in low-income nations with inadequate delivery of care (Najam et al., 2019). The first training for the Mental Health Gap Action Program (mhGAP) in Pakistan was held in 2014. This was not a government or institutionally led project but was instead organized by a team of mental health experts who volunteered their time and resources. The second initiative in August 2017, however, was a pilot project at the federal and provincial levels that introduced mhGAP training in primary healthcare through five districts in Pakistan.

Community mental health services in Pakistan have made headway in the last few years. There have been some improvements in the psychiatric facilities provided by the public sector where apart from the standard psychiatric and pharmacological management, crisis management centers, drug rehabilitation facilities, vocational centers, mental health helplines, and mental health applications are also available. Patients in private psychiatric facilities and non-governmental organizations receive far more specialized services in addition to those mentioned above like counseling, cognitive behavior therapy, occupational therapy, behavior therapy, art therapy, and tele-psychiatric and tele counseling services.

In 2021, in response to COVID-19, the Ministry of Planning, Development, and Special Initiatives (M/o PD&SI) launched the Mental Health and Psychosocial Support (MHPSS), a cutting-edge digital and virtual mental healthcare system (Humayun & Asif, 2021). The project marks the first instance of an evidence-driven model being used to address public health emergencies in Pakistan. This is accessed through a robust web portal integrated with a learning management system (LMS) and three mobile applications. Through data collection, enhanced psychosocial support services for vulnerable populations, and training and supervision of mental health workers, this model supports the integration of mental health services into primary and secondary care. The MPHSS concept was partially piloted in the province of Khyber Pakhtunkhwa in 2023 when 70 primary care physicians and 30 clinical psychologists were trained and supervised for a period of 6 months. Following this, similar initiatives are being launched in other provinces to implement MPHSS.

The United Nations Office on Drugs and Crime estimates that 6.7 million people, which makes 6% of the country's total population, were drug addicts in Pakistan in the year 2013. It is reasonable to assume that these figures have only gone up over the last ten years, given the misuse of heroin, cannabis, and other narcotics. To provide quality treatment and meet the growing deficiency of rehabilitation facilities, the Anti-Narcotics Force (ANF) of Pakistan has established six Model Addiction Treatment and Rehabilitation Centers (MATRCs). 2464 people received care at these facilities in FY 2024. Besides these facilities, several private drug rehabilitation and treatment facilities are spread out nationwide. The majority of these private treatment centers and rehabilitation facilities are run by allied health professionals and not by psychiatrists and provide detoxification services only.

In a society like Pakistan, which is predominantly patriarchal in nature, women and children are the most vulnerable. More than 10,000 incidences of violence against women were reported in 2020, according to the National database and Registration authorities. Taking these figures into consideration, there has been an upsurge in victim support programs in the past several years. According to a national directory of service providers, victims of abuse, harassment, and assault, especially women and children, have now access to a variety of services. Currently, 532 victim support services—from the governmental and private sectors as well as NGOs—are in operation. These consist of housing, accommodations, food, clothing, counseling, psychological support, rehabilitation, emergency finances, and assistance with medical and mental health issues, and legal challenges.

Mental health awareness programs are much more crucial in a developing nation like Pakistan since they not only help to lessen stigma but also inform people about the resources that are available and inspire and encourage them to use them. The first community-based action was a joint effort between the Pakistani government and WHO to improve mental health in schools, emphasizing the use of technology to increase mental health access. Any single regulating authority in Pakistan does not supervise public education and awareness initiatives about mental health illnesses. Nonetheless, for the past five years, government agencies, non-governmental organizations, and international organizations have supported public awareness and education programs. Vulnerable populations, including women, children, adolescents, trauma survivors, and other minority groups, have been the focus of the campaigns. The majority of mental health programs are started by NGOs and the private sector, including British Asian Trust, Taskeen Health Initiative, Umang Pakistan, Sehat Kahani, Agha Khan University, and Saya Health.

## 6 Mental Health Needs of Special Vulnerable Populations

Certain groups in Pakistan face heightened vulnerabilities when it comes to mental health due to socio-cultural, economic, and political factors.

**Women**, for instance, are disproportionately affected by depression and anxiety, often linked to gender-based violence, societal pressures, and economic dependence (Niaz, 2004). Limited access to education and employment opportunities further exacerbates their mental health struggles. In conservative settings, stigma may prevent women from seeking professional help, entrenching their distress, and limiting their access to care. (Ahmad & Koncsol, 2022)

**Children and adolescents** also experience significant mental health challenges. Exposure to domestic violence, academic pressure, child labor, and socio-economic instability can have lasting impacts on their psychological well-being (Niaz, 2004). Suicide rates among young people are rising, yet mental health support in schools is nearly non-existent. Additionally, rapid urbanization and modernization have led to increased migration and displacement, placing young individuals in fragile situations that heighten their risk of mental health disorders. A pressing need exists for child-specific mental health interventions according to their developmental needs (Choudhry et al., 2023).

**Minority communities**, including ethnic and religious minorities, may face discrimination and marginalization, intensifying feelings of isolation and distress (Dilawri et al., 2014). The compounded effects of social exclusion and economic hardship contribute to chronic stress, PTSD, and anxiety disorders (Ahmad &

Koncsol, 2022). These populations require culturally tailored mental health services that acknowledge their unique experiences and challenges.

**Refugees and internally displaced persons (IDPs)**, particularly those from conflict zones such as Afghanistan and Pakistan's tribal areas, experience high rates of PTSD, depression, and anxiety. Many have endured war and violence. Displacement, separation from family, and loss of livelihood contribute to severe psychological distress (Minas & Lewis, 2017). While humanitarian organizations and government agencies are beginning to address these needs, much remains to be done to ensure mental health interventions are both accessible and culturally appropriate (Ahmad & Koncsol, 2022).

**Elderly** individuals face increasing mental health challenges as traditional family structures shift due to urbanization. Loneliness, neglect, and a lack of geriatric mental healthcare contribute to undiagnosed conditions such as dementia and late-life depression. With limited specialized services for older adults, mental health concerns in this demographic often go unnoticed and untreated (Choudhry et al., 2023).

**LGBTQ + individuals**, though largely invisible in public discourse, experience severe mental health distress due to rejection by family and society, discrimination, and even violence. They may face depression, anxiety, and suicidal ideation (Minas & Lewis, (Minas et al., 2017). The absence of safe spaces and mental health resources specific to their needs leaves them particularly vulnerable (Ahmad & Koncsol, 2022).

Despite the urgent needs of these populations, Pakistan's mental health policies and services remain largely generalized, failing to address the specific challenges faced by different demographic groups. Targeted, inclusive, and culturally sensitive mental health interventions are crucial to bridging these gaps and ensuring adequate support for the country's most vulnerable communities.

## 7 Cultural Norms and Mental Illness

The culture of Pakistan is shaped by centuries-old traditions, religious influences, social hierarchy, and family structure. Mental illness has always been recognized in Pakistan. However, its interpretation is often interwoven with spiritual, moral, and social dimensions which makes the clinical picture far more complex than a mere biomedical condition.

Pakistani society is a collectivist society where the family unit is of paramount importance. (Ahmad & Koncsol, 2022) As a result, mental health issues are not solely understood as individual struggles but as challenges that affect the entire family. This means that the patients can count on their families to provide emotional and practical support while they recover. However, the same structure can hinder the expression of struggle and suffering for the fear of causing distress to the family. Moreover, the family may choose to distance themselves from the individual if the condition is viewed as a threat to their reputation (Farooqi, 2006).

In addition, the culture guides the specific roles in the family based on gender. For men, this means that they must display a persona of stoicism and leadership in a household. For women, it often translates into self-sacrifice and prioritization of familial responsibilities over personal well-being (Karim et al., 2004). When individuals fail to meet these expectations due to mental illness, they may face social isolation, judgment, or even outright rejection (Shafiq, 2020).

Cultural norms also dictate acceptable expressions of emotion and distress. For example, displays of vulnerability, particularly in men, are frequently discouraged. This may lead individuals to internalize stress, resulting in somatic complaints or other physical manifestations of mental distress (Shafiq, 2020).

Additionally, the understanding of causes and remedies for psychological distress is molded by culture. It is frequently linked to supernatural causes in cultural narratives. Concepts such as the "evil eye" (nazar) or spirit possession (jinn influence) are commonly cited as reasons for mental illness (Ahmad & Koncsol, 2022; Zulfiqar et al., 2019). As a result, instead of seeking professional psychiatric care, many individuals and families turn to religious or spiritual remedies (Zulfiqar et al., 2019).

## 8 Culture-Bound Syndromes

Culture-bound syndromes are psychological phenomena that manifest in culturally specific ways. The specific cultural interpretations, social norms, and belief systems in Pakistan shape the expression of psychological distress. This leads to unique presentations that differ from Western psychiatric classifications.

A prominent feature of culture-bound syndromes in Pakistan is the expression of mental distress through somatic complaints (Husain et al., 2020). Many individuals, particularly women, report chronic pain, fatigue, headaches, or gastrointestinal discomfort without any identifiable medical cause (Niaz, 2004). This tendency toward somatization is deeply rooted in cultural perceptions of the mind–body relationship, making it a socially acceptable way to communicate psychological distress (Shafiq, 2020). However, it also complicates clinical assessments, as mental health professionals must carefully evaluate the culturally influenced symptoms to reach the diagnosis of an underlying psychiatric condition. (Irfan et al., 2017)

Spiritual and supernatural beliefs further influence how mental health issues are understood and addressed. Mental illnesses and unexplained health conditions are often attributed to supernatural causes such as **black magic (*Kala Jadoo*)**. Many cases of dissociative disorders, psychosis, or epilepsy are interpreted as **Jinn/Churail possession**, leading individuals to seek treatment at shrines or from spiritual healers rather than psychiatric professionals (Irfan et al., 2017; Zulfiqar et al., 2019). Similarly, conversion symptoms especially among rural women, often involve trance-like states, uncontrollable crying, or reported visions, which are sometimes viewed as spiritual encounters rather than signs of psychological distress. **Evil Eye (*Buri Nazar*)** indicates a widespread belief that jealousy can harm individuals, particularly children, causing illness. Protective measures include reciting Qur'anic verses, wearing amulets, and offering charity (*sadaqah*) (Zulfiqar et al., 2019)

**Athra** is a belief prevalent in rural Punjab where women who suffer repeated miscarriages are thought to have a spiritual affliction called Athra. This is believed to be transferred to another women, which may be diagnosed if a baby is born weak (*kamzor*). (Zulfiqar et al., 2019)

**Dhat Syndrome** is a condition predominantly affecting men, characterized by anxiety over semen loss, believed to cause weakness. (Zulfiqar et al., 2019)

These culture-bound syndromes highlight the need for culturally sensitive mental healthcare in Pakistan. Western psychiatric models emphasize biomedical explanations but dismissing cultural interpretations outright can alienate patients and hinder effective treatment. Recognizing and respecting these cultural nuances is crucial for developing effective, culturally appropriate mental health interventions.

## 9 Community Attitudes toward Mental Health

The general public in Pakistan views mental health issues with a blend of ignorance, indifference and fear. Public discourse on mental health is often hushed. Conversations about emotional distress are cloaked in silence and misconception. Inadequate awareness of the scientific foundations of mental diseases leads to myriads of explanations ranging from supernatural afflictions to divine punishment (Husain et al., 2020).

One of the most damaging attitudes is that mental illness is a sign of weak faith (Husain et al., 2020). It may be assumed that a person struggling with psychological distress is not praying enough or is being punished for past sins. This creates an added burden for those suffering, making them feel ashamed or unworthy of seeking help.

Similarly, anxiety, depression, and trauma-related disorders may go unnoticed or be dismissed as personal failings rather than health conditions requiring intervention. Patients do not talk about their struggles as they fear being judged negatively or labelled insane ('pagal') (Javed et al., 2020). Families prefer to hide affected individuals rather than risk social disgrace (Shafiq, 2020). Moreover, psychiatric facilities (which are traditionally branded 'pagal-khanay'/madhouses) are often perceived as places of abandonment rather than healing (Karim et al., 2004; Minas & Lewis, 2017). In some situations, the patient's family does not access professional treatment as this can damage marriage prospects, especially for a woman (Causier et al., 2024).

Urban areas with higher literacy rates have begun to show some awareness on the topic. Younger people with access to global discourse via social media are gradually changing their perspectives. However, in rural and conservative communities, mental health remains a taboo subject (Ahmad & Koncsol, 2022).

## 10 Stigma toward Mental Health

Stigma is one of the biggest barriers to mental healthcare in Pakistan. It exists in multiple forms:

Individuals feel shame about their struggle. Within families, stigma manifests as secrecy and denial (Ahmad & Koncsol, 2022; Zehra et al., 2023). Parents may avoid admitting that their child has schizophrenia, bipolar disorder, or severe depression out of fear that it will harm their family's reputation and social status. This leads to poor access to care for those who can benefit from it (Husain et al., 2020). Especially in rural areas, where traditional values are more rigidly adhered to, stigma may result in social isolation, loss of marital prospects, or diminished social standing. For women, in particular, the stigma associated with mental illness can exacerbate gender inequalities, often leading to further marginalization, neglect and violence (Causier et al., 2024).

At the social level, people with mental illnesses are often ridiculed, feared or taken pity on. Labels such as crazy (pagal) or "possessed" (majnoon) are used.

At the institutional level, discrimination is evident in workplaces, schools, and even healthcare settings. There are no legal protections in place. Hence, employers can refuse to hire individuals with a history of mental illness, and schools lack mental health programs to support students (Karim et al., 2004). In healthcare, practitioners often have limited training as psychiatry is not a separate subject in the medical college professional examinations. Doctors and medical students tend to share negative attitudes toward the mentally ill with the broader society (Hussain et al., 2018; Zafar et al., 2024). The lack of awareness results in limited appropriate referrals to specialists, misdiagnoses, or unsuitable treatments. Even where psychiatric services exist, they are scarce, underfunded, and stigmatized (Hussain et al., 2018).

Media portrayals often reinforce negative stereotypes. People with mental illness may be shown to be unpredictable, dangerous, or violent in TV and film (Husain et al., 2020). Newspapers are no different in terms of the language they use in perpetuating stereotypes (Zehra et al., 2023).

## 11 Local Religion, Spirituality, and Mental Health

The majority of the people in Pakistan are Muslims. Other faiths practiced in the region include Christianity and Hinduism among others. Religion is deeply embedded in the Pakistani way of life. Its role in mental health cannot be ignored. The concept of the divine may provide solace by framing suffering as part of a larger cosmic plan. Religious faith can therefore become a source of strength providing a sense of hope and resilience in difficult times. Religious coping mechanisms such as prayer, fasting, and Quranic recitation are commonly used to deal with distress (Zulfiqar et al., 2019).

This can be a double-edged sword: while it might encourage acceptance and endurance, it may also deter individuals from seeking modern psychiatric interventions since people may believe that increased religious observance will cure mental illness (Javed et al., 2020).

## 12 Cross-Religion Help-Seeking and Faith Healers

Despite being a predominantly Muslim country, Pakistan has a rich tradition of interfaith spiritual healing. The cross-religious nature of faith healing is reflective of a broader cultural consensus that values spiritual intervention in times of distress. People from diverse backgrounds, whether Muslim, Hindu, or belonging to other minority faiths, frequently consult these healers. The shared cultural belief in the power of spiritual intervention fosters a sense of trust and legitimacy around these practices. Sufi shrines are widely visited by people looking for spiritual healing (Farooqi, 2006).

Faith healers or spiritual practitioners are widely respected across different religious communities. Their services are sought by individuals who might be wary of conventional medical treatments. These healers use a variety of methods including prayer, amulets, and rituals to address what they interpret as spiritual afflictions or curses. This phenomenon is particularly notable in rural areas where access to modern health care facilities is limited and traditional healers often serve as the primary source of mental health support (Irfan et al., 2017; Saeed et al., 2000).

While faith healing provides an accessible and culturally acceptable avenue for many, it can also delay the diagnosis and treatment of psychiatric conditions. The reliance on spiritual remedies may cause individuals to forego or postpone seeking help from mental health professionals. (Ahmad & Koncsol, 2022). In addition, their practices sometimes involve questionable methods, including physical punishments, dietary restrictions, or expensive talismans (Gadit, 2003). Some fraudulent healers exploit desperate families, charging exorbitant fees for their services (Javed et al., 2020).

Nevertheless, there is potential for a collaborative approach wherein traditional healers with appropriate training work in conjunction with medical practitioners (Choudhry et al., 2023). Such integration could harness the community's trust in traditional practices while ensuring that individuals receive comprehensive care that addresses both spiritual and clinical dimensions of mental illness (Gadit, 2003).

Furthermore, spiritual leaders and religious scholars hold significant influence within communities. Their interpretation of mental health issues can shape public opinion. They can be pivotal in bridging the gap between traditional and modern approaches to mental healthcare (Hussain et al., 2018). By endorsing integrative practices that combine spiritual support with psychiatric care, they can help mitigate the stigma and encourage more holistic treatment pathways.

## 13 Role of Traditional Healing Practices and Integration with Modern Psychiatric Care

Modern psychiatric care in Pakistan has made significant strides over recent decades. However, the shortage of trained professionals and limited resource allocation to mental healthcare limits its availability, especially in the rural areas. Where it is available, it may not be fully acceptable to the users based on the cultural barriers discussed above. In this context, traditional healing practices offer a complementary alternative that is more readily accepted by the community (Javed et al., 2020).

These practices include herbal medicine, homeopathy, and spiritual healing. Ayurvedic and Unani medicine blend Islamic and South Asian healing traditions. They are widely practiced in Pakistan, sometimes in conjunction with spiritual rituals. These have been passed down through generations and continue to coexist with modern psychiatric care (Farooqi, 2006; Gadit, 2003). People trust these methods more than Western medicine as they are believed to be natural and free from harmful side effects. While some mental health professionals acknowledge the cultural significance of faith-based healing, others dismiss it entirely.

The integration of traditional healing with contemporary mental health services can be a promising avenue for improving mental health outcomes in Pakistan in a culturally sensitive manner. For instance, traditional healers provide counseling that is embedded within the cultural and religious narratives familiar to patients. This approach can help in building trust and easing the stigma associated with mental illness (Gadit, 2003). Some mental health set-ups have begun to incorporate religious counseling with modern treatments to encourage acceptance of medical interventions (Farooqi, 2006). However, the gap between traditional and modern approaches remains vast, requiring more dialogue and collaboration.

Collaborative initiatives are the need of the hour, for example, training traditional healers in basic mental health literacy and establishing referral systems between healers and psychiatric clinics.

## 14 Poverty, Unemployment, and Mental Health

Historically, Pakistan's economy has faced significant challenges. These challenges owe to a variety of contributory factors including political issues, as well as a longer-standing history of colonial rule which only recently abated. Though progress has been made since the establishment of Pakistan as an independent country, this progress is tempered by continued experience of poor socio-economic conditions by a substantial proportion of the population. Indeed, using the lower- and middle-income poverty rate of $3.65 USD per day, the World Bank calculated that 40.5% of Pakistanis were poor in 2024. Other measures incorporating other dimensions of poverty (multidimensional poverty) based on slightly older data from 2018 to 19 placed the estimate even higher at close to 50% (Haq et al., 2024). As always when it comes to data on LMICs, the true burden of poverty in Pakistan cannot be captured by a single number. The extent of poverty can be dramatic.

Poverty and the risks that travel with it—such as lack of access to basic resources and increased exposure to adversities in LMICs—is perhaps among the most powerful toxic stressors (Blair & Raver, 2016). Studies largely based in higher-income countries such as the United States unequivocally demonstrate that growing up in poverty disrupts brain development and stress signaling. Environmental unpredictability (such as not knowing where the next meal will come from or not trusting that the surrounding community is safe or trustworthy) and impaired caregiving by overburdened parents may be some of the key mechanisms involved in this relationship. Empirical research from LMICs is comparatively limited, though it is likely that the harms are even more severe considering an extent of poverty which is rarely seen in higher-income countries. In LMICs, a "vicious cycle" may ensue in which poverty sets the stage for poor mental health which, in its debilitating effects on functioning, prevents the individual from escaping from the poor socio-economic position (Patel & Kleinman, 2003). In Pakistan, youth suicide cases have recently been attributed to poverty in the newspapers. With inflation (25%) and unemployment (31%) on the rise, youth may be especially pre-disposed to poor mental health as the pathways to a stable future appear narrower and fewer in number (Siddiqui et al., 2024).

Housing shortages coupled with poverty lead to a significant burden of homelessness in Pakistan, though it is difficult to find data documenting the true extent of the problem. Recently, the government has started the Pannah Gah (shelter home) initiative to establish shelters for those with nowhere to go. Interestingly, a survey of people living in Pannah Gah in Lahore found that though most did not bring their families with them, almost all of them maintained a connection with them, with almost two-thirds contacting them daily (Hameed et al., 2025). When asked where they would live if not for Pannah Gah, they provided a variety of answers including footpaths and parks.

This form of homelessness may be slightly different than that in other countries such as the United States. For example, many of the people living in this shelter had a primary household elsewhere but established a state of "homelessness" in order to seek employment in Lahore. Clearly, though, the homeless population in Pakistan is heterogeneous and would benefit from targeted supports for mental health. An option could be to pilot integrating mental healthcare to the services provided by these establishments.

How can the problem of poverty be tackled in Pakistan, a nation which as a whole is facing such significant macroeconomic challenges? Though it is clear that the burden of mental suffering in Pakistan needs to be addressed across all levels of societal organization up to national policy, smaller ways to start involve efforts to support the functioning of individuals and families living in poverty. Direct cash transfer efforts as well as caregiving interventions may be more easily deployed first steps to attempt to remediate family functioning, considering the core role of family in Pakistani society and its intimate linkage to individual mental health. Cash transfer has already been implemented through the Benazir Income Support Programme (BISP) which provides cash assistance (Rs. 6000) to women below a poverty threshold (Sarfraz et al., 2022). The North East England South Asia Mental Health Alliance recently documented that Pakistan has no social pension system in place (Matthews et al., 2023). As already mentioned, there are some other social protection systems such as BISP for cash transfer or the Sehat Sahulat programme for improved healthcare coverage. Though, overall, there is clearly more to be done to improve social security in Pakistan.

## 15 Income Equity and Mental Health Services

Not only is poverty a critical risk factor to address in efforts to improve mental health in Pakistan, but it also plays a role in the accessibility of treatment for individuals who are seeking help. In a recent Internet survey of over 5,000 Pakistanis, we (SM) found that over 70% of respondents viewed seeing a mental health professional as "not accessible for most people," and over 50% saw it as "something most people can't afford" (Mirza et al., 2024). Departments of psychiatry based in teaching hospitals are overwhelmingly based in urban centers, choking off access for the large (~60%) rural population (Main Thompson & Saleem, 2025). The alternative option is private institutions with out-of-pocket expenses (Dayani et al., 2024). A study over 15 years ago documented a significant cost of treatment for deliberate self-harm in private hospitals, at that time up to USD $255 (Shahid et al., 2008). Coupled with the tremendous income inequality that is intimately woven into the Pakistani social fabric, this set-up essentially renders the poor of Pakistan largely helpless to access mental health services at all.

There is one possible avenue that is being presently tested as a more easily disseminated vehicle for mental healthcare in communities which have limited access. The already existing Lady Health Worker Programme is a community health worker system which aims to promote maternal and child health across Pakistan. Lady health workers are trained to provide primary care and are embedded within communities. Recently, a digital app, mPareshan, was developed to deliver psychosocial counseling via lady health workers in rural Sindh (Akhtar et al., 2025). Based on a qualitative analysis, the intervention appears to be a feasible, acceptable, and appropriate approach to scaling up mental health interventions in more resource-deprived areas of Pakistan.

Notably, Pakistan is taking steps toward universal health coverage. Starting in 2015, the Sehat Sahulat ("Health Facility") Programme has been implemented to cover treatment up to Rs. 1 million per family per year for families living below the poverty line. The program started in KP but is being expanded to other provinces (Hasan et al., 2022). There are many issues with the program including that cost of treatment may still be too expensive even with the provision of these funds. Also, mental health is basically excluded from this program (Riaz et al., 2022). Expansion of universal health coverage efforts to also include mental health will be an important frontier for reducing the inequalities in access.

## 16 Impact of Rapid Urbanization on Mental Health

In South Asia, the rapid pace of urbanization, though improving countries' economies, can come at the cost of a deteriorating social fabric and new ways of life which introduce novel challenges (Trivedi et al., 2008). Among the new issues faced by Pakistani society is a breakdown in the family fabric including an increasing pattern of the elderly being left behind in rural areas while youth make their way to urban areas. Though the struggles of the elderly are not relegated to rural areas: a high prevalence of depression (41%) was documented among the elderly living in Karachi, with the belief that their children would not support them in the future conferring two-fold increased odds of depression (Bhamani et al., 2013). Children may also be exposed to significant harms in cities such as trafficking and homelessness. Women may be at higher risk for violence in urban settings.

Urban centers are also nuclei for provision of mental healthcare. The concentration of mental health services in urban areas intensifies the disparities between urban and rural areas, rendering rural Pakistanis an especially vulnerable population of key focus.

Critical foci for addressing this issue include bolstering mental health care tailored toward older individuals, women, and children, with a focus on improving access to care in rural areas.

## 17 Human Rights: Focus on Women and Children

A key contributor to mental health in LMICs is human rights violations. There are many threats to human rights in Pakistan. One of the foremost is gender-based violence (Sarfraz et al., 2022). In 2021, Pakistan was ranked as the fourth most dangerous country for women. Up to 90% of married women in Pakistan experienced abuse by their spouses. Further, conviction rate in rape cases was only 4% in 2016. Convergent evidence shows that married women are at elevated risk for a variety of mental health problems, including self-harm (Niaz, 2004).

Multiple adverse experiences within the household can be detrimental to mental health. Stress within families can contribute to intimate partner violence and child abuse. A particularly pernicious form of violence is honor killing. Men are typically the perpetrators of honor killing, including close family members such as fathers and brothers. These killings are so-called efforts to restore honor to the family after it has been dishonored in some way. Honor killings are part of a fabric of violence that must be eradicated from Pakistani society in order for it to progress. Fortunately, efforts have been made to this end, including policy which increases the consequences for honor killings (Fatima et al., 2017).

Lady health workers are part of the response to these issues with the hope that women can be met with trained peers who could offer support. There are also government efforts such as the Pakistan's Domestic Violence Act and non-governmental organizations which prioritize the well-being of women and children (Karmaliani et al., 2012). Though, considering that the mistreatment of women stems from deeper cultural attitudes, it is unlikely that these interventions on their own will completely solve the issue. Continued efforts to change the culture and improve treatment of women by multiple avenues are needed.

Children are also victims of violence in Pakistan. Sahil is a non-profit organization which documents the epidemiology of child sexual abuse in Pakistan and releases a publication known as "Cruel Numbers." The organization documented that in 2023, 11 children were abused per day. Stronger child protection efforts and interventions delivered to families are needed to reduce the burden of violence experienced by Pakistan's children. Children who experience violence are likely to grow up with serious mental health problems, and unfortunately these experiences may propagate across generations considering that children who have experienced violence may be more likely to inflict violence themselves.

## 18 Electronic Media

Like other countries, social media use is prevalent in Pakistan. In 2021, 28% of Pakistani population was using the Internet and 78% had mobile devices (Ittefaq et al., 2022). YouTube, Facebook, WhatsApp, and Twitter are commonly used platforms. These platforms have at times been used to organize political movements or disseminate news by alternative channels. It has been documented that Pakistanis use social media to discuss health including to access knowledge and interact with online communities. Younger individuals may be more likely to use social media in this way. In this way, social media may be helpful in terms of providing knowledge on mental health as well as connecting individuals with others who are experiencing similar issues. Digital health approaches may capitalize on the widespread use of social media, especially among youth, to deliver scalable preventions and interventions. The mPareshan app is not directly used by vulnerable individuals, but rather community health workers—but it may serve as a model example demonstrating that apps can be used to improve mental health in Pakistan.

A recent study of adolescents in Punjab found a positive association between social media screen-exposure time and suicidal ideation (Alyas et al., 2025), suggesting that, like elsewhere, social media may sometimes present harms. The issue is complex as time spent on social media captures other forms of risk (such as isolation) rather than that of social media content itself. Coaching youth on appropriate and inappropriate uses for social media will be paramount as social media and digital technology use continue to increase in Pakistan.

One important media avenue in Pakistan is the television drama. Dramas are regularly aired televised series which often depict the struggles of everyday and family life in Pakistani society. They are widely watched and touch on important topics including mental health. Some recent dramas have sensibly approached issues such as child abuse, substance use, and parenting challenges. Though, overall mental illness is still highly stigmatized. Stigmatizing stereotypes still find avenues for perpetuation in television dramas, despite recent positive examples. There is an opportunity for organizations hoping to improve awareness of mental health problems and the treatment options to partner with these media avenues.

Consulting newspaper articles which discuss mental illness is one way to better understand the views on mental illness in Pakistani society. We already noted that stigmatization continues in many newspaper articles (Zehra et al., 2023). In Dawn, the largest English-language newspaper, there are a number of articles recently published which discuss the need for improved mental health treatment and the de-stigmatization of mental illness. Though importantly, newspapers such as Dawn are not regularly read by all of the Pakistani population.

In a country such as Pakistan where there are numerous obstacles to receiving treatment, telehealth approaches may be effective. We have already seen an example of such in mHealth interventions such as mPareshan which are delivered by community health workers. In rural northern Pakistan, telepsychiatry was practiced after a flood and earthquake left individuals with post-traumatic stress symptoms; though outcomes were not documented, the project appeared feasible (Qadir et al., 2016). Telepsychiatry may reduce stigma and improve access to care. For telepsychiatry to be an effective medium for mental health care, though, it will need to be standardized and efforts will need to be taken to make sure it is accessible across strata of society, rather than only those who are privileged enough to access it (Asad et al., 2024).

## 19 Role of Family in Mental Illness, Treatment, and Management

Considering the importance of the family in Pakistani society, the family can be leveraged as a source of support for vulnerable individuals. However conversely, family can also present unique risk factors which drive an individual to poor mental health. For example, we have already noted that married women appear to be at elevated risk for mental health problems, likely because they are frequently subordinated by their spouses and limited in their autonomy as well as exposed to violence and abuse. Notable research on targeting the family to support mental health has focused on children. Maternal (or paternal) depression is a salient risk factor for the development of mental illness. Children in two rural subdistricts of Rawalpindi were assessed for emotional and behavioral problems and the contributing impact of maternal depression. Children whose mothers were depressed prenatally and at the time of assessment showed elevated burdens of problems (Maselko et al., 2016). A peer-delivered psychosocial depression intervention was tested, but it did not show any significant difference from placebo in a cluster randomized trial (Maselko et al., 2020).

Interestingly, a more recent cluster randomized trial of a group parenting intervention for fathers showed significant improvements in a variety of domains including paternal depression, parenting stress, and intimate partner violence; and improvements in early child development (Husain et al., 2025). The intervention, LTP + Dads, was a combination of Learning Through Play (LTP), a guide on parent–child play to support child development, and Focus on Fathers, a skills-focused program geared toward fathers. Community health workers delivered the intervention across 12 group sessions over 4 months.

Multi-family intervention groups have been explored in the treatment of depression and anxiety in Korangi district of Karachi. Patients along with their family members engaged in group-based therapy once per month over six months. They showed significant improvements in quality of life, symptom levels, and social situation (Saleem et al., 2021). Further, culturally adapted family intervention is being tested for patients with schizophrenia and has shown promise of feasibility (Husain et al., 2021).

## 20 Mental Health Legislation in Pakistan

From its independence until 2001, the Islamic Republic of Pakistan followed the Indian Lunacy Act of 1912 as mental health legislation, which it acquired from British colonial overlords. In 2001, local Pakistani psychiatrists and UK-trained Pakistani psychiatrists produced a draft that later became the Mental Health Ordinance of 2001. The United Kingdom's Mental Health Act of 1983 served as a major reference for this mental health legislation of 2001 (Malik et al., 2021) Although this Mental Health Ordinance (MHO) was eventually issued as a presidential decree, its practical implementation was lacking despite advancements in the legislative framework. (Malik et al., 2021). Following the 18th constitutional amendment in 2011, the provinces were given the authority to enact mental health laws and carry out their regulations. The province of Sindh took the lead in changing over from the Mental Health Act of 2001 to the Sindh Mental Health Act of 2013 and in line with this act, they established a Sindh Mental Health Authority composed of prominent psychiatrists and policymakers. This authority was involved in drafting the Sindh Mental Health Policy 2023–2030, the first at the provincial and federal level. Following this, the Punjab Mental Health Act of 2014, the Khyber Pakhtunkhwa Mental Health Act of 2017, and the Baluchistan Mental Health Act of 2019 were passed (Malik et al., 2021) but the mental health authorities of these provinces are yet to be established.

## 21 The Criminal Justice System

The Criminal Justice System of Pakistan comprise of five components: Police, Prosecution, Courts, Prisons, and Correctional Services. These distinct agencies operate together as the principal means of maintaining the rule of law within society.

Up until 2002, the Pakistan Police Department continued to operate under the outdated Police Act of 1861. Eventually, the 1861 Police Act was replaced by the 2002 Pakistan Police Order. In accordance with this order, police officers are instructed to apprehend the mentally ill in order to stop them from endangering themselves, other people, or their property. However, this police order makes no mention of the requirement for police officers to receive basic training in mental health illnesses as part of their training in order to identify offenders who may be suffering from mental health issues (Malik et al., 2021). Since the first contact an offender has with the criminal justice system is usually with the police it is crucial that police officers are trained to recognize a mentally ill offender and involve a forensic psychiatrist in order to correctly assess, support, and safeguard the rights of mentally ill offenders.

Pakistan's criminal justice system operates under the Pakistan Penal Code of 1860 (PPC), which is the countrys official criminal code. Sections 82, 83, and 84 of chapter IV of the Pakistan Penal Code contain provisions that abolish the attribution of criminal liability in cases when an offender is deemed to be mentally ill (Malik et al., 2021). Despite this law, Pakistani jails currently house a disproportionately large percentage of mentally ill inmates.

The principles governing criminal procedures in Pakistani courts are established by the Criminal Procedure Code of 1898 (CrPC). This Code provides formal guidelines for the legal repercussions of criminal offenses specified in the PPC1860. In the event that the alleged is insane, the process of holding a trial or inquiry is outlined in Chapter XXIV of the CrPC, titled "Lunatics" (Malik et al., 2021). It is interesting to note that the CrPC appoints a medical officer rather than a psychiatrist to assess the mental state of the accused. More notably the CrPc still refers to the mentally ill offender as lunatics and mental health institutes as lunatic asylum and is still following the outdated lunacy act of 1912.

Justice Project Pakistan (JPP) is a non-profit organization that works for the rights of prisoners in Pakistan. According to statistics shared by JPP, there were a total of 100,366 inmates in Pakistani prisons in the year 2023 (*FACT SHEET 2023—Prison Population of Pakistan*, 2023). To date, there are no officially documented figures of mentally ill convicts in Pakistani jails. Due to limited resources available for rehabilitation and absence of forensic units, post-conviction sentencing for mentally ill offenders focuses mostly on incarceration and, occasionally, on therapy. In certain central prisons, inmates with behavioral or mental health issues are housed in a separate block. In the past two decades there have been significant reforms in Pakistan's prison system, including the establishment of prison drug rehabilitation facilities for drug addicts housed there; the statistics of which stand at 6355 until now. A medical officer is assigned to periodically check these drug users and provide them with specialist medical care.

## 22 Breakthrough in Forensic Psychiatry

The Pakistani justice system has not been kind to those who suffer from mental health issues. Due to underdevelopment of forensic psychiatry, many who suffered from mental disorders were denied the essential assistance they needed for mental health treatment and proper legal proceedings. The historic verdict by the Supreme Court of Pakistan in the Imdad Ali's case is considered a turning point for forensic psychiatry in Pakistan. In an effort to uphold the rights of mentally ill prisoners in the criminal justice system, the Supreme Court of Pakistan remitted the death sentences of two mentally ill people. The court ordered that the terms "unsoundness of mind," "unsound mind," and "lunatic" be replaced with the terms mental disease or mental illness. Additionally, the court also ruled that the accused be examined by a Medical Board, instead of a medical officer as previously mentioned in the CrPC. This medical board, notified by the provincial government, shall comprise qualified and experienced psychiatrists and psychologists to determine the mental state of the accused at the time of crime and assess whether he is fit to stand trial. The report must be detailed and structured that specifically addresses psychopathology (if any) in the mental functions of consciousness, intellect, thinking, mood, emotions, perceptions, cognition, judgment, and insight. In order to assess, treat, and rehabilitate inmates awaiting trial and convicted individuals who have developed mental illnesses while incarcerated, the court further mandated that the federal and provincial governments build High Security Forensic Mental Health Facilities in teaching and training institutions of mental health. The federal and provincial governments were also ordered by the court to establish training programs and set up courses on mental illnesses and forensic mental health assessment for trial court judges, prosecutors, lawyers, psychiatrists, clinical psychologists, social workers, police, prison staff, and court employees. In addition to this, the court has maintained that the rights of individuals with psychosocial disabilities be protected throughout the criminal justice system. This case marks the first time in Pakistan's history that the Supreme Court has given serious consideration to rights of mentally ill offenders.

Nevertheless, there are still numerous voids that must be filled before forensic psychiatry can be firmly established in Pakistan. To guarantee that laws pertaining to mentally ill offenders be implemented, new advancements in the field of forensic psychiatry are crucial. A greater degree of cooperation between the judiciary, courts, prison system, the psychiatric community, and non-governmental organizations (NGOs) is necessary for this. The psychiatric community, police, and judiciary must undergo continual education and training in order to be aware of and carry out the laws pertaining to mentally ill offenders.

## 23 Juvenile Justice System

In 2018, Pakistan changed its legislation concerning young individuals who faced the criminal justice system by amending the Juvenile Justice System Order (JJSO) 2000 into the Juvenile Justice System Act (JJSA) 2018. This statute outlines the process for safeguarding the impressionable minds of minors and assisting in their reintegration into society (Malik et al., 2021). Notwithstanding its existence, the government has yet to put it into effect entirely. There is currently no proper implementation of the Juvenile Justice System Act (JJSA), which clearly stipulates that juvenile offenders must be identified prior to trial, they must be tried in juvenile courts, they must receive adequate legal representation from a state attorney, and that rehabilitation and observation centers must be established. As of 2025, Group Development Pakistan reports that there are nine juvenile courts in Pakistan, one each in the Islamabad Capital Territory, Punjab, and Baluchistan, two in Sindh, and four in Khyber Pakhtunkhwa, each of which is governed by its respective district and session courts. Nevertheless, neither the magistrates nor the police have been sending cases to the relevant juvenile courts. Additionally, in places where juvenile courts have not yet been formed, the vast majority of minors are still tried in adult courts and receive adult punishments.

For Juvenile offenders to become law-abiding citizens of Pakistan, it is crucial to provide them with proper rehabilitation and educational opportunities. Although every province has a Borstal Act in place that mandates the establishment of five different kinds of juvenile institutions including remand homes, industrial and certified schools, reform schools, and borstals—only four borstals/remand homes have been made thus far. There are still relatively few of these establishments clearly evident from the statistics given by Justice Project Pakistan, that in the year 2023 only 30.7% of juveniles were housed in juvenile institutions and the majority of juvenile offenders, 69.5%, were housed in regular prison. Additionally, there are not enough facilities at these juvenile institutions to help rehabilitate juvenile offenders. Instead, they have to deal with severe conditions, overcrowding, and a dearth of recreational and educational options.

It is imperative that Pakistan amends its laws and see to it that the Juvenile Justice System Act is being properly implemented, in addition to making certain that the police, prosecutor, investigator, probation officer, medico legal officer, psychologist, and child rights experts perform their jobs effectively. The goal is to help the offender understand the reasons behind their offense and reintegrate them into society with an appropriate sense of accountability and self-worth. This will enable them to make wise decisions and stay away from future offenses.

## 24 Closing the Mental Health Gap

With limited involvement from general practitioners, community health workers, and other non-specialist providers, the current mental health delivery system mostly depends on psychiatrists and clinical psychologists. There is a noticeable lack of mental health education in the school curricula and workplace healthcare programs are basically non-existent and the public sector has yet to tap into digital mental health solutions (Main Thompson & Saleem, 2025).

There is a dire need for a comprehensive plan to improve community mental health in Pakistan. This would include increasing the public health spending, integrating mental health into primary care, incorporating mental health literacy into school curricula, teacher training for mental health, launching anti-stigmatization campaigns, maintaining political commitment, quality assurance, and continuous research for contextual interventions. Despite enormous obstacles, putting community-driven, decentralized mental health systems first can guarantee that no one is left behind on the journey to improved well-being.

## 25 Conclusions

Pakistan is a young country with great promise for the future. Though, like any other growing country, the society faces significant challenges which contribute to a mental health burden which must be addressed promptly and appropriately. Multi-level efforts, from national policy to family-centered interventions, must be innovatively combined to promote well-being. The foundation of improved mental health in Pakistan will be improved data. Without high-quality data, the true extent of the mental health burden and the possible prevention and intervention avenues will remain unknown. Government must recognize mental health as a national priority and take efforts to invest in the future of this young country. Allocating funds toward mental health research and social support programs could be the first step toward making Pakistan a healthier country.

## References


*7th Population and Housing Census—Detailed Results*. (n.d.). Retrieved March 23, 2025, from https://www.pbs.gov.pk/digital-census/detailed-results

Ahmad, S. S., & Koncsol, S. W. (2022). Cultural Factors Influencing Mental Health Stigma: Perceptions of Mental Illness (POMI) in Pakistani Emerging Adults. *Religions, 13*(5), 401. https://doi.org/10.3390/rel13050401

Akhtar, S., Rabbani, F., Nafis, J., Siddiqui, A., & Merali, Z. (2025). A qualitative study assessing acceptability and appropriateness of a technology-assisted mental health intervention by community frontline workers: mPareshan implementation research in rural Pakistan. *BMC psychiatry, 25*(1), 16. https://doi.org/10.1186/s12888-024-06459-8

Alvi, M. H., Ashraf, T., Kiran, T., Iqbal, N., Gumber, A., Patel, A., & Husain, N. (2023). Economic burden of mental illness in Pakistan: an estimation for the year 2020 from existing evidence. *BJPsych International, 20*(3), 54–56. https://doi.org/10.1192/bji.2023.4

Alyas, M., Mahesar, R. A., Shoib, S., Khan, M. B., Ali, S. A., & Ventriglio, A. (2025). The impact of social media screen-exposure time on suicidal ideation among Pakistani adolescents. *The International Journal of Social Psychiatry, 71*(1), 149–158. https://doi.org/10.1177/00207640241285133

Asad, N., Pirani, S., Osama, K., & Nadeem, T. (2024). Patients' experiences with tele-mental health services during COVID-19 in Pakistan. *Eastern Mediterranean Health Journal = La revue de sante de la Mediterranee orientale = al- Majallah al-sihhiyah li-sharq al-mutawassit, 30*(4), 283–291. https://doi.org/10.26719/2024.30.4.283

Bhamani, M. A., Karim, M. S., & Khan, M. M. (2013). Depression in the elderly in Karachi, Pakistan: A cross sectional study. *BMC psychiatry, 13,* 181. https://doi.org/10.1186/1471-244X-13-181

Blair, C., & Raver, C. C. (2016). Poverty, stress, and brain development: New directions for prevention and intervention. *Academic Pediatrics, 16*(3 Suppl), S30–S36. https://doi.org/10.1016/j.acap.2016.01.010

Causier, C., Johns, L., Radez, J., Hassan, H., Maughan, D., & Waite, F. (2024). Experiences of help-seeking for severe mental health problems in young Pakistani women: A preliminary qualitative study. *Journal of Cross-Cultural Psychology, 55*(4), 429–443. https://doi.org/10.1177/00220221241236944

Choudhry, F. R., Khan, N., & Munawar, K. (2023). Barriers and facilitators to mental health care: A systematic review in Pakistan. *International Journal of Mental Health, 52*(2), 124–162. https://doi.org/10.1080/00207411.2021.1941563

Dayani, K., Zia, M., Qureshi, O., Baig, M., & Sabri, T. (2024). Evaluating Pakistan's mental healthcare system using World Health Organization's Assessment Instrument for Mental Health System (WHO-AIMS). *International Journal of Mental Health Systems, 18*(1), 32. https://doi.org/10.1186/s13033-024-00646-6

Dilawri, S., Salim, A., Ishfaq, H., & Saleem, M. (2014). The rising marginalization of religious communities in Pakistan. https://minorityrights.org/app/uploads/2024/01/mrg-searching-for-security-pakistan-report.pdf

*FACT SHEET 2023—Prison Population of Pakistan.* (2023, December 30). JPP. https://jpp.org.pk/report/fact-sheet-2023-prison-population-of-pakistan/

Farooqi, Y. N. (2006). Traditional healing practices sought by Muslim psychiatric patients in Lahore, Pakistan. *International Journal of Disability, Development and Education, 53*(4), 401–415. https://doi.org/10.1080/10349120601008530

Fatima, H., Qadir, T. F., Hussain, S. A., & Menezes, R. G. (2017). Pakistan steps up to remove "honour" from honour killing. *The Lancet. Global Health, 5*(2), e145. https://doi.org/10.1016/S2214-109X(16)30359-X

Gadit, A. A. (2003). Ethnopsychiatry—A review. *Journal of the Pakistan Medical Association, 53*(10), 483–490.

*GHO | By category | Life expectancy and Healthy life expectancy—Data by country.* (n.d.). Retrieved March 24, 2025, from https://apps.who.int/gho/data/node.main.688

Hameed, R., Aslam, A. B., & Khan, M. S. U. (2025). How Pannah Gahs (shelter homes) are helping the homeless people in Lahore, Pakistan. *Journal of Housing and the Built Environment, 40,* 417–439. https://doi.org/10.1007/s10901-025-10175-4

Haq, W., Azam, M., Babar, Z. (2024). Investigation of multidimensional poverty in Pakistan at the national, regional, and provincial level. *Humanities & Social Sciences Communications, 11,* 517. https://doi.org/10.1057/s41599-024-03005-5

Hasan, S. S., Mustafa, Z. U., Kow, C. S., & Merchant, H. A. (2022). "Sehat Sahulat Program": A Leap into the Universal Health Coverage in Pakistan. *International Journal of Environmental Research and Public Health, 19*(12), 6998. https://doi.org/10.3390/ijerph19126998

Humayun, A., & Asif, M. (2021, July 15). Mental health goals. *Dawn.* https://www.dawn.com/news/1635182/mental-health-goals

Husain, M. I., Kiran, T., Sattar, R., Khoso, A. B., Wan, M. W., Singla, D. R., Umer, M., Mangrio, R., Bassett, P., Chaudhry, I. B., Zafar, S. N., Jafri, F. A., Chaudhry, N., & Husain, N. (2025). A group parenting intervention for male postpartum depression: A cluster randomized clinical trial. *JAMA Psychiatry, 82*(1), 22–30. https://doi.org/10.1001/jamapsychiatry.2024.2752

Husain, M. O., Zehra, S. S., Umer, M., Kiran, T., Husain, M., Soomro, M., Dunne, R., Sultan, S., Chaudhry, I. B., Naeem, F., Chaudhry, N., & Husain, N. (2020). Stigma toward mental and physical illness: Attitudes of healthcare professionals, healthcare students and the general public in Pakistan. *BJPsych Open, 6*(5), e81. https://doi.org/10.1192/bjo.2020.66

Husain, M. O., Khoso, A. B., Renwick, L., Kiran, T., Saeed, S., Lane, S., Naeem, F., Chaudhry, I. B., & Husain, N. (2021). Culturally adapted family intervention for schizophrenia in Pakistan: a feasibility study. *International Journal of Psychiatry in Clinical Practice, 25*(3), 258–267. https://doi.org/10.1080/13651501.2020.1819332

Hussain, S. S., Khan, M., Gul, R., & Asad, N. (2018). Integration of mental health into primary healthcare: Perceptions of stakeholders in Pakistan. *Eastern Mediterranean health journal = La revue de sante de la Mediterranee orientale = al-Majallah al-sihhiyah li-sharq al-mutawassit, 24*(2), 146–153.

*Integration of mental health into primary healthcare: perceptions of stakeholders in Pakistan.* (n.d.). World Health Organization—Regional Office for the Eastern Mediterranean. Retrieved March 24, 2025, from http://www.emro.who.int/emhj-volume-24-2018/volume-24-issue-2/integration-of-mental-health-into-primary-healthcare-perceptions-of-stakeholders-in-pakistan.html

Irfan, M., Saeed, S., Awan, N. R., Gul, M., Aslam, M., & Naeem, F. (2017). Psychological healing in Pakistan: From sufism to culturally adapted cognitive behaviour therapy. *Journal of Contemporary Psychotherapy, 47*(2), 119–124. https://doi.org/10.1007/s10879-016-9354-3

Ittefaq, M., Seo, H., Abwao, M., & Baines, A. (2022). Social media use for health, cultural characteristics, and demographics: A survey of Pakistani millennials. *Digital Health, 8,* 20552076221089454. https://doi.org/10.1177/20552076221089454

Javed, A., Khan, M. N. S., Nasar, A., & Rasheed, A. (2020). Mental healthcare in Pakistan. *Taiwanese Journal of Psychiatry, 34*(1), 6–14. https://doi.org/10.4103/TPSY.TPSY_8_20

Karim, S., Saeed, K., Rana, M. H., Mubbashar, M. H., & Jenkins, R. (2004). Pakistan mental health country profile. *International Review of Psychiatry, 16*(1–2), 83–92. https://doi.org/10.1080/09540260310001635131

Karmaliani, R., Pasha, A., Hirani, S., Somani, R., Hirani, S., Asad, N., Cassum, L., & McFarlane, J. (2012). Violence against women in Pakistan: Contributing factors and new interventions. *Issues in Mental Health Nursing, 33*(12), 820–826. https://doi.org/10.3109/01612840.2012.718046

Main Thompson, A., & Saleem, S. M. (2025). Closing the mental health gap: Transforming Pakistan's mental health landscape. *Frontiers in Health Services, 4,* 1471528. https://doi.org/10.3389/frhs.2024.1471528

Malik, W. A., Arnold, C., Vithiananthan, A., & Hassan, T. (2021). Forensic psychiatry in Pakistan: An update. *International Journal of Risk and Recovery, 4*(2), 42–50. https://doi.org/10.15173/ijrr.v4i2.4622

Maselko, J., Sikander, S., Bangash, O., Bhalotra, S., Franz, L., Ganga, N., Rajan, D. G., O'Donnell, K., & Rahman, A. (2016). Child mental health and maternal depression history in Pakistan. *Social Psychiatry and Psychiatric Epidemiology, 51*(1), 49–62. https://doi.org/10.1007/s00127-015-1143-x

Maselko, J., Sikander, S., Turner, E. L., Bates, L. M., Ahmad, I., Atif, N., Baranov, V., Bhalotra, S., Bibi, A., Bibi, T., Bilal, S., Biroli, P., Chung, E., Gallis, J. A., Hagaman, A., Jamil, A., LeMasters, K., O'Donnell, K., Scherer, E., … Rahman, A. (2020). Effectiveness of a peer-delivered, psychosocial intervention on maternal depression and child development at 3 years postnatal: A cluster randomised trial in Pakistan. *The Lancet Psychiatry, 7*(9), 775–787. https://doi.org/10.1016/S2215-0366(20)30258-3

Matthews, N. R., Porter, G. J., Varghese, M., Sapkota, N., Khan, M. M., Lukose, A., ... & Walker, R. (2023). Health and socioeconomic resource provision for older people in South Asian countries:

Bangladesh, India, Nepal, Pakistan and Sri Lanka evidence from NEESAMA. *Global health action, 16*(1), 2110198. https://doi.org/10.1080/16549716.2022.2110198

*Mental Health Atlas 2020 Country Profile: Pakistan.* (n.d.). Retrieved March 24, 2025, from https://www.who.int/publications/m/item/mental-health-atlas-pak-2020-country-profile

Minas, H., & Lewis, M. (Eds.). (2017). *Mental health in Asia and the Pacific: Historical and cultural perspectives.* Springer US. https://doi.org/10.1007/978-1-4899-7999-5

Ministry of national health services regulations and coordination. (n.d.). *Ministry of national health services regulations and coordination.* Retrieved March 24, 2025, from https://www.nhsrc.gov.pk/Detail/YjIxNDkyYWQtNzcxNi00NTNmLThiNzItYWI3YzY0ZGYxZmYx

Mirza, I., & Jenkins, R. (2004). Risk factors, prevalence, and treatment of anxiety and depressive disorders in Pakistan: Systematic review. *BMJ, 328*(7443), 794. https://doi.org/10.1136/bmj.328.7443.794

Mirza, S., Rehman, A., Haque, J., & Khan, M. M. (2024). Perceptions of suicide among Pakistanis: Results of an online survey. *Archives of Suicide Research: Official Journal of the International Academy for Suicide Research, 28*(4), 1350–1367. https://doi.org/10.1080/13811118.2024.2305397

Najam, S., Chachar, A. S., & Mian, A. (2019). The mhgap; will it bridge the mental health Treatment gap in Pakistan? *Pakistan Journal of Neurological Sciences (PJNS), 14*(2), 28–33. https://ecommons.aku.edu/pjns/vol14/iss2/6

*National Health Accounts.* (n.d.). Retrieved March 24, 2025, from https://www.pbs.gov.pk/content/national-health-accounts

*National Vision 2016–2025.* (n.d.). Retrieved March 24, 2025, from https://www.unicef.org/pakistan/reports/national-vision-2016-2025

Niaz, U. (2004). Women's mental health in Pakistan. *World Psychiatry.*

Patel, V., & Kleinman, A. (2003). Poverty and common mental disorders in developing countries. *Bulletin of the World Health Organization, 81*(8), 609–615.

Qadir, T. F., Fatima, H., Usmani, M. H., & Hussain, S. A. (2016). Telepsychiatry in Pakistan after natural disasters. *The Lancet Psychiatry, 3*(11), 1016. https://doi.org/10.1016/S2215-0366(16)30323-6

Rahman, R., Sheehan, D., Javed, A., Ahmad, S., Shafiq, K., Kanwal, U., Afridi, M., Nizami, A., Rasool, G., Taj, R., Ansari, M., Naim, M., Farooq, S., Memon, A., Karim, M., Hana, Y., & Ayub, M. (2024). The national psychiatric morbidity survey of Pakistan (2022): Prevalence, socio-demographic and disability correlates. *medRxiv.* https://doi.org/10.1101/2024.07.08.24310056

Riaz, M. M. A., Nayyer, B., & Alkasaby, M. A. (2022). No social security without mental health security. *The Lancet Regional Health. Southeast Asia, 8,* 100125. https://doi.org/10.1016/j.lansea.2022.100125

Saeed, K., Gater, R., Hussain, A., & Mubbashar, M. (2000). The prevalence, classification and treatment of mental disorders among attenders of native faith healers in rural Pakistan. *Social Psychiatry and Psychiatric Epidemiology, 35*(10), 480–485. https://doi.org/10.1007/s001270050267

Saleem, S., Baig, A., Sajun, S., Bird, V., Priebe, S., Pasha, A. (2021). A mixed methods exploration of the role of multi-family groups in community treatment of patients with depression and anxiety in Pakistan. *International Journal of Mental Health Systems 15*(1), 78. https://doi.org/10.1186/s13033-021-00500-z

Sarfraz, A., Sarfraz, Z., Sarfraz, M., & Qarnain, Z. (2022). Gender-based violence in Pakistan and public health measures: A call to action. *Bulletin of the World Health Organization, 100*(7), 462–464. https://doi.org/10.2471/BLT.21.287188

Shafiq, S. (2020). Perceptions of Pakistani community towards their mental health problems: A systematic review. *Global Psychiatry, 3*(1), 28–50. https://doi.org/10.2478/gp-2020-0001

Shahid, M., Khan, M. M., Naqvi, H., & Razzak, J. (2008). Cost of treatment of deliberate self-harm. A study from Pakistan. *Crisis, 29*(4), 213–215. https://doi.org/10.1027/0227-5910.29.4.213

Siddiqui, T., Saadat, A., Zubair, R., & Taseen, S. (2024). The contemporary economic breakdown of Pakistan and its consequences on the mental health of inflation-stricken nation. *Health Science Reports, 7*(9), e70094. https://doi.org/10.1002/hsr2.70094

Trivedi, J. K., Sareen, H., & Dhyani, M. (2008). Rapid urbanization—Its impact on mental health: A South Asian perspective. *Indian Journal of Psychiatry, 50*(3), 161–165. https://doi.org/10.4103/0019-5545.43623

*UNDP's 2023–2024 Human Development Report points to a global 'gridlock' of increased inequality and political polarization.* (n.d.). UNDP. Retrieved March 24, 2025, from https://www.undp.org/pakistan/press-releases/undps-2023-2024-human-development-report-points-global-gridlock-increased-inequality-and-political-polarization

World Health Organization. (n.d.). *Universal health coverage benefit package of Pakistan: Essential package of health services with localized evidence.* Retrieved March 24, 2025, from https://www.dcp-3.org/resources/universal-health-coverage-benefit-package-pakistan-essential-package-health-services

Zafar, M., H Zaidi, T., Zaidi, N. H., Ahmed, M. W., Memon, S., Ahmed, F., Siddiqui, A., Fatima, A., Shahid, A., Hussain, B., & Salam, A. (2024). Attitude towards seeking professional help for mental health among medical students In Karachi, Pakistan. *Future Science OA, 10*(1), FSO916. https://doi.org/10.2144/fsoa-2023-0114

Zehra, M., Khan, F., & Naureen, S. (2023). Exploring stigmatizing discourses of mental illness in Pakistani newspapers through CDA lens in psychology. *Sjesr, 6*(2), 1–10. https://doi.org/10.36902/sjesr-vol6-iss2-2023(1-10)

Zulfiqar, L., Idrees, N., & Rafiq, M. (2019). Culture bound syndromes in Pakistan: Implications and strategic vision for health management. *Pakistan Journal of Neurological Sciences, 14*(4).

# Chapter 7
# Social Psychiatry in Sri Lanka

**Anuradha Baminiwatta and Shehan Williams**

**Abstract** Sri Lanka's unique sociocultural milieu has been shaped by South Asian influences, mainly from India, as well as Western colonial legacies. Its social landscape continues to evolve with shifting cultural norms, changes in social class and structure, and the growing impact of social media. Although research on the social determinants of mental health is limited, existing epidemiological data indicate a high prevalence of mental health issues linked to factors such as poverty, lack of social protection, war-related trauma and displacement, gender inequality, and the marginalization of minority groups. Stigma, low mental health literacy, and cultural beliefs about mental illness continue to hinder service provision and access. Conversely, strong family and community support, religious coping mechanisms, and resilience serve as protective factors deeply embedded in Sri Lankan society. Mental health legislation remains out-dated, while recent policy recommendations face logistical and administrative challenges to implementation. Mental health services are still largely hospital-based, and the development of community-based services must be aligned with the strengths and opportunities of the existing healthcare system. There is a pressing need for more research to explore the relevance and application of social psychiatry in the Sri Lankan context and to inform culturally responsive mental health strategies.

**Keywords** Society · Culture · Norms · Community · Religion · Poverty · War · Family · Stigma

## 1 Introduction

Sri Lanka, an island nation in South Asia, has a population of 22 million, primarily comprising Sinhala (75%), Tamil (15%), and Moor (9%) ethnic groups. It has nine administrative provinces. It is classified as a lower middle-income country, and the Gini index of 37.7 reflects a significant income disparity (World Bank Group,

A. Baminiwatta (✉) · S. Williams
Department of Psychiatry, Faculty of Medicine, University of Kelaniya, Ragama, Sri Lanka
e-mail: baminiwatta@kln.ac.lk



S. M. Y. Arafat et al. (eds.), *Social Psychiatry in South Asia*, South Asian Perspectives in Mental Health and Psychology , https://doi.org/10.1007/978-981-96-8078-8_7

2019). However, Sri Lanka's Human Development Index (HDI) was 0.78 in 2022, ranking 78th globally and placing it in the high human development category (United Nations Development Programme, 2022). The country outperforms other South Asian nations with similar population densities and exceeds the regional average in HDI, life expectancy, and education. Sri Lanka has grappled with tumultuous periods, including the 26-year civil war (1983–2009), the 2004 tsunami, the Easter bomb attacks, the COVID-19 pandemic, and the economic collapse that followed. Social determinants of mental health are understandably very important in this context, signifying the potential role for social psychiatry in Sri Lanka.

### 1.1 Historical Background of Sri Lanka

Sri Lanka has been inhabited by humans for 75,000–125,000 years (Prematilleke et al., 2007). Buddhist chronicles like the *Dipavamsa* and *Mahavamsa* trace the Sinhalese to northern Indian migrants around the fifth-century BCE, while the Tamil population likely arrived later from southern India (De Silva, 2005). Despite historical ties with India, Sri Lanka developed a distinct cultural identity due to its geographical separation. Buddhism flourished here even as it declined in India, and the Sinhalese language evolved into a unique literary tradition.

The island's strategic location made it a key hub in maritime trade, linking Europe, the Middle East, and Asia. Colonial rule began with the Portuguese in 1505, followed by the Dutch (1658) and British (1796). Sri Lanka, then called Ceylon, gained independence on February 4, 1948, and officially became the Democratic Socialist Republic of Sri Lanka in 1972.

### 1.2 History of Mental Health Services

Sri Lanka's healthcare history dates back around 5,000 years, with legends of King Ravana describing him as a skilled physician (Nirekha De Silva, 2015). The *Mahavamsa* records hospitals in the fourth-century BCE, while King Buddhadasa's *Sarartha Sangrahaya* (398 CE) described traditional treatments, including for mental illness (Silva, 2024). The traditional healthcare system evolved from Ayurveda, Siddha, Unani, and indigenous medicine.

Western-based mental health services began under British rule with lunatic asylums in 1839 (Harischandra Amarasinghe & Rajapakse, 2024; Gambheera, 2011; Kathriarachchi et al., 2019). Patients were initially housed in Hendala and later transferred to the Borella Lunatic Asylum in 1847, but overcrowding led to patients being detained in prisons. In 1926, the Angoda asylum opened but remained overcrowded. A 1928 review by Edward Mapother exposed inhumane conditions of the Angoda asylum, prompting reforms, decentralization, and specialist psychiatric care. The first outpatient psychiatric clinic opened in 1939, with the first Ceylonese psychiatrist appointed in 1940.

Since the 1990s, mental health services have rapidly expanded with the training of Board-Certified Psychiatrists through the Postgraduate Institute of Medicine. Specialist training is now offered in general adult, forensic, old age, and child and adolescent psychiatry. However, workforce shortages persist, with around 0.47 psychiatrists per 100,000 people and limited coverage in regions like the Northern Province (Pathirathne & Kulathilake, 2024).

## *1.3 Role of Social Psychiatry*

Social psychiatry is currently not recognized as a separate entity within psychiatric practice in Sri Lanka. Postgraduate training in psychiatry emphasizes the importance of social factors in the aetiology and management of psychiatric patients, but there is no separate training on social psychiatry. Although a member of the World Association of Social Psychiatry, the Sri Lankan branch has not been active in related academic activities.

## *1.4 Social Structure*

Sri Lankan society has been stratified by class and caste, with variations across ethnic groups and regions (Ekanayake & Guruge, 2016; Riswan, 2014). Traditionally, Sinhalese society was segmented by occupation-based castes, though less rigid than in India. The hierarchy included the aristocratic *Radala*, *Govigama* peasants, service castes, and lower groups like *Kinnara*, *Ahikuntika*, and *Rodee*.

Over time, the system evolved into a class structure based on wealth and influence, with upper, middle, and lower classes. Occupation remains a key marker of social status, with professions like doctors, engineers, and lawyers enjoying higher recognition. However, in some regions, the caste still influences marriage arrangements.

## *1.5 Cultural Norms*

Sri Lanka's cultural norms are shaped by its diverse ethnic and religious traditions, with strong influences from Buddhism, but also from Hinduism, Islam, and Christianity. Collectivism is a key feature, with family, community, and social harmony prioritized over individualism. Respect for elders, hierarchical social structures, and deference to authority are deeply ingrained. Gender roles tend to be traditional, though evolving, and arranged or semi-arranged marriages remain common. Religious and spiritual beliefs play a significant role in health and illness perceptions, often influencing help-seeking behaviours, including mental health.

### *1.6 Political and Human Rights*

Sri Lanka has a democratic political system, but its history has been marked by periods of civil conflict, political instability, and human rights challenges. The 26-year civil war between the government and the Liberation Tigers of Tamil Eelam deeply affected social cohesion and mental health, particularly among war-affected communities (Jayasuriya et al., 2016). Political patronage and hierarchical power structures influence access to resources, including healthcare. While constitutional protections exist for human rights, issues such as discrimination and challenges faced by marginalized groups, including those with mental illness, persist.

### *1.7 Mental Health Law*

Sri Lanka's Mental Health Act, originally established under the Lunacy Ordinance of 1873 and revised in 1956, provides the legal framework for the care and treatment of individuals with mental illness. However, it remains out-dated, with a primary focus on institutionalization rather than community-based care and patient rights (Hapangama et al., 2023). The law permits involuntary admission under specific conditions but lacks strong protections for patient autonomy, informed consent, and rehabilitation. With expansion of mental health services to all the districts of the country, the mental health law in existence is redundant. Admissions and discharges are done under common law, based on risk and patients are often detained involuntarily with no legal framework for review and discharge. However, all consultant psychiatrists are trained for one to two years in developed countries such as the United Kingdom or Australia and base their practice on accepted ethical norms. Almost all units are based in general hospitals and only admit involuntarily for short periods lasting two to four weeks for acute treatment. Efforts have been made to modernize mental health legislation in line with international human rights standards, emphasizing deinstitutionalization, community-based services, and reducing stigma.

## 2 Social Epidemiology of Mental Illness

Epidemiological data on mental illness in Sri Lanka are limited. A national mental health survey in 2007 with 6120 participants using PRIME-MD/PHQ and the Psychosis Screening Questionnaire reported a one-month prevalence of mental disorders at 15% (Institute for Research and Development, 2007). Major depressive syndrome was 2.1%, other depression 7.1%, somatoform disorder 3%, PTSD 1.7%, panic syndrome 0.5%, anxiety syndrome 0.9%, binge eating disorder 0.02%, and psychotic symptoms 3.6% (any one symptom). Disorders were more common among females and those aged 35–65. A meta-analysis of 33 studies estimated the pooled point prevalence of depressive symptoms at 19.4% (Alwis et al., 2023). Prevalence was highest among young individuals (39%), while rates were 8.7% in adults, 18.4% in older adults, and 16.9% in maternal populations. Screening instruments yielded higher prevalence (21.2%) than diagnostic interviews (4.3%).

A large epidemiological study conducted on depression and anxiety across 18 districts in post-conflict Sri Lanka suggests that the prevalence of these conditions is greater in war-affected areas (Jayasuriya et al., 2016). Data on ethnic differences in depression prevalence have been inconclusive, but Jayasuriya et al. (2016) suggest that ethnic minorities are at greater risk.

### *2.1 Mental Health Literacy*

Despite having a literacy rate of 93.3% in 2021, Sri Lankans appear to be lacking "mental health literacy". Mental health being ignored in school-based education may be an important contributor to this lack of mental health literacy. A survey of the public's ability to recognize mental health disorders and their awareness of treatment avenues has revealed that among the conditions, depression was the most recognized, followed closely by schizophrenia (Abesinghe et al., 2023). In contrast, recognition was lower for dementia and social phobia, indicating that certain mental health conditions may be less well understood within the community. Awareness regarding professional services was generally low, suggesting a gap in knowledge regarding available mental health support systems. Similar deficits in mental health literacy have been observed among adolescents, undergraduates, and caregivers (Amarasuriya, Jorm, & Reavley, 2015; Attygalle et al., 2017; Ediriweera et al., 2012). Training programs are sometimes conducted to improve mental health literacy, and some of them have been empirically studied (Ginige et al., 2021).

## 2.2 *Mental Health Stigma and Cultural Beliefs*

Stigma, prejudice, and discrimination against people with mental illness are widespread in Sri Lanka, manifesting as public, self, secondary, and structural stigma.

A qualitative study in rural Sri Lanka found that poverty, relationship issues, and religious beliefs are viewed as causes of mental illness, with cultural explanations including spells, the evil eye, and bad karma (Guruge et al., 2021). Derogatory terms like *pissa* (mad person) are common, and those with mental illness often face social exclusion. Stigma appears more pronounced in rural areas, though data on rural–urban differences is limited.

Stigmatizing attitudes have been reported among undergraduates (Amarasuriya, Jorm, Reavley, et al., 2015; Chandrasekara, 2020), medical students (Baminiwatta et al., 2020), nurses (Baminiwatta et al., 2023a), doctors (Fernando et al., 2010), adolescents (Attygalle et al., 2020), and caregivers (Fernando et al., 2017a). Higher stigma is linked to conditions like substance use and schizophrenia. Among associated factors, female gender, and personal exposure to mental illness were noteworthy. Clinical attachments in psychiatry have been shown to improve medical students' attitudes (Alwis et al., 2013; Rodrigo et al., 2012).

From the perspective of people with mental illness, common stigma experiences include isolation, inability to have a satisfactory marital life, discrimination, and avoiding disclosure (Fernando et al., 2017b). However, more than half reported increased family support.

Mental health professionals and caregivers experience *courtesy stigma*, where others view them less favourably due to their association with mental illness (Liyanage et al., 2018). Stigma among caregivers is linked to greater caregiver burden.

## 2.3 *Culture-Bound Syndromes and Cultural Idioms of Distress*

Culture-bound syndromes observed in other parts of Asia have been reported in Sri Lanka reflecting cultural similarities. Among them, *Dhat* syndrome has been reported frequently in the 1980s, at a time when attributing health problems to semen loss appears to have been relatively common (de Silva & Dissanayake, 1989; Dewaraja & Sasaki, 1991). The main source of these beliefs appears to be the Ayurvedic medical tradition. Although clinical experience suggests that the incidence has dwindled over time, cases of *Dhat* syndrome have been reported recently (Alles et al., 2023).

Koro, a culture-bound syndrome initially described among people of Chinese origin, has also been reported in Sri Lanka (Ellepola, 2021; Perera, 1988). Reports from both the 1980s and 2020s can be found, evincing that the syndrome has not yet disappeared.

Some cultural idioms of distress have been described among Tamil survivors of mass trauma. One of them, known as "walking corpse syndrome", is characterized by cognitive difficulties, dissociative attacks, and sensation of empty-headedness (Affleck et al., 2022). Tamil psychiatrists in Sri Lanka have described several other head- or mind-related cultural idioms of distress among Tamil people as expressions of war trauma (Sivoyokan, 2011; Somasundaram, 2010).

Although eating disorders were originally considered a cultural syndrome of the West, they are increasingly reported in Asian contexts, including in Sri Lanka, probably because of the Western influence on cultural perceptions of body image. However, the presentations may be different, with atypical eating disorders more common, and "fat phobia" less commonly associated (Rodrigo & Hewawitharana, 2017). However, typical presentations are also reported (Perera et al., 2002).

As observed in other Asian countries, depression often manifests as non-specific somatic complaints in Sri Lanka. Direct expressions of sadness and guilt are less common. Common idioms of distress include *bade gindara* (fire in the abdomen), and *vaatha amaru* (a term from Ayurvedic tradition referring to generalized discomfort in the body). Taking note of these cultural idioms of distress and clinical experience with depressed patients, Abeyasinghe et al. (2012) developed a culturally relevant tool to screen for depression.

## 2.4 Gender and Mental Health

The status of women in the Sri Lankan society is mixed (Gunawardena, 2015). While the society has been traditionally patriarchal, women have reached high positions in political and other spheres; notably, Sri Lanka boasts of having the world's first female Prime Minister—Sirimavo Bandaranaike. However, women from lower social strata have had fewer opportunities. Sri Lanka ranks 90th out of 166 countries on the Gender Inequality Index with a score of 0.376 in 2022, performing better than most South Asian countries (United Nations Development Programme, 2022).

Despite progress, women still face disadvantages. Family estates are passed down patrilineally, with daughters receiving dowries and sons inheriting property. Historically, women were financially dependent on men and stayed home to raise children, while men made family decisions. Over time, women have increasingly joined the workforce, but many still balance employment with childcare, a challenging task. Employment has been linked to depression among women with lower living standards (Ball et al., 2010). In recent years, men have begun sharing household responsibilities.

Gender-based violence is widespread, with 40% of women aged 15 or older having experienced violence from a partner (Department of Census and Statistics, 2020). Domestic violence affects both men and women, with some studies demonstrating similar prevalence among genders. Such violence is associated with depression, suicidal thoughts, and mental illness (Bandara et al., 2022). Gender-based violence is a significant contributor to mental health issues, especially among women and perinatal mothers. Depression rates are higher among women in Sri Lanka, and the aforesaid psychosocial stressors may be important etiologic factors (Alwis et al., 2023).

LGBTQ + individuals in Sri Lanka face significant social, cultural, and legal challenges, including human rights violations, despite some recent progress (EQUAL GROUND, 2013). Homosexuality remains highly stigmatized in the conservative society, leading to discrimination and family rejection. Same-sex relations are still criminalized under colonial-era laws (Sect. 365A of Penal Code), though discussions on decriminalization have emerged. Mental health issues are common among sexual minorities due to stigma, discrimination, and lack of social support (Karunanayake, 2024; Manchanayake et al., 2023). Transgender individuals face barriers to social acceptance and equal opportunities. Since 2016, they can change their gender on identity documents following psychiatric assessment and gender-affirming treatment, but unclear guidelines complicate access to care (Ariyarathne, 2023).

## 2.5 The Role of the Family in Mental Illness

Family plays a key role in both the aetiology and management of mental illness in Sri Lanka. Family-related factors such as intimate partner violence, parenting styles, child abuse, and elder abuse are common contributors to mental illness. Parental migration for overseas employment, especially by mothers, poses psychological risks to children (Senaratne et al., 2011). However, Sri Lanka's collectivistic culture often provides strong family support and social capital, serving as protective factors.

Families typically take responsibility for caregiving, with members accompanying patients to clinics and ensuring treatment adherence (Guruge et al., 2021). Extended family often provides additional support, though disputes can arise over primary caregiving responsibilities. Parental overinvolvement is culturally sanctioned, and such family dynamics create high expressed emotions that could be counterproductive. Nevertheless, better outcomes have been reported in Sri Lanka for psychotic disorders, such as schizophrenia, compared to Western countries, possibly due to cultural beliefs, family norms, and the treatment system (Waxler, 1979).

## 2.6 Poverty, Social Security, and Mental Health

Poverty is a major contributor to mental health problems in Sri Lanka (Alwis et al., 2023). People with mental illness are often from lower socio-economic backgrounds, with severe conditions like schizophrenia leading to "social drift" and homelessness. Employment is difficult due to stigma and lack of relevant supports.

Despite free government healthcare, shortages of essential medications often force patients to buy them privately, adding to financial burdens (Jayasinghe, 2013). Limited social security options include a small monthly allowance of 5000 Sri Lankan rupees for those unable to work, along with minimal housing and medical aid. Welfare schemes like *Samurdhi* offer additional support but are often insufficient. The recent economic recession has worsened these issues (Matthias & Jayasinghe,

2022). Poor coordination between health and social services further limits access to social protection. Furthermore, private health insurance schemes do not cover mental illness.

## 2.7 *Religion and Spirituality*

Religion and spirituality are deeply intertwined with mental health in Sri Lanka, shaping both individuals' experiences of psychological distress and their pathways to recovery. The country's rich religious landscape—dominated by Buddhism, alongside Hinduism, Islam, and Christianity -permeates everyday life and offers culturally embedded coping mechanisms. Buddhist teachings on impermanence (*anicca*), suffering (*dukkha*), and non-attachment (*anatta*) provide individuals with frameworks to understand and accept life's adversities, which can foster resilience. However, when interpreting the negative cognitions of depression in this setting, which share some outward similarities with Buddhist ideas of suffering, a sound understanding of these cultural nuances is required (Obeyesekere, 1985). Practices such as meditation, chanting, and visiting temples offer not only spiritual comfort but also social connectedness. Some Buddhist approaches to problems share similarities with Western models of psychotherapy (Chandradasa & Kuruppuarachchi, 2019; Somasundaram, 2013). Similarly, Hindu rituals, Islamic prayer, and Christian community gatherings can serve as sources of support and coping.

However, religion and spirituality sometimes present challenges for mental health in Sri Lanka. Certain beliefs, such as attributing mental illness to karma, spirits, or divine punishment, delay help-seeking and lead individuals to prioritize faith healers or traditional practices over medical treatment. While these systems offer valuable cultural healing practices, their exclusive reliance sometimes results in worse outcomes. *Bali Thovil* are common healing rituals that involve drumming, dancing, wooden masks, and chanting by shamans, and usually aim to combat illnesses supposedly caused by demonic interference (Nirekha De Silva, 2015). Some Buddhists engage in religious rituals such as *Bodhi pooja*, and *Pirith* chanting to achieve good health or to ward off evil forces.

## 2.8 *Social Media and Mass Media*

Advent of social media has been rapidly changing the dynamics of social interactions in Sri Lanka. About two-thirds of the Sri Lankan population use the internet and one-third are active social media users (Asia Pacific Institute of Digital Marketing & Department of Marketing Management, 2023). Facebook, YouTube, and Instagram are the most popular social media platforms, accounting for 87%, 41%, and 23% of active users, respectively. Recent research among children and young populations in Sri Lanka suggests that excessive social media use may be linked to depression, stress, and reduced emotional intelligence (Hazzana, 2024; Keara & De Zoysa, 2022; Manori et al., 2024). However, beneficial effects or absent negative effects have been suggested by some studies (De Zoysa et al., 2015; Sandupama De Silva et al., 2023; Sathurusinghe, 2024). Since most of the extant research is cross-sectional in design, whether social media use predates mental health outcomes or vice versa has not been established. Screen media use among children rose steeply during the pandemic and may have has significant mental health effects (Baminiwatta et al., 2023b; Manori et al., 2024).

## 2.9 Disasters, Pandemics, Conflict, Trauma, and Resilience

Sri Lanka has faced numerous disasters, both natural and man-made, that have had profound psychological and social consequences. The 2004 tsunami caused immense loss of life and displacement, leaving lasting trauma among survivors (Galappatti, 2005; Henderson & Elsass, 2015). Religion and cultural coping methods have been protective against mental health problems following tsunami exposure (de Silva, 2006; Wickrama et al., 2024). Floods, landslides, and droughts also affect vulnerable communities, exacerbating mental health challenges. In addition, the COVID-19 pandemic placed unprecedented strain on individuals and healthcare systems, increasing anxiety, depression, and economic distress (Baminiwatta et al., 2021).

Decades of civil conflict resulted in significant trauma, particularly among war-affected populations in the North and East. The prolonged exposure to violence, displacement, and loss led to widespread psychological distress, including PTSD, depression, and substance abuse (Husain et al., 2011; Siriwardhana et al., 2013). The 2019 Easter attacks further underscored the psychological impact of terrorism on national security and collective well-being. However, resilience remains a defining feature of Sri Lankan society. Cultural and religious practices, community solidarity, and grassroots mental health initiatives have been instrumental in promoting healing. Efforts to integrate trauma-informed care into psychiatric services and community-based interventions continue to evolve, aiming to address both immediate and long-term psychological needs.

## 2.10 Impact of Migration and Displacement on Mental Health

Migration and displacement in Sri Lanka, driven by economic hardship, conflict, and natural disasters, have significant mental health consequences. Many Sri Lankans migrate for employment, particularly to the Middle East, facing stressors such as social isolation, exploitative working conditions, and separation from family, which increase the risk of anxiety, depression, and substance use. Internal displacement, particularly due to the decades-long civil war and recurrent natural disasters, has left many struggling with PTSD, depression, and prolonged grief. Limited access to mental health services, stigma, and economic instability further exacerbate psychological distress among these populations.

## 2.11 *Suicidal Behaviour*

Sri Lanka had the second highest suicide rate in the world in 1995. However, the rates came down drastically afterwards, probably reflecting the steps implemented by the Presidential Task Force on Suicide Prevention, which included banning import of lethal pesticides (Gunnell et al., 2007; Rajapakse, 2017). Suicide rates have been higher in Northern and Eastern parts of the island, which were more severely affected by the civil war (Baminiwatta & Ediriweera, 2022). A reduction in suicide rates was observed after the war ended (Rodrigo et al., 2013). Suicides are reported more frequently from rural areas (Knipe et al., 2017). Many other sociocultural factors appear to influence suicide and self-harm. Childhood adversities including childhood abuse, witnessing household violence, having a household member with mental illness or suicidal behaviour, and parental death/separation/divorce have been implicated (T. Rajapakse et al., 2020). Intimate partner violence has shown a clear link with self-harm (Bandara et al., 2024). As reasons for suicide among the elderly, physical illness, mental illness, spousal violence, economic problems, and drug addiction have been reported (Baminiwatta A, 2024).

## 2.12 *Vulnerable Populations*

Certain groups in Sri Lanka face heightened mental health risks due to socioeconomic, cultural, and systemic factors. Women, particularly those experiencing domestic violence or economic hardship, are at greater risk of depression and anxiety. Children, especially those affected by poverty, abuse, or conflict, often struggle with developmental and psychological challenges. The elderly, facing social isolation and health-related concerns, frequently experience depression and cognitive decline, yet their mental health needs remain largely overlooked. Prisoners, many of whom have a history of trauma, substance use, or mental illness, encounter inadequate psychiatric care within the correctional system. Currently, there are very few psychiatrists who have sub-specialized in child and adolescent, forensic, and old age psychiatry to plan and implement relevant mental health interventions (Pathirathne & Kulathilake, 2024).

## 2.13 Community-Based Mental Health Interventions

Sri Lanka has strengthened its community-based mental health initiatives since the 2004 tsunami. The mental health policy 2005–2015 and the recently revised policy 2020–2030 have placed significant emphasis on the development of community-based services. In the south Asian region, Sri Lanka perhaps has the best coverage of the whole country, with mental health services in all the districts. A hub-and-spoke model is being developed with every district having a dedicated psychiatric unit in a general hospital setting from which community initiatives are developed. Efforts are targeted towards collaborative care and to integrate community-based care into the existing healthcare system (Rajasuriya et al., 2021). The hospital-based mental health teams, with the support of community psychiatry nurses and psychiatry social workers, conduct outreach clinics and home visits to administer long-acting injectables for patients at risk of relapse. In some districts especially in the Northern Province, community support workers (CSW) do home visits and support patients and caregivers. Several NGOs too, including the Nest, Sumithrayo, Lanka Alzheimer's Foundation, Sahanaya, Escape, and Women in Need, provide important services in the community. Nevertheless, the community services are still lacking in breadth and depth and leave much to be improved.

Weerasundera (2010) advocated for a practical approach to community psychiatry where the specific advantages and limitations of each locality are taken into consideration. This approach is particularly feasible given the fact that health services are devolved to the nine provinces in Sri Lanka, and every province has the freedom to identify its unique needs and adapt as necessary. It has been suggested that Sri Lanka's strong primary healthcare system can be leveraged to enhance mental healthcare delivery (Rodrigo, 2017). This hopefully will be the next step in mental healthcare delivery where primary healthcare clusters will have primary care clinics which will provide mental health services. Initial pilots show promise particularly in the context of all Sri Lankan medical graduates receiving extensive training in psychiatry with psychiatry being a separate stand-alone subject in the final MBBS examinations.

## 2.14 Telepsychiatry

Telehealth services are not widely available in Sri Lanka at present (Kulatunga et al., 2020). Although there was a rise in the availability of telepsychiatry services following the COVID-19 pandemic, only a limited number of psychiatrists provide telepsychiatry services (Perera et al., 2020). A survey among caregivers of children and adolescents receiving specialized treatment services showed that the majority wished to be contacted by video call (Rohanachandra et al., 2022). Although telepsychiatry has the potential to enhance access to mental health services particularly in areas where psychiatrists are scarce, inadequacy of internet access and technical know-how in rural areas remains a challenge in implementing this.

### 2.15 Social Prevention and Social Management of Mental Illness

Social prevention of mental illness in Sri Lanka should address aforesaid social factors contributing to mental health problems. Prevention efforts need to focus on reducing poverty, domestic violence, and social isolation through welfare schemes, mental health literacy programs, and community support networks. NGOs and community organizations that provide crisis support and suicide prevention services need to be strengthened.

Social management involving community-based care through outreach clinics, home visits, and support from community workers needs to be supported. Family involvement, peer support groups, and vocational rehabilitation should be leveraged for recovery and social integration. Expanding community services and strengthening collaboration between health and social service sectors are key to improving outcomes.

## 3 Conclusion

Sri Lanka's mental health landscape is deeply intertwined with its sociocultural, economic, and political fabric. The impact of war, poverty, disaster, and displacement underscores the importance of social psychiatry in understanding and addressing mental health needs in the Sri Lankan context. While the country has made significant progress in expanding hospital-based mental health services, numerous challenges remain—from stigma and low mental health literacy to inadequate legislation and limited community-based services. Strong family structures, cultural beliefs, and religious coping mechanisms serve as both protective and, at times, obstructive influences. Vulnerable populations, including women, children, ethnic minorities, and the LGBTQ + community, face unique psychosocial risks that must be addressed through targeted interventions. Strengthening research, policy implementation, and intersectoral collaboration will be essential to transforming mental healthcare. As the country moves forward, leveraging its strong primary care infrastructure offers an opportunity to integrate social psychiatry into community mental health services, fostering resilience and equity in mental healthcare delivery.

## References

Abesinghe, A. M. I. D., Katuwawela, K. P. D. K. I., Lakmali, K. P. W., Jayanetti, N. L., Munidasa, K. G. P. K., De Silva, B. S. S., & Marikar, F. M. M. T. (2023). Mental health literacy: A survey of the public's ability to recognize mental disorders and their knowledge about the effectiveness of helpful interventions to help the victims. *Journal of Evidence-Based Psychotherapies, 23*(2), 173–202. https://doi.org/10.24193/jebp.2023.2.16

Abeyasinghe, D. R. R., Tennakoon, S., & Rajapakse, T. N. (2012). The development and validation of the Peradeniya Depression Scale (PDS)—A culturally relevant tool for screening of depression in Sri Lanka. *Journal of Affective Disorders, 142*(1–3), 143–149. https://doi.org/10.1016/j.jad.2012.04.019

Affleck, W., Thamotharampillai, U., & Hinton, D. (2022). Walking Corpse Syndrome: A trauma-related idiom of distress amongst Sri Lankan Tamils. *Transcultural Psychiatry, 59*(4), 448–460. https://doi.org/10.1177/13634615211001701

Alles, P. S., Akurana, C., Amarakoon, D. L. U., & Rohanachandra, Y. M. (2023). An elderly man presenting with symptoms suggestive of Dhat syndrome. *Sri Lanka Journal of Psychiatry, 14*(1), 50–52. https://doi.org/10.4038/sljpsyc.v14i1.8409

Alwis, I., Baminiwatta, A., & Chandradasa, M. (2023). Prevalence and associated factors of depression in Sri Lanka: A systematic review and meta-analysis. *Social Psychiatry and Psychiatric Epidemiology.* https://doi.org/10.1007/s00127-023-02495-z

Amarasinghe, S. C., Rajapakse, T. N. (2024). Psychiatric Morbidity and Mental Health Services in Sri Lanka. In S. M. Y. Arafat & S. K. Kar (Eds.), *Access to Mental Health Care in South Asia.* Springer. https://doi.org/10.1007/978-981-99-9153-2_8

Amarasuriya, S. D., Jorm, A. F., & Reavley, N. J. (2015). Quantifying and predicting depression literacy of undergraduates: A cross sectional study in Sri Lanka. *BMC Psychiatry, 15*(1), 269. https://doi.org/10.1186/s12888-015-0658-8

Amarasuriya, S. D., Jorm, A. F., Reavley, N. J., & Mackinnon, A. J. (2015). Stigmatising attitudes of undergraduates towards their peers with depression: A cross-sectional study in Sri Lanka. *BMC Psychiatry, 15,* 129. https://doi.org/10.1186/s12888-015-0523-9

Ariyarathne, K. (2023). Test for real life? The gender transition process in Sri Lanka. *Polity.*

Asia Pacific Institute of Digital Marketing & Department of Marketing Management, U. of K. (2023). *Digital outlook Sri Lanka 2023: The annual market insight report.*

Attygalle, U. R., Perera, H., & Jayamanne, B. D. W. (2017). Mental health literacy in adolescents: Ability to recognise problems, helpful interventions and outcomes. *Child and Adolescent Psychiatry and Mental Health, 11*(1), 38. https://doi.org/10.1186/s13034-017-0176-1

Attygalle, U. R., Perera, H., & Jayamanne, B. D. W. (2020). Stigma related to mental health issues—A study among adolescents in Sri Lanka. *Sri Lanka Journal of Psychiatry, 11*(1), 8–13. https://doi.org/10.4038/sljpsyc.v11i1.8243

Ball, H. A., Siribaddana, S. H., Kovas, Y., Glozier, N., McGuffin, P., Sumathipala, A., & Hotopf, M. (2010). Epidemiology and symptomatology of depression in Sri Lanka: A cross-sectional population-based survey in Colombo District. *Journal of Affective Disorders, 123*(1–3), 188–196. https://doi.org/10.1016/j.jad.2009.08.014

Baminiwatta A. (2024). Changing patterns of suicide among the elderly in Sri Lanka from 2015 to 2022: An analysis based on national suicide statistics. *Annual Academic Sessions of the Sri Lanka College of Psychiatrists.*

Baminiwatta, A., Alahakoon, H., Herath, N. C., Kodithuwakku, K. M., & Nanayakkara, T. (2023a). Trait mindfulness, compassion, and stigma towards patients with mental illness: A study among nurses in Sri Lanka. *Mindfulness, 14*(4), 979–991. https://doi.org/10.1007/s12671-023-02108-5

Baminiwatta, A., De Silva, S., Hapangama, A., Basnayake, K., Abayaweera, C., Kulasinghe, D., Kaushalya, D., & Williams, S. (2021). Impact of COVID-19 on the mental health of frontline and non-frontline healthcare workers in Sri Lanka. *The Ceylon Medical Journal, 66*(1), 16–31. https://doi.org/10.4038/cmj.v66i1.9351

Baminiwatta, A., & Ediriweera, D. (2022, September 28). *Changes in the geospatial distribution of suicides in Sri Lanka during the COVID-19 pandemic: An analysis of police data.* https://doi.org/10.13140/RG.2.2.27623.73123

Baminiwatta, A. K. A. B., Bandara, W. A. V. S., Athurugiriya, A. A. I. D., Yangdon, T., Cader, G. R., Bokalamulla, L. A. B., Bandara, W. R. R. D., Bandara, W. M. K. M., Chandradasa, K. A. S. I. P., Athukorala, H. P., & Dias, G. S. S. R. (2020). A nationwide survey of attitudes towards psychiatry among final-year medical students in Sri Lanka. *Asian Journal of Psychiatry,* 102101. https://doi.org/10.1016/j.ajp.2020.102101

Baminiwatta, A., Nanayakkara, T. D., Fernando, A., & Wijethunga, S. (2023b). Screen addiction among children and adolescents and the self-efficacy of mothers in screen use management during the COVID-19 lockdown in Sri Lanka. *Sri Lanka Journal of Psychiatry, 14*(1), 36–43. https://doi.org/10.4038/sljpsyc.v14i1.8407

Bandara, P., Page, A., Rajapakse, T., & Knipe, D. (2024). Intimate partner violence, suicide and self-harm in Sri Lanka: Analysis of national data. *PLOS ONE, 19*(3), e0298413. https://doi.org/10.1371/journal.pone.0298413

Bandara, P., Page, A., Senarathna, L., Wijewardene, K., Silva, T., Gunnell, D., Knipe, D., & Rajapakse, T. (2022). Clinical and psychosocial factors associated with domestic violence among men and women in Kandy, Sri Lanka. *PLOS Global Public Health, 2*(4), e0000129. https://doi.org/10.1371/journal.pgph.0000129

Chandradasa, M., & Kuruppuarachchi, K. A. L. A. (2019). Confluence of western psychotherapy and religious teachings in mental healthcare of an Asian Buddhist community: Sri Lanka. *Journal of Religion and Health, 58*(5), 1471–1476. https://doi.org/10.1007/s10943-018-0674-3

Chandrasekara, S. (2020). *Beyond stigma: Perceived barriers and enablers for help seeking for mental health issues in undergraduate students in Sri Lanka.*

de Alwis, A., Perera, R., Vasantha, H. L., Henegama, T., & Fernando, S. (2013). The attitude of medical students towards the mental mentally ill: The impact of a clinical attachment in Psychiatry. *Sri Lanka Journal of Psychiatry.* https://doi.org/10.4038/sljpsyc.v3i2.5132

De Silva, K. M. (2005). *A history of Sri Lanka.* Vijitha Yapa Publications. https://books.google.com.au/books?id=PWbRAqsIJgIC

de Silva, P., & Dissanayake, S. A. (1989). The loss of semen syndrome in Sri Lanka: A clinical study. *Sexual & Marital Therapy, 4*(2), 195–204. https://doi.org/10.1080/02674658908408337

De Zoysa, P., Wickrama, T., & Wickramasuriya, T. (2015). Online social networking and its perceived life satisfaction among Sri Lankan medical students. *South-East Asian Journal of Medical Education, 9,* 33. https://doi.org/10.4038/seajme.v9i2.81

Department of Census and Statistics, S. L. (2020). *Women's wellbeing survey—2019: Fndings from Sri Lanka's first dedicated national survey on violence against women and girls.*

Dewaraja, R., & Sasaki, Y. (1991). Semen-loss syndrome: A comparison between Sri Lanka and Japan. *American Journal of Psychotherapy, 45*(1).

Ediriweera, H. W., Fernando, S. M., & Pai, N. B. (2012). Mental health literacy survey among Sri Lankan carers of patients with Schizophrenia and depression. *Asian Journal of Psychiatry, 5*(3), 246–250. https://doi.org/10.1016/j.ajp.2012.02.016

Ekanayake, E., & Guruge, C. (2016). *Social stratification, modernization and restructuring of Sri Lankan society* (vol. 5, pp. 96–107).

Ellepola, A. (2021). Koro, psychological retraction of the genitalia: A case series. *Sri Lanka Journal of Psychiatry.* https://doi.org/10.4038/sljpsyc.v12i2.8304

EQUAL GROUND, S. L. (2013). *Human Rights Violations against Lesbian, Gay, Bisexual, and Transgender (LGBT) People in Sri Lanka: A Shadow Report.*

Fernando, A. M., Godavitharana, A. M. M., Pathirana, S., Tennakoon, S., Ariyasinghe, D., & Rajapakse, T. N. (2017a). Stigma experienced by persons diagnosed to have a mental illness—A descriptive study. *Sri Lanka Journal of Psychiatry, 8*(2), 24. https://doi.org/10.4038/sljpsyc.v8i2.8157

Fernando, S. M., Deane, F. P., & McLeod, H. J. (2010). Sri Lankan doctors' and medical undergraduates' attitudes towards mental illness. *Social Psychiatry and Psychiatric Epidemiology, 45*(7), 733–739. https://doi.org/10.1007/s00127-009-0113-6

Fernando, S. M., Deane, F. P., McLeod, H. J., & Davis, E. L. (2017b). A carer burden and stigma in schizophrenia and affective disorders: Experiences from Sri Lanka. *Asian Journal of Psychiatry, 26,* 77–81. https://doi.org/10.1016/j.ajp.2017.01.023

Galappatti, A. (2005). Psychosocial work in the aftermath of the tsunami: Challenges for service provision in Batticaloa, Eastern Sri Lanka. *Intervention Journal of Mental Health and Psychosocial Support in Conflict Affected Areas, 3*(1). https://journals.lww.com/invn/fulltext/2005/03010/psychosocial_work_in_the_aftermath_of_the_tsunami_.8.aspx

Ginige, P., Perera, I. B. R. U., Arambepola, S. C. A., Kuruwita, K. A. P. R., & Gunawardena, E. R. N. D. (2021). The impact of a specialized training programme on teacher mental health literacy in Central Sri Lanka. *Sri Lanka Journal of Medicine, 30*(1), 34. https://doi.org/10.4038/sljm.v30i1.243

Gunawardena, N. S. (2015). Women in Sri Lanka: Achievements and challenges. *Journal of the College of Community Physicians of Sri Lanka, 20*(1), 4. https://doi.org/10.4038/jccpsl.v20i1.8067

Gunnell, D., Fernando, R., Hewagama, M., Priyangika, W. D. D., Konradsen, F., & Eddleston, M. (2007). The impact of pesticide regulations on suicide in Sri Lanka. *International Journal of Epidemiology, 36*(6), 1235–1242. https://doi.org/10.1093/ije/dym164

Guruge, N., Dahlström, C., Perera, M., & Andersson, L. (2021). Views and perceptions toward mental illness: A qualitative study from a rural, agricultural community in Anuradhapura, Sri Lanka. *Asian Pacific Journal of Health Sciences, 8*. https://doi.org/10.21276/apjhs.2021.8.2.9

Hapangama, A., Mendis, J., & Kuruppuarachchi, K. A. L. A. (2023). Why are we still living in the past? Sri Lanka needs urgent and timely reforms of its archaic mental health laws. *Bjpsych International, 20*(1), 4–6. https://doi.org/10.1192/bji.2022.26

Harischandra Gambheera. (2011). The evolution of psychiatric services in Sri Lanka. *South Asian Journal of Psychiatry, 2*(1).

Hazzana H.S.F, B. R. M. P. M. R. W. R. G. S. D. S. T. (2024). Social media addiction and depression during healthcare professional education at Eastern University, Sri Lanka. *Journal of HealthCare Education, 1*(1).

Henderson, S. E. K., & Elsass, P. (2015). Predictors of trauma and distress in Sri Lanka five years after the Indian Ocean tsunami: A cross-sectional study. *International Journal of Disaster Risk Reduction, 14,* 438–444. https://doi.org/10.1016/j.ijdrr.2015.09.010

Husain, F., Anderson, M., Lopes Cardozo, B., Becknell, K., Blanton, C., Araki, D., & Kottegoda Vithana, E. (2011). Prevalence of war-related mental health conditions and association with displacement status in Postwar Jaffna district, Sri Lanka. *JAMA, 306*(5), 522. https://doi.org/10.1001/jama.2011.1052

Institute for Research and Development. (2007). *National Survey on Mental Health in Sri Lanka.*

Jayasinghe, S. (2013). Illness and social protection: An agenda for action in Sri Lanka. *Sri Lanka Journal of Social Sciences.* https://doi.org/10.4038/sljss.v33i1-2.5455

Jayasuriya, D., Jayasuriya, R., Tay, A. K., & Silove, D. (2016). Associations of mental distress with residency in conflict zones, ethnic minority status, and potentially modifiable social factors following conflict in Sri Lanka: A nationwide cross-sectional study. *The Lancet Psychiatry, 3*(2), 145–153. https://doi.org/10.1016/S2215-0366(15)00437-X

Karunanayake, D. (2024). *The Role of Family Support on the Mental Health of Gay Men in Sri Lanka.*

Kathriarachchi, S. T., Seneviratne, V. L., & Amarakoon, L. (2019). Development of mental health care in Sri Lanka: Lessons learned. *Taiwanese Journal of Psychiatry, 33*(2), 55. https://doi.org/10.4103/TPSY.TPSY_15_19

Keara, D., & De Zoysa, P. (2022). The association between the use of selected forms of social media and the emotional intelligence of undergraduates of a state university in Sri Lanka. *Sri Lanka Journal of Psychiatry, 13*(2), 13–17. https://doi.org/10.4038/sljpsyc.v13i2.8396

Knipe, D. W., Padmanathan, P., Muthuwatta, L., Metcalfe, C., & Gunnell, D. (2017). Regional variation in suicide rates in Sri Lanka between 1955 and 2011: A spatial and temporal analysis. *BMC Public Health, 17*(1), 193. https://doi.org/10.1186/s12889-016-3961-5

Kulatunga, G. G., Hewapathirana, R., Marasinghe, R. B., & Dissanayake, V. H. W. (2020). A review of Telehealth practices in Sri Lanka in the context of the COVID-19 pandemic. *Sri Lanka Journal of Bio-Medical Informatics, 11*(1), 8. https://doi.org/10.4038/sljbmi.v11i1.8090

Liyanage, U. L. N. S., Rowel, W. W. J. S. M., Hewawitharana, U. H., De Silva, V., & Dissanayake, D. M. T. (2018). Stigma due to their work in mental health, among mental health professionals in Sri Lanka. *Sri Lanka Journal of Psychiatry, 9*(1), 4. https://doi.org/10.4038/sljpsyc.v9i1.8174

Manchanayake, D., Baminiwatta, A., Delpachitra, M., & Wijesinghe, C. (2023). *Internalized homonegativity, self-esteem and depression among individuals who identify as gay, lesbian and bisexual in Sri Lanka.*
Manori D. M., S., Bowatta P. G., S., Basnayaka, U. P., Fernando, J. M. W., Nishshanka, N. T., Pathirana, K. S. H. P., & Senarathna, D. N. A. M. (2024). Screen addiction and associated factors among grade-10 school children in Nuwaragampalatha— east educational zone in Anuradhapura, Sri Lanka. *International Journal of Community Medicine And Public Health, 11*(12), 4804–4810. https://doi.org/10.18203/2394-6040.ijcmph20243647
Matthias, A. T., & Jayasinghe, S. (2022). Worsening economic crisis in Sri Lanka: Impacts on health. *The Lancet Global Health, 10*(7), e959. https://doi.org/10.1016/S2214-109X(22)00234-0
Nirekha De Silva. (2015). Sri Lanka's Traditional Knowledge about Health and Wellbeing: History, Present Status and Need for Safeguarding. In S. Garg (Ed.), *Traditional Knowledge and Traditional Cultural Expressions of South Asia.* SAARC Cultural Centre.
Obeyesekere, G. (1985). 4. Depression, Buddhism, and the work of culture in Sri Lanka. In *Culture and Depression* (pp. 134–152). University of California Press. https://doi.org/10.1525/9780520340923-007
Pathirathne, W. P. K. G. & Kulathilake, S. (2024, July 26). Survey on available numbers of consultant psychiatrists in the government sector of Sri Lanka [Conference Presentation]. Annual Academic Sessions of the Sri Lanka College of Psychiatrists 2024, Colombo, Sri Lanka.
Perera, H., Wickramasinghe, V., Wanigasinghe, K., & Perera, G. (2002). Anorexia nervosa in early adolescence in Sri Lanka. *Annals of Tropical Paediatrics, 22*(2), 173–177. https://doi.org/10.1179/027249302125000904
Perera H.V. (1988). Two cases of koro-like states occurring in Sri Lanka. *Journal of the Ceylon College of Physicians, 21.*
Perera, S., Gambheera, H., & Williams, S. (2020). "Telepsychiatry" in the time of COVID-19: Overcoming the challenges. *Indian Journal of Psychiatry, 62*(9), 391. https://doi.org/10.4103/psychiatry.IndianJPsychiatry_848_20
Prematilleke, L., S. Bandaranayake, S.U. Deraniyagala, & R. Silva. (2007). *The Art and Archaeology of Sri Lanka.* Central Cultural Fund.
Rajapakse, T. N. (2017). A review of the changing patterns of suicide and deliberate self-harm in Sri Lanka. *Sri Lanka Journal of Psychiatry, 8*(1), 3. https://doi.org/10.4038/sljpsyc.v8i1.8132
Rajapakse, T., Russell, A. E., Kidger, J., Bandara, P., López-López, J. A., Senarathna, L., Metcalfe, C., Gunnell, D., & Knipe, D. (2020). Childhood adversity and self-poisoning: A hospital case control study in Sri Lanka. *PLOS ONE, 15*(11), e0242437. https://doi.org/10.1371/journal.pone.0242437
Rajasuriya, M., Hewagama, M., Ruwanpriya, S., & Wijesundara, H. (2021). Community-Based Psychiatric Services in Sri Lanka: A Model by WHO in the Making. *Consortium Psychiatricum, 2*(4), 40–52. https://doi.org/10.17816/CP106
Riswan, M. (2014). A Historical Survey of Social Class and Caste System in Sri Lanka. *"KALAM" International Journal of Faculty of Arts and Culture, VIII*(1).
Rodrigo, A., & Hewawitharana, U. (2017). Variant of anorexia nervosa in Sri Lanka: A case series. *Ceylon Medical Journal, 62*(2), 104. https://doi.org/10.4038/cmj.v62i2.8476
Rodrigo, A., Owada, K., Wainer, J., Baker, R., & Williams, S. (2013). Comparison of suicide rates in Sri Lanka during and after the civil war. *Australasian Psychiatry, 21*(4), 410–410. https://doi.org/10.1177/1039856213486218
Rodrigo, A., Wijesinghe, C. & Kuruppuarachchi, K. (2012). Changes in attitudes toward psychiatry with introduction of a new curriculum: Experiences of a Sri Lankan medical school. *Sri Lanka Journal of Psychiatry, 3*(1), pp.14–16.
Rodrigo, E. K. (2017). Community psychiatry, community mental health services or primary care psychiatry? *Sri Lanka Journal of Psychiatry, 8*(2), 1. https://doi.org/10.4038/sljpsyc.v8i2.8152
Rohanachandra, Y. M., Nanayakkara, K. A. S. D., Vipulanandan, S., & Yoheswaran, A. (2022). Impact of the COVID-19 pandemic on treatment adherence and the caregivers' preference regarding telepsychiatry services at a specialized child and adolescent mental health service in

a teaching hospital in Sri Lanka. *Sri Lanka Journal of Psychiatry, 13*(2), 18–20. https://doi.org/10.4038/sljpsyc.v13i2.8362

Sandupama De Silva, S. K. N., Tzenios, N., & Salibi, G. (2023). Relationship between the use of social media and the effects on the sleep cycle among Sri Lankan undergraduate students. *Special Journal of the Medical Academy and Other Life Sciences, 1*(7). https://doi.org/10.58676/sjmas.v1i7.42

Sathurusinghe, R. (2024). An analysis on the impact of social media on the children's minds in modern Sri Lankan society. *Brazilian Journal of Development, 10,* e71087. https://doi.org/10.34117/bjdv10n7-015

Senaratne, B., Perera, H., & Fonseka, P. (2011). Mental health status and risk factors for mental health problems in left-behind children of women migrant workers in Sri Lanka. *Ceylon Medical Journal, 56*(4), 153. https://doi.org/10.4038/cmj.v56i4.3893

Silva, P. de. (2006). The tsunami and its aftermath in Sri Lanka: Explorations of a Buddhist perspective. *International Review of Psychiatry, 18*(3), 281–287. https://doi.org/10.1080/09540260600658270

Silva, S. (2024). The Physician King Buddhadasa: A Mine of Virtues, as the Sea is of Jewels. *Cureus*. https://doi.org/10.7759/cureus.71416

Siriwardhana, C., Adikari, A., Pannala, G., Siribaddana, S., Abas, M., Sumathipala, A., & Stewart, R. (2013). Prolonged internal displacement and common mental disorders in Sri Lanka: The COMRAID Study. *PLOS ONE, 8*(5), e64742. https://doi.org/10.1371/journal.pone.0064742

Sivoyokan, S. (2011). Meanings beyond words: Expressions of distress in three communities in the North. In S. Fernando & C. Weerackody (Eds.), *Aspects of mental health in Sri Lanka*. People's Rural Development Association.

Somasundaram, D. (2010). Collective trauma in the Vanni—A qualitative inquiry into the mental health of the Internally Displaced due to the civil war in Sri Lanka. *International Journal of Mental Health Systems, 4*(1), 22. https://doi.org/10.1186/1752-4458-4-22

Cultural relaxation methods for minor mental health disorders. *Sri Lanka Journal of Psychiatry, 3*(2), 3. https://doi.org/10.4038/sljpsyc.v3i2.5130

United Nations Development Programme. (2022). *Human development reports*. https://hdr.undp.org/data-center/country-insights#/ranks

Waxler, N. E. (1979). Is outcome for schizophrenia better in nonindustrial societies? *The Journal of Nervous and Mental Disease, 167*(3), 144–158. https://doi.org/10.1097/00005053-197903000-00002

Weerasundera, R. (2010). Community psychiatry in a Sri Lankan setting: Should we rush to push the boundaries? *Sri Lanka Journal of Psychiatry, 1*(2), 27. https://doi.org/10.4038/sljpsyc.v1i2.2568

Wickrama, T., Merten, M. J., Wickrama, K. A. S., & Terrell, A. (2024). Adolescents' tsunami exposure and mental health consequences: Protective role of cultural coping strategies. *International Journal of Environmental Research and Public Health, 21*(6), 756. https://doi.org/10.3390/ijerph21060756

World Bank Group. (2019). *Gini Index—Sri Lanka*. Gini Index.

# Chapter 8
# Social Psychiatry in Bhutan and the Maldives

**Amit Singh**

**Abstract** Social psychiatry in Bhutan and the Maldives plays a crucial role in addressing mental health challenges within their unique socio-cultural contexts. Both nations face mental health issues influenced by traditional beliefs, stigma, and evolving societal changes. Despite progress, including the establishment of dedicated mental health centres and integration of services into primary healthcare, challenges such as stigma and discrimination, lack of resources, and limited mental health professionals persist. Both countries face challenges related to gender-based violence, climate change, migration, and evolving societies. They should work towards strengthening community-based mental health programmes, integrating traditional healing with modern psychiatry, and enhancing disaster response mechanisms. By adopting a holistic and culturally sensitive approach, Bhutan and the Maldives can further enhance the acceptability of the services, and ensure inclusive and sustainable mental healthcare for their populations.

**Keywords** South Asia · Bhutan · Maldives · Mental Health · Social Psychiatry

## 1 Introduction

Bhutan and the Maldives are small nations in South Asia in terms of land area and population. Bhutan is a landlocked country with a population of about 7.86 lacs. The Maldives is a chain of 1,192 coral islands in the Indian Ocean, 188 of which are currently inhabited. It has a population of 5.86 lacs. While Bhutan is a lower middle income country, the Maldives is an upper middle income country (World Bank Group, 2025). Both nations have a life expectancy of around 75 years (WHO, 2025). Religion has a huge influence on the culture and practices in these nations. In Bhutan, Buddhism is the official and the most practiced religion (74.7%), followed by Hinduism (22.6%). Bhutan's socio-cultural landscape is deeply rooted in its Buddhist heritage, which shapes the country's traditions, values, and way of

A. Singh (✉)
Department of Psychiatry, King George's Medical University, Uttar Pradesh, Lucknow, India
e-mail: amitsingh0612@gmail.com



S. M. Y. Arafat et al. (eds.), *Social Psychiatry in South Asia*, South Asian Perspectives in Mental Health and Psychology , https://doi.org/10.1007/978-981-96-8078-8_8

life. In the Maldives, Islam is the official religion and is practiced by about 99% of the population.

Bhutan has a society deeply rooted in hierarchical values (Pelzom, 2024). Despite globalization, it strives to maintain a harmonious balance between tradition and modernity, making it one of the world's most culturally distinct nations. The commitment to preserving its culture is evident in policies that limit the drawbacks associated with modernization, ensuring that Bhutanese customs remain integral to daily life (Schuelka et al., 2021). Bhutan has also been the nation that prioritizes gross national happiness (GNH) over economic growth as a measure of development. It was the fourth king of Bhutan who coined the term "Gross National Happiness" in the 1970s (Givel, 2022). GNH represents the overall happiness and well-being of the nation. The underlying message was that the development measures should take a holistic approach encompassing happiness and well-being as key measures and be limited to economic aspects of development. The policies inspired by GNH attempt to address the basic reasons for stress and mental disorders and help create a supportive society. It strives to ensure access to holistic healthcare, support systems, and stress-reducing environments. Also, a lot of emphasis in policies and programmes is put on spiritual practices including mindfulness and meditation, cultural preservation and environmental conservation. The cultural values foster emotional resilience and a sense, of purpose among citizens. Meanwhile, a good natural environment helps reduce stress. Thus, the GNH approach was crucial in promoting mental health in Bhutan. However, with society constantly evolving, Bhutan grapple with the challenge of striking a balance between preserving traditional values and embracing innovative approaches, and modern instruments to stay aligned with the changing world.

The Maldives has a society deeply rooted in community values, Islamic traditions, and a close connection to the sea (Mohamed, 2015b). As a small island nation, social bonds are strong, with family and community playing a central role in daily life. Islam, the state religion, influences social norms, customs, and governance, shaping the moral and ethical framework of the country (Cui & Li, 2025). With more women taking part in public life and decision-making, gender roles in the Maldives have progressively evolved towards higher gender equality. The rapid growth of tourism and urbanization, especially in the capital Malé, has introduced new cultural and economic influences, leading to a blend of tradition and modernity. Despite these changes, Maldivian society remains deeply connected to its heritage, valuing a strong sense of national identity.

## 2 Social Epidemiology

### *2.1 Psychiatric Disorders*

The overall prevalence of mental disorders (in 2019) in Bhutan and the Maldives was 12.25% and 11.4%, respectively.

**Table 1** People with mental disorders consulting health facilities in Bhutan

| Type of mental disorders | 2021 | 2022 | 2023 |
|---|---|---|---|
| Dementia | 34 | 59 | 144 |
| Alcohol use disorder | 1906 | 2157 | 2825 |
| Substance use disorder | 579 | 702 | 871 |
| Psychosis | 971 | 707 | 1109 |
| Depression | 2410 | 2082 | 2687 |
| Anxiety | 4140 | 3441 | 3765 |
| Other mental disorders | 1716 | 1891 | 1708 |

Annual Health Bulletin 2024, Ministry of Health, Royal Government of Bhutan

In Bhutan, a recent national health survey found symptoms of moderate to severe depression in about 0.4% of the population, and mild depression in 12.1% (Ministry of Health, 2024). Self-harming behaviours in the past month were present in about 2.1% of the population (Ministry of Health, 2024). The recent figures for mental disorders in Bhutan are presented in Table 1.

In the Maldives, there is limited recent data regarding the current prevalence of mental disorders. It was in 2003 that a comprehensive nation-wide survey of mental disorders was conducted. The overall prevalence of mental disorders was 29.1%. The prevalence of neurotic disorders, anxiety and depression, and somatic disorders were 23.3%, 5%, and 4%, respectively. Psychotic disorders were present in 1% of the individuals (WHO, 2022). The WHO STEPS survey, a study conducted nationwide, found moderate to severe depression in 3.8% of the population aged 15–69, with rates higher among females (5.3%) compared to males (2.5%). Regarding symptoms of depression, 17.7% of the respondents reported feeling low, and 17.1% reported sleeping difficulties (Raheem & Moosa, 2022).

## 2.2 *Suicide*

Suicide is a key health challenge in Bhutan. There were 103 reported suicides in 2024, and 96 suicides in 2023 (Choden, 2025). A large proportion of dying people were economically active individuals between the age group of 20 to 59. However, children and adolescents also died by suicide (Choden, 2025). A survey of the nationally representative population found that 0.6% of the population (0.8% women, 0.4% men) seriously considered death by suicide in the past 12 months (Ministry of Health, 2024). Suicidal attempt in lifetime was reported by about 1.6% of the population (2.0% women, 1.2% men). Meanwhile, a history of close family members dying by suicide was present in 2.3% of the population. The factors implicated in suicide include family issues and domestic violence, unemployment, societal pressures, and substance use (UNICEF Bhutan, 2021). A hospital-based study found that the factors contributing to suicide attempts include pre-existing psychiatric disorders (55.5%),

**Table 2** Age-standardized suicide rates (per 100 000 population)

| Country | Sex | 2019 | 2018 | 2017 | 2016 | 2015 |
|---|---|---|---|---|---|---|
| Bhutan | Both | 5.1 [2.7–8.5] | 5.1 [2.8–8.6] | 5.1 [2.8–8.7] | 5.1 [2.8–8.5] | 5.2 [2.8–8.7] |
| | Male | 6.8 [3.6–11.5] | 6.8 [3.6–11.6] | 6.8 [3.7–11.7] | 6.7 [3.7–11.5] | 6.9 [3.8–11.8] |
| | Female | 3.1 [1.7–5.0] | 3.1 [1.7–5.1] | 3.2 [1.8–5.1] | 3.1 [1.8–5.0] | 3.1 [1.8–5.1] |
| Maldives | Both | 2.8 [1.7–4.1] | 2.9 [1.9–4.3] | 3.1 [2.0–4.6] | 3.2 [2.0–4.6] | 3.0 [1.9–4.3] |
| | Male | 4.1 [2.6–6.1] | 4.3 [2.7–6.4] | 4.6 [2.9–6.8] | 4.7 [3.1–6.9] | 4.4 [2.9–6.5] |
| | Female | 0.9 [0.5–1.3] | 0.9 [0.5–1.3] | 0.8 [0.5–1.3] | 0.8 [0.5–1.3] | 0.9 [0.5–1.3] |

Global Health Observatory Data Repository (South-East Asia Region)

stressful life events (19.5%), relationship issues (13.9%), and the presence of other health conditions (11.1%) (Letho et al., 2021). Major depressive disorder was implicated in 27.8% of the suicide attempts. The predominant method used for attempted suicide was self-poisoning on medication (76.3%) (Letho et al., 2021). The rates of people seeking professional help for suicidal ideations are low. Only a third of the people with serious ideas of suicide in the past year sought professional help (Ministry of Health, 2024).

In Maldives, a recent nationwide study found that 4.3% of people considered self-harm, 1.95% planned self-harm and 1.9% of the population attempted it (Raheem & Moosa, 2022).

The age-standardized suicide rates in Bhutan and Maldives is depicted in Table 2 (WHO, 2021a).

## 2.3 *Gender-Based Violence*

Gender-based violence, especially towards women and sexual minorities, is an important issue with huge mental health implications (WHO, 2024). It has been variously categorized; however, some common forms include physical violence, psychological violence, verbal violence, sexual violence, and socio-economic violence (Council of Europe, 2025). In a survey conducted in Bhutan, a substantial proportion of female respondents aged 15–64 reported experiencing violence (Ministry of Health, 2024). 16.4% experienced physical violence, 6.9% suffered sexual violence, and 17.5% had undergone emotional violence at some point in their lives. In the past 12 months, 4.4% experienced physical violence, 2.6% faced sexual violence, and 8.5% endured emotional violence. Controlling behaviours were experienced by 29.0% of women sometime in their lives. 18.3% faced such behaviours in the past year. Overall, 39.7%

of ever-partnered women aged 15 to 64 years reported some form of violence anytime in their lives. 23.6% experienced violence in the past year (Ministry of Health, 2024). Intimate partner violence was also a common occurrence, with 24.9% of women facing it at the hands of their partner at some point in their lives, with 10.8% experiencing it in the past 12 months (Ministry of Health, 2024). In the Maldives, 11% of women aged 15–49 experience sexual violence at some point in their lives. 1% of women experienced sexual violence in the preceding year. It was more common in divorced/separated/widowed women (26%) compared to those who have never married (13%) or those who are currently married (9%). Intimate partner violence was experienced by 24% of the ever-married women, with 17% experiencing it in the past one year. Overall, 22% of women in the 15–49 age group experienced either physical or sexual violence, or both (Ministry of Health & ICF, 2018). Tragically, 12.2% of women aged 15–49 reported having experienced childhood sexual abuse (Shuhad, 2019).

Gender-based violence stems from deeply rooted societal norms, power imbalances, and systemic inequalities. It may be attributed to the beliefs that perpetuate stereotypes about gender roles, where one gender is seen as dominant over another. A hint of cultural normalization and tolerance of gender-based violence is evident in the responses of women surveyed in Bhutan where 43.9% of women justified women getting hit by men in the suggested circumstances (Ministry of Health, 2024). Also, in the Maldives, 26% of women (aged 15–49) compared to 21% of men, justified the beating of a wife by their husbands for specified circumstances (WHO, 2023a). Economic disparities, lack of education, and limited access to resources exacerbate gender-based violence.

## 3 Climate Change and Mental Health

Both Bhutan and the Maldives are at particular risk when it comes to the impact of climate change. The health of the population, including mental health, is affected by extreme weather events, rising temperatures, pollution, and the psychological distress caused by the threat to ecosystems and livelihoods. This can potentially lead to anxiety, depression, and even post-traumatic stress (Marty et al., 2025).

Bhutan maintains a high forest cover (over 70%). Green spaces have been found to keep temperatures low, enhance air quality, and lower people's stress levels (Chhetri et al., 2024). However, infrastructure development, agriculture expansion, and illegal logging have put pressure on forests. Land degradation due to overgrazing and soil erosion has impacted agriculture and biodiversity (WHO, 2011). Rapid urbanization, especially in Thimphu and Paro, has led to increasing waste and posed challenges related to waste management (Yangden, 2024). Water resource management is an upcoming challenge in Bhutan. While urban areas face water supply issues, rural areas struggle with irrigation. Though Bhutan has abundant water resources, seasonal water shortages occur due to uneven distribution and overuse. Climate change can potentially reduce water flow and hydropower production putting a strain on the economy and human lives. Climate change and migration from rural areas have affected agricultural productivity. It needs Bhutan to import a significant proportion of its food despite having fertile land. Also, the glaciers in the nation are melting at an alarming rate, leading to glacial lake outburst floods (GLOFs), which threaten settlements downstream. A partial burst of a glacial lake in Lunana in 1994 resulted in 21 people losing their lives and left about 90 houses and other infrastructure damaged (UNDP Bhutan, 2022). Rising temperatures have affected Bhutan's biodiversity and water resources. Also, Bhutan is prone to environmental disasters in the form of earthquakes, landslides, and flash floods, which affect livelihoods and infrastructure (Dorji & Lucero-Prisno, 2022; Yangden, 2024). These events not only cause damage to lives and infrastructure but disrupt the social and mental health of the people. Environmental conservation is one of the cornerstones of GNH and is mandated through Bhutan's constitution. However, no study has yet assessed the impact of climate change on mental health in Bhutan (Chhetri et al., 2024).

The Maldives is the world's lowest-lying country, with an average elevation of 1.5 m. Due to rising sea levels, it is at high risk of submersion. Also, it can affect human health through coastal erosion, flooding, damaging homes and infrastructure, contamination of soil and drinking water, vector- and water-borne disease, and mental health impacts. People living less than one metre above sea level are especially vulnerable (Romanello et al., 2023). Rising sea levels and coastal erosion force internal migration, leading to overcrowding in the capital Malé, contributing to mental health morbidity and adversely affecting the mental health infrastructure (Mohamed, 2015a). Besides, the Maldives is highly vulnerable to extreme weather events such as storm surges, cyclones, and flooding, which damage infrastructure and displace people. The average summer temperature has increased in recent years so has the frequency of heatwaves. Exposure to extreme heat not only adversely impacts physical health, sleep quality, and well-being but also labour productivity and functioning and average income, key determinants of mental health (Romanello et al., 2024).

Freshwater scarcity in the Maldives for which it relies on rainwater and desalination is another major challenge. Coral bleaching caused by rising sea temperatures threatens the Maldives' rich marine life and tourism industry. Overfishing and plastic pollution further harm coral ecosystems. Maldives developed its Health National Adaptation Plan (HNAP) in 2020, with assistance from WHO, to improve the resilience of health facilities in the face of climate change. It also aimed to bring into focus the management of hazards to health and healthcare facilities from climate change through a multisectoral response, foster healthcare capacity, and raise public awareness regarding the impact of climate change (WHO, 2023b).

## 4 Migration

In 2017, about half of the population of Bhutan moved from their usual place of residence (Tobden et al., 2025). It resulted from both internal migration (between urban and rural areas) as well as external migration to other countries, including India, the USA, Australia, and other international destinations. Education was positively associated with international migration. The individuals with higher degrees and qualifications were substantially more likely to emigrate than those lacking formal education, leading to a brain drain (Tobden et al., 2025). Many young Bhutanese have migrated to cities in search of jobs and other opportunities, leaving rural areas underdeveloped and increasing urban congestion. The consequences of large-scale migration could be profound for a country, impacting the quality of services delivered.

In the Maldives about 26% of the population are foreigners. About 90% of all the international migrants are from Bangladesh (56%), India (25%), and Sri Lanka (9%) (Riyaza, 2023). Also, internal migration from the atolls to the capital Male' is common, especially for medical treatments. There is no comprehensive policy to regulate migration.

Migration results in mismanagement, overwhelming the receiving end and putting excessive strain on limited infrastructure and social service systems. Moreover, migrants encounter difficulties in accessing healthcare services, including mental issues throughout the migration process—before departure, during transit, at their destination, and upon return. The harsher the working and living conditions, the greater the likelihood that migrants and host communities will face health risks. Migrants may also refrain from seeking help for their health problems out of stigma and fear of getting replaced at the workplace. This only increases the overall mental health burden (Plewa, 2018).

## 5 Stigma and Traditional Beliefs

Like other South Asian nations, mental health issues in Bhutan and the Maldives are often stigmatized. Derogatory terms like "choelom," or "psycho," are used for people exhibiting oddities in their thinking or behaviours. Even if inadvertently used, these words hurt the individuals and can be considered linguistic microaggression, which undermines a person's identity. Stigma and shame negatively influence the help-seeking behaviour of the people affected with mental disorders and their families. Due to lack of awareness Even people with severe mental illnesses are expected to self-amend their thinking and behaviour, leading to delays in help seeking (Calabrese & Dorji, 2014; Gyeltshen et al., 2024). Stigma has been extensively studied among Bhutanese refugees and in other countries. A study conducted among Bhutanese refugees in the United States found that over 71% believed that others might look down on the person who sought out a counsellor (MacDowell et al., 2020). Many individuals associate mental illness with spiritual issues or karma, leading them to seek help from monks or traditional healers instead of mental health professionals (Calabrese & Dorji, 2014).

Similarly, in the Maldives mental illnesses are often interpreted through a spiritual lens—viewing them as consequences of supernatural influences or divine displeasure. Thus, people are expected to bear the punishment given by God in the form of mental health problems and pray to them for their forgiveness rather than seeking treatment. This belief often leads to a reliance on traditional healers rather than modern psychiatric services, delaying proper treatment. In some instances, it is also viewed as a personal weakness or spiritual weakness. This stigma is compounded by traditional views that discourage open discussion about mental health, which hinders early diagnosis and treatment.

Also, in these countries, there is a strong family system; individuals are viewed as reflections of their family, and their laurels or dishonours are associated with their family. Consequently, people tend to hide their mental health struggles to avoid bringing shame to their families.

People with mental illnesses often face discrimination and violence. Despite the availability of treatment, owing to the stigma and discrimination attached to mental disorders, nearly two-thirds of people in Bhutan never seek help from health professionals (Nirola, 2019). A study conducted in the Maldives found that about half (46.5%) of people with mental health conditions experience violence (Banks et al., 2020). Its prevalence was significantly higher in patients with mental disorders compared to people with other impairments. Moreover, the odds of experiencing a health problem by people with mental health difficulties were twice as compared to people with other disabilities (Banks et al., 2020).

## 6 Mental Health Services and Psychiatric Care

Bhutan and the Maldives have recently intensified efforts to enhance mental health services. There were no mental health professionals in Bhutan until a WHO-sponsored psychiatrist started psychiatric services in 1997. Thus, the modern mental healthcare ecosystem developed after 1997. Also, the National Mental Health Programme was launched in 1997 by the Ministry of Health. It formulated plans and programmes for implementation through the district hospitals and Primary Healthcare Centres (PHCs). Thus, the programme emphasized the integration of mental healthcare delivery to the PHC network for a wider availability of services. In consonance with this plan, doctors were trained to identify, diagnose, and manage common mental disorders, including anxiety, depression, psychosis, and substance use disorders, along with the nurses, and other health professionals. Various psychotropic medications, including antipsychotics, antidepressants, mood stabilizers, and sedative drugs, were made available at the PHCs (Sharma & Joshi, 2024).

The government of Bhutan offers all citizens and residents free medical care, including mental healthcare. Though specialized mental health services are available only at the JDW National Referral Hospital, which has a limited bed strength of 20, psychiatric services are provided through more than 60 outpatient health facilities in district hospitals and PHCs. However, there is a huge shortage of specialist manpower to deal with psychiatric issues comprehensively in the population, with just five psychiatrists, five postgraduate Master level clinical counsellors, 24 clinical counsellors with basic training, and five trained psychiatric nurses. There are no trained clinical psychologists (Dorji, 2023).

Bhutan has instigated several initiatives to ensure the delivery of high-quality mental health services. In 2022, her Majesty the Gyaltsuen Jetsun Pema's Secretariat established a high-level mental health steering committee to unite all pertinent stakeholders, including various government departments and civil society organizations, under a single umbrella body for improved coordination and collaboration to offer comprehensive mental health services as a single package (Gyeltshen et al., 2024). Also, there is a plan to establish a state-of-the-art 60-bed mental health facility called the PEMA Center as the apex referral, research and training centre for mental health (The Pema Secretariat, 2023).

In the Maldives, in total, there were 33 mental health professionals, including 17 psychiatrists (3.2 per lakh population), 7 psychologists (1.32 per lakh population), 2 social workers, and 7 other specialized mental health workers (like occupational therapists). Integration of mental health into primary care is lacking. There is a single mental health outpatient facility and an inpatient facility in the general hospital setting. There are 0.75 general hospital psychiatric unit beds per lakh population (WHO, 2021b). In 2019, the Maldives launched its first Mental Health Centre, marking a significant milestone in strengthening mental healthcare infrastructure. In line with the WHO guidelines, a collaborative network was established in 2020, bringing together private sector organizations and NGOs to provide mental health support and services. Key participants include the National Drug Agency (NDA), Society for Women Against Drugs (SWAD), Society for Health Education (SHE), Care Society, Maldives Autism Association, Beautiful Eyes—Down Syndrome Association, Hand in Hand Health Awareness Program (MHAF), and the Maldivian Red Crescent (MRC) (Kariyawasam, 2024). In June 2023, the Maldives Government, in collaboration with UNICEF and WHO, inaugurated a psychological first aid helpline, to provide guidance and help to students seeking mental health assistance (Kariyawasam, 2024). Despite these advancements, a key challenge to the provision of services is that the majority of these services are limited to Greater Male but are not available in outlying islands and atolls (Kariyawasam, 2024).

## 7 Mental Health Programmes and Policies

Bhutan formulated its mental health policy and plan in 1997. The key components of the policy included building a system of community mental health services through integration into primary healthcare ensuring its availability and accessibility, developing human resources, engaging users and other stakeholders, mental health advocacy, and a monitoring system for quality improvement (Pelzang, 2012; WHO & Ministry of Health, 2006). In 2015, the Ministry of Health also formulated the National Suicide Prevention Programme to address this significant public health issue. Strategies to improve the detection of suicidal ideation and respond to suicidal ideation and attempts are part of the nation's Suicide Prevention Action Plan (2018–2023). A national suicide registry was established, along with training for a new cadre of mental health specialists known as "clinical counsellors" (Dorji, 2023; WHO, 2021b). Also, Bhutan adopted a National Policy for Persons with Disabilities (NPPD) in 2019. It was a signatory to the UN Convention on the Rights of Persons with Disabilities (UNCRPD) since 2010 and ratified it in October 2023 to formally protect the human rights of people with disabilities (Social & Cultural Affairs Committee, 2024). The Integrated Management of Newborn and Childhood Illness (IMNCI) and Reproductive Health (RH) programmes focus on early childhood development and promotion of maternal/parental mental health, while the National School Health Programme and Youth/Adolescent Friendly Health Services (YFHS) focus on promoting health including mental health and prevention of substance use. Furthermore, a dedicated department under the Ministry of Home and Cultural Affairs manages the mental health and psychosocial aspects of disaster preparedness and risk reduction.

The Maldives also has a policy for mental health, the National Mental Health Policy—2015–2025, formulated in 2015 with a vision to promote the mental health of the people, focused on mental illness prevention and providing high-quality care to support people with mental illnesses in their recovery and well-being, without any stigma or prejudice (Ministry of Health, 2017). Also, it recently launched its National Mental Health Strategic Action Plan 2025–2029, a comprehensive roadmap designed to improve mental healthcare services, integrate mental health into primary care, and reduce the stigma associated with mental illness (Anwar, 2025). The Disability Act of Maldives (2010) and Health Services Act covers areas for the provision and accessibility of health services required for the community. However, mental health legislation is lacking. Maldives also lacks a policy for suicide prevention. In the Maldives, school-based mental health prevention and promotion are run by the Ministry of Education in coordination with the UNICEF. Also, psychosocial support programmes for mental health and psychosocial support as component of disaster preparedness and disaster risk reduction are in place.

## 8 Family System and Support

In both Bhutan and the Maldives, family plays a vital role as a primary support system for mental health, providing emotional, social, and financial care for individuals facing psychological challenges. Rooted in strong cultural and communal values, families in both countries often serve as the first line of support, offering comfort and guidance to those experiencing distress. Due to the stigma surrounding mental health issues, individuals may be more likely to seek help from family members rather than professional services.

In Bhutan, family support is often intertwined with Buddhist principles, encouraging mindfulness and spiritual healing. 80.9% of respondents in a nationwide survey admitted having supportive family members who were always ready to provide help, while only 2.9% reported not receiving any support from their family members during challenging times. The survey also revealed that about 80% of the population seeks support from their family members during serious emotional distress, followed by friends (25.5%) and professionals (16.8%) (Ministry of Health, 2024).

Similarly, in the Maldives, where Islamic traditions emphasize family cohesion, individuals with mental health conditions rely heavily on their relatives for care and support. Also, it is well known that a healthy marital relationship is associated with the well-being of the concerned individuals, family, and society at large. However, the nuclear family system is gradually increasing here. Besides, the divorce rates are relatively higher in the Maldives. 70% of the individuals between the ages 18 and 39 in the population are divorced. The divorce rates among females and males aged 26 to 39 are 58% and 59%, respectively (Ahmed & Riyaz, 2024). The issue of high divorce rates is so concerning that it led the government to take steps to reduce it in the form of the Family Act 2000, which made the divorce procedure tougher. Nevertheless, it was unable to lower the divorce rates significantly. Divorce adversely affects the mental health of the couple. High psychological stress has been reported in 46.7% of divorced women (Aboobakuru & Riyaz, 2021). Also, it is associated with the physical and sexual abuse of women.

As mental health services expand in both countries, preserving the family system and empowering families with education and resources is crucial in fostering a more supportive and understanding environment for those in need. Some families become burned out in trying to manage them, and may even seek to abandon their ill relative, while some families show great compassion in continuing to seek treatment (Calabrese & Dorji, 2014).

## 9 Future Directions

The efforts to integrate mental health services into primary healthcare, expand community-based support, and reduce stigma through education and awareness campaigns should continue (Sharma & Joshi, 2024). Strengthening collaborations between modern psychiatric care and traditional or religious healing practices can enhance acceptance and accessibility. Addressing youth mental health through school-based programmes will increase awareness, reduce stigma, and promote early identification of mental health issues. Similarly, workplace mental health initiatives will be essential in promoting well-being. Given both countries' vulnerability to climate-related disasters, developing strong psychosocial response mechanisms is crucial. Expanding training for healthcare workers, increasing mental health and substance use related research, and leveraging telepsychiatry and digital interventions will further enhance service accessibility, especially for remote and rural populations. These strategies can help create a more inclusive and community-driven mental health system, aligning with the unique socio-cultural contexts in these countries.

## 10 Conclusion

Over the past few decades, Bhutan and the Maldives have made significant strides in reducing mental disorders' burden and improving their populations' well-being. However, various social factors—such as stigma, unemployment, poverty, urbanization, environmental disasters, migration, and substance use—continue to pose evolving challenges to mental healthcare. Persistent gaps in healthcare systems highlight the need for expanded and strengthened services to enhance mental health support. Addressing these challenges requires a collaborative effort from policymakers, healthcare professionals, civil society, and individuals affected by mental disorders. A unified approach is essential to ensuring accessible, high-quality mental health services that promote overall well-being and provide effective treatment for those in need.

## References


Aboobakuru, S., & Riyaz, A. (2021). Stress and coping resources of divorced women in the Maldives. *The Maldives National Journal of Research, 9*(1), Article 1. https://doi.org/10.62338/pmqaes13

Ahmed, F., & Riyaz, A. (2024). Causes of divorce in the Maldives: An in-depth socio-economic analysis. *The Maldives National Journal of Research, 12*(2), Article 2. https://doi.org/10.62338/mtxwrp36

Anwar, J. (2025). *Maldives launches mental health strategic action plan 2025–2029*. MM. http://en.mmtv.mv/2525

Banks, L. M., Hameed, S., Kawsar Usman, S., & Kuper, H. (2020). No one left behind? comparing poverty and deprivation between people with and without disabilities in the Maldives. *Sustainability, 12*(5), Article 5. https://doi.org/10.3390/su12052066

Calabrese, J. D., & Dorji, C. (2014). Traditional and modern understandings of mental illness. *Journal of Bhutan Studies, 30*.

Chhetri, B., Zangpo, D., & Gyeltshen, D. (2024). Climate change and mental health in Bhutan. *Bhutan Health Journal, 10*(2), Article 2. https://doi.org/10.47811/bhj.174

Choden, D. (2025). *Suicide cases rise among Bhutan's economically-active population.* https://asianews.network/suicide-cases-rise-among-bhutans-economically-active-population/

Council of Europe. (2025). *Types of gender-based violence—Gender Matters*—www.coe.int. Gender Matters. https://www.coe.int/en/web/gender-matters/types-of-gender-based-violence

Cui, J., & Li, T. (2025). Religion, power, and national identity: The dual role of Islam in the history and modernization of the Maldives. *Religions, 16*(2), Article 2. https://doi.org/10.3390/rel16020201

Dorji, C. (2023). Addressing Mental Health in Bhutan. *The Druk Journal, 9*(1), 4–14.

Dorji, T., & Lucero-Prisno, D. E. I. (2022). Climate change and its implications on health in Bhutan. *Bhutan Health Journal, 8*(2), Article 2. https://doi.org/10.47811/bhj.142

Givel, M. (2022). Gross national happiness policy outputs in Bhutan from 1972 to 2014. *Journal of Bhutan Studies, 47*.

Gyeltshen, K., Chhetri, B., & Gyeltshen, D. (2024). Delivery of mental health services in Bhutan: Challenges and way forward. *Public Health Challenges, 3*(3), Article 3. https://doi.org/10.1002/puh2.211

Kariyawasam, I. (2024). Exploring mental health awareness and stigma in the Maldives—Ishani Kariyawasam. *The Maldives National University.* https://www.academia.edu/123242578/Exploring_Mental_Health_Awareness_and_Stigma_in_the_Maldives_Ishani_Kariyawasam

Letho, Z., Wangmo, N., & Kuenzang, K. (2021). Characteristics of attempted suicide patients admitted in Jigme Dorji Wangchuck national referral hospital from January 2014 to September 2018. *Bhutan Health Journal, 7*(1), Article 1. https://doi.org/10.47811/bhj.112

MacDowell, H., Pyakurel, S., Acharya, J., Morrison-Beedy, D., & Kue, J. (2020). Perceptions toward mental illness and seeking psychological help among Bhutanese refugees resettled in the U.S. *Issues in Mental Health Nursing, 41*(3), 243–250. https://doi.org/10.1080/01612840.2019.1646362

Marty, C., Amghar, S., Barrera Patlan, A., & Adams, A. (2025). The psychosocial impacts of slow onset climate change events among youth in LMICs: A rapid evidence review. *The Journal of Climate Change and Health, 22,* 100416. https://doi.org/10.1016/j.joclim.2025.100416

Ministry of Health. (2017). *National mental health policy—2015–2025.* Ministry of Health Maldives & World Health Organization.

Ministry of Health. (2024). *5th national health survey: integrated stepwise household survey 2023.* Ministry of Health, Royal Government of Bhutan. https://moh.gov.bt/wp-content/uploads/2025/01/Final_National-Health-Survey-2023-1.pdf

Ministry of Health, & ICF. (2018). *Maldives demographic and health survey 2016–17.* Ministry of Health (MOH) [Maldives] and ICF. https://dhsprogram.com/pubs/pdf/FR349/FR349.pdf

Mohamed, A. (2015a). Resuscitating the national mental health policy in the Maldives. *Australasian Psychiatry, 23*(6_suppl), 26–28. https://doi.org/10.1177/1039856215609766

Mohamed, M. (2015b). Historical changes in human-nature interactions in island communities of the Maldives. *Rural South Asian Studies, 1,* 22–36.

Nirola, D. K. (2019). Mental health matters: Everyone's responsibility. *Bhutan Health Journal, 5*(1), Article 1. https://doi.org/10.47811/bhj.72

Pelzang, R. (2012). Mental health care in Bhutan: Policy and issues. *WHO South-East Asia Journal of Public Health, 1*(3), Article 3. https://doi.org/10.4103/2224-3151.207030

Pelzom, K. (2024). Social hierarchy and citizen engagement in Bhutan. *The Druk Journal, 10*(2), 95–105.

Plewa, P. (2018). *Migration in Maldives a country profile 2018.* International Organization for Migration (IOM). https://maldives.iom.int/sites/g/files/tmzbdl1666/files/documents/mp_maldives_2018.pdf

Raheem, R. A., & Moosa, S. (2022). *WHO STEP survey on risk factors for noncommunicable diseases Maldives 2020–2021.* The Maldives National University, Health Protection Agency, and World Health Organization.

Riyaza, F. (2023). *Human mobility and migration dynamics an analysis from census 2022*. Maldives Bureau of Statistics (MBS), Ministry of National Planning, Housing & Infrastructure. https://census.gov.mv/2022/wp-content/uploads/2024/02/Migration-Report-Census-2022.pdf

Romanello, M., Napoli, C. D., Green, C., Kennard, H., Lampard, P., Scamman, D., Walawender, M., Ali, Z., Ameli, N., Ayeb-Karlsson, S., Beggs, P. J., Belesova, K., Berrang Ford, L., Bowen, K., Cai, W., Callaghan, M., Campbell-Lendrum, D., Chambers, J., Cross, T. J., … Costello, A. (2023). The 2023 report of the lancet countdown on health and climate change: The imperative for a health-centred response in a world facing irreversible harms. *The Lancet, 402*(10419), 2346–2394. https://doi.org/10.1016/S0140-6736(23)01859-7

Romanello, M., Walawender, M., Hsu, S.-C., Moskeland, A., Palmeiro-Silva, Y., Scamman, D., Ali, Z., Ameli, N., Angelova, D., Ayeb-Karlsson, S., Basart, S., Beagley, J., Beggs, P. J., Blanco-Villafuerte, L., Cai, W., Callaghan, M., Campbell-Lendrum, D., Chambers, J. D., Chicmana-Zapata, V., … Costello, A. (2024). The 2024 report of the lancet countdown on health and climate change: Facing record-breaking threats from delayed action. *Lancet (London, England), 404*(10465), 1847–1896. https://doi.org/10.1016/S0140-6736(24)01822-1

Schuelka, M. J., Braznell, M., Leavesley, M., Dorji, S., Dorji, K., Nidup, K., & Latsho, P. (2021). Happiness, wellbeing, and mental health in Bhutanese higher education: Exploring student and staff experiences and perceptions within a framework of Gross National Happiness. *Journal of International and Comparative Education (JICE)*, 33–50.

Sharma, P., & Joshi, D. (2024). Access to mental health care in Bhutan: current status, potential challenges, and ways out. In S. M. Y. Arafat & S. K. Kar (Eds.), *Access to mental health care in South Asia: Current status, potential challenges, and ways out* (pp. 57–69). Springer Nature. https://doi.org/10.1007/978-981-99-9153-2_4

Shuhad, A. (2019). Violence against women in Maldives. *Resource Material Series, 108*, 114–118.

Social and Cultural Affairs Committee. (2024). *A review report on the state of persons with disabilities*. National council of Bhutan. https://dpobhutan.org/wp-content/uploads/2024/07/A-Review-Report-on-the-State-of-Persons-with-Disabilities.pdf

The Pema Secretariat. (2023). The Institution of "The PEMA" for mental health care for Bhutan. *The Druk Journal, 9*(1), 15–22.

Tobden, T., Ugyel, L., & Dorjee, T. (2025). Characteristics and determinants of international migration: The recent phenomenon of migration of Bhutanese to international destinations. *Journal of Bhutan Studies, 49*. https://doi.org/10.62104/jbs.06

UNDP Bhutan. (2022). *Living in constant fear of glacial lake outburst flood by UNDP Bhutan on exposure*. Exposure. https://undp-bhutan.exposure.co/living-in-constant-fear-of-glacial-lake-outburst-flood

UNICEF Bhutan. (2021). *Promoting mental health and well-being deserves our undivided attention and long-term investment | UNICEF Bhutan*. https://www.unicef.org/bhutan/stories/promoting-mental-health-and-well-being-deserves-our-undivided-attention-and-long-term?utm_source=chatgpt.com

WHO. (2011). *Climate change adaptation to protect human health Bhutan*. World Health Organization. https://cdn.who.int/media/docs/default-source/climate-change/adaptation-report-bhutan-2010.pdf

WHO. (2021a). *GHO | Global Health Observatory Data Repository (South-East Asia Region) | Suicide rate estimates, age-standardized—Estimates by country*. WHO; World Health Organization. https://apps.who.int/gho/data/node.main-searo.MHSUICIDEASDR?lang=en

WHO. (2021b). *Mental health atlas 2020*. World Health Organization.

WHO. (2022). *Addressing mental health in Maldives*. World Health Organization, Regional Office for South-East Asia.

WHO. (2023a). *Deinstitutionalization of people with mental health conditions in the WHO South-East Asia Region*. World Health Organization, Regional Office for South-East Asia. https://www.who.int/publications/i/item/9789290211211

WHO. (2023b). *Maldives: Leading the way to sustainable environmental health*. https://www.who.int/southeastasia/news/feature-stories/detail/sustainable-environmental-health-maldives

WHO. (2024). *Violence against women.* https://www.who.int/news-room/fact-sheets/detail/violence-against-women

WHO. (2025). *Bhutan.* Datadot. https://data.who.int/countries/064

WHO & Ministry of Health. (2006). *WHO-AIMS report on mental health system in Bhutan.* World Health Organization and Ministry of Health.

World Bank Group. (2025). *World bank open data.* World Bank Open Data. https://data.worldbank.org

Yangden, T. (2024). Impact of climate change on communities in phobji and gangtey valley in Bhutan. *Journal of Bhutan Studies, 48,* 93–112. https://doi.org/10.62104/jbs.04

# Chapter 9
# Social Determinants of Mental Health in South Asia

**Arghya Pal, Arpit Parmar, and Pawan Sharma**

**Abstract** South Asia comprises a socio-culturally and economically homogenous group of countries with complex geo-political relationships. These countries are the home to a sizeable population. The current chapter introduces the uniqueness of this region and the unique attributes regarding their vulnerabilities and healthcare outcomes. The factors that govern these vulnerabilities are not merely the direct effect of the causative factors but also due to the complex interplay with other related stakeholders. A similar pattern was also observed while reviewing this population's potential social determinants of mental health. We could identify certain factors that are known to play a role universally across all population groups (like age, gender, educational status, and socio-economic status). Additionally, we could identify further determinants that are pertinent to this region owing to its geo-political situation (e.g., migration, minority affiliation, socioeconomic deprivation, etc.). The current state of research points to a need for intervention measures to target the determinants to improve the mental health conditions of the residents. Both governmental and non-government sectors have initiated a number of measures in this regard. However, there is still a need for better appreciation of the situation and the introduction of newer strategies with more intersectoral collaboration backed by political will.

**Keywords** South Asia · Social determinants · Mental health · Migration · Conflict · Suicide

A. Pal (✉)
Department of Psychiatry, All India Institute of Medical Sciences, Kalyani, West Bengal, India
e-mail: arghya.psy@aiimskalyani.edu.in

A. Parmar
Department of Psychiatry, All India Institute of Medical Sciences, Bhubaneswar, Odisha, India

P. Sharma
Department of Psychiatry, School of Medicine, Patan Academy of Health Sciences, Lalitpur, Nepal



S. M. Y. Arafat et al. (eds.), *Social Psychiatry in South Asia*, South Asian Perspectives in Mental Health and Psychology , https://doi.org/10.1007/978-981-96-8078-8_9

## 1 Introduction

The World Health Organization (WHO) conceptualizes mental health as a state of mental well-being that enables individuals to mitigate day-to-day stressors and realize their potential by meaningfully contributing to society (*Mental Health*, 2025). It is important for us to understand that mental health is not just an absence of disorder and that the fine line between the absence of illness and wellness is contributed by various determinants. Throughout our lives, multiple factors can play a role. This can be broadly classified as biological, psychological, and social determinants. Biological and psychological determinants include various pre-existing attributes that govern the initiation and perpetuation of mental health issues. They can be unmodifiable (e.g., gender, genetics, age, etc.) and may be modifiable as well (e.g., diet, addictions, etc.).

Social determinants is a term used in the context of public health matters. It refers to the set of factors that result in the social patterning of health, disease, and illness. The WHO established a Commission of Social Determinants of Health (CSDH) in March 2005 to assist countries in identifying and initiating research on the social factors contributing to health, disease, and illnesses (World Report on Social Determinants of Health Equity, 2025). The commission recommended improving the daily living conditions, tackling the inequitable distribution of resources, measuring and understanding the problem, and assessing the impact. The recommendations were executed by supporting certain countries in developing policies, creating and sharing contextual knowledge, and obtaining vital inputs of the society on the commission's work.

## 2 South Asia as a Unique Geographical Territory

South Asia is a group of countries that have been politically defined and share ethno-cultural similarities. The World Bank has defined South Asia as comprised of Afghanistan, Bangladesh, Bhutan, India, Maldives, Nepal, Pakistan, and Sri Lanka (Arafat & Kar, 2024). However, all these countries seem to share similar profiles in terms of their gross domestic product (GDP) and challenges on the healthcare front. This region is also home to about one-fifth of the population of the world, and the commonality in their profile could be attributable to their integrated and overlapping socio-economic factors (Coker et al., 2011; Irwin et al., 2006). However, this region arguably hosts 40% of the world's poor population, and hence, various recognized challenges like unemployment, gender inequalities, migration, and unequal access to healthcare could pose significant challenges to the mental health of the region.

This subsection of the chapter will try to illustrate why it is important to consider this region as a unique geographical territory and, hence, also provide background about the various attributes that need to be kept in mind while studying or designing mental healthcare interventions for the region.

## 2.1 Differential Outcomes

The South Asian countries have been identified as a paradox by the World Bank. These countries have been recognized for their rapid economic growth and potential for the transition from low-income to middle-income status. However, in contrast to this development, this region continues to be home to a substantial amount of people with social deprivation and poverty. The World Bank claims that the South Asian countries have more people suffering from poverty than the Sub-Saharan African countries (*The South Asian Paradox*, n.d.). Experts in the field could identify that in this region, the economic growth rate has not been translated to a proportionate reduction of poverty. Similarly, the pace of human development and gender equality matrices have also not been at par with the economic growth in the region. This report from the World Bank claims that South Asian Countries like Bangladesh, India, and Sri Lanka have matched the global trends in reducing poverty in line with their economic growth. Indeed, the poverty rate (defined as a person with a per capita income of less than $1.25 per day) for the South Asian region fell from 60% in 1981 to 40% in 2005. However, that fall did not translate to a fall in the number of persons living in poverty due to population growth. Experts believe that merely matching global trends may not be sufficient for this region to alleviate the issues arising out of poverty for this region.

## 2.2 Differential Vulnerability

The South Asian population is also postulated to have a different vulnerability profile. This population tends to have a high propensity for intra-country and inter-country migration. In addition to the climate and environmental changes, the caste system and separation lead to higher vulnerability (Rajan, 2023). Other than that, the South Asian population has also been found to be unique in terms of their vulnerability to various mental health conditions. For example, in a study, it was seen that the risk of developing various oral cancers were unique among the South Asian population, and their risk could be ascertained based on their religious beliefs because they also governed their inclination to use a substance (Csikar et al., 2013; Vora et al., 2000). It was found that since Hindus tended to use alcohol, paan, and tobacco, they had the highest risks among all the religions, While Jains and Muslims, who had a relatively lower risk of using alcohol, also tended to have a lesser prevalence of oral cancers compared to Hindus. This risk, attributable to their change in social practices, has also led to changes in the prevalence pattern of other disorders. It has been seen that the prevalence of breast cancer is also on the rise among South Asian females and their rise in alcohol use has been one of the causative factors (Karasz et al., 2019). Furthermore, this vulnerability is manifested differently across various age groups. For example, in the youth, high parental expectations can lead to higher stress (Bhattacharya & Schoppelrey, 2004). In older adults, South Asian people, especially women, remain at a higher risk of neglect, which could contribute to the development of psychiatric illness (Diwan, 2008).

## 2.3 *Differential Healthcare Outcomes*

Like most ethnic backgrounds, South Asian patients also tend to have a distinct outcome pattern in the context of mental healthcare. In a study by Chiu et al., conducted in a Canadian setting, it was found that South Asian ethnicity was associated with higher severity of mental health problems (Chiu et al., 2016). This result was obtained after controlling for the effects of various relevant clinical and sociodemographic factors. Similarly, these patients also tend to respond to the effects of various psychotropic medications. As an example, it can be stated that people of South Asian descent tend to present with the CYP2C19*2 allele, which posits them to develop adverse effects of various antidepressants and antipsychotics (including Clozapine), and the clinical response to these drugs can be seen at a lower dose than their European counterparts (Leung, 2023). Such considerations become very important in the context of clinical prescription of the patients, and the repercussions of the decision can have far-reaching social effects (adverse effects of drugs leading to discrimination and stigmatization).

## 2.4 *Differential Consequences*

It has been seen that the South Asian population tends to interpret various health conditions very differently from the way it is dealt with in other ethnic groups. For example, the Caucasian population tends to analyze their mental health conditions in a biological framework. In the South Asian population, they are attributed to the accumulated life stressors. A qualitative study conducted to understand the patients' perceived causes of depression among women of South Asian descent reported that these females tended to associate their symptoms with relationships, culture, migration, and socioeconomic factors. Interestingly, this study did not attribute their symptoms to religious or supernatural factors (Ekanayake et al., 2012). However, similar research in the context of psychotic disorders has illustrated the preponderance of this population to attribute their symptoms to supernatural causes, and that was associated with a delay in their help-seeking or reliance on using other traditional faith healers before arriving at mental health professionals for healthcare (Mirza et al., 2019). South Asian population, owing to their alternative explanation of mental health conditions, also tended to have a more stigmatizing and discriminatory outlook towards the problem, and that has led to more barriers to seeking help, lesser community participation, and more detrimental long-term consequences like poor quality of life (Pal et al., 2021).

# 3 Social Determinants of Mental Health in South Asia

There is a definite role and impact of social factors and contextual variables on the etiology and evolution of mental disorders (Fig. 1). These factors also play an important role in treatment and its outcome (Silva et al., 2016). The South Asian region faces multiple challenges like poverty, education, unemployment, gender inequalities, and poor access to basic amenities of life, migration, urbanization, and globalization that affect the overall mental health (Dhillon et al., 2012).

## *3.1 Adult Population*

A systematic review among South Asian general or hospital populations showed that there were higher odds of depression among people who had financial difficulty and subjective economic status (Barrass et al., 2024). A systematic review of studies from southeast Asia showed that socioeconomic position measured as education, measures of financial difficulty, and subjective measures of financial circumstance had a greater than threefold increased risk of suicide. The most consistent and largest association was seen with subjective measures of financial circumstance (Knipe et al., 2015). The research on the Indian population has shown that depression is more common in poor people with poor economic backgrounds and poor nutritional status, Muslims, divorced or widowed, residing in nuclear families, unemployed, low educational

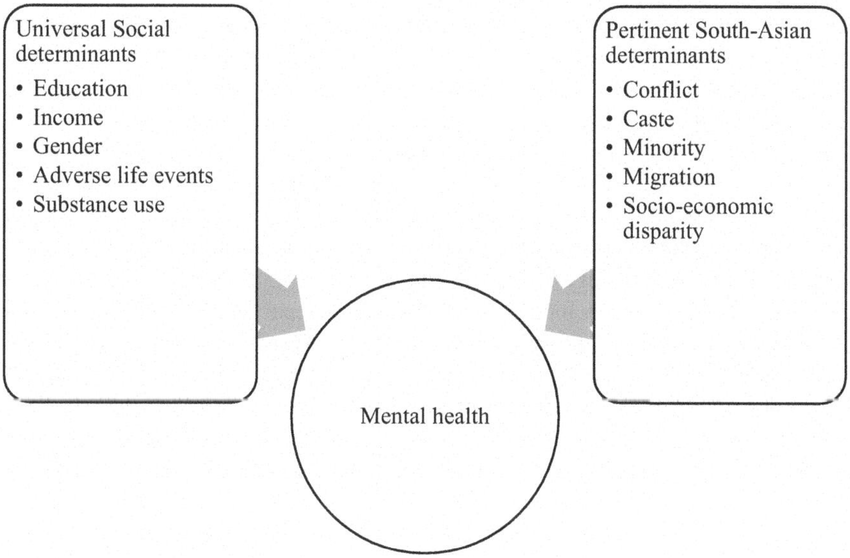


**Fig. 1** Overview of social determinants of mental health in South Asia

level, in subjects living in a nuclear family or in those living alone (Grover et al., 2010). A study from India showed that factors like female gender, economic stress, stress due to life events involving religious violence in the community, and life events involving caste conflicts or caste discrimination were factors that predicted suicidal ideation (Nath et al., 2011). A study from Bangladesh found that poor economic background, older age, i.e., 45 years or above, and large family size were associated with mental disorders (Monawar Hosain et al., 2007). Poverty, torture, and violence were also linked with poor mental health status as per a review of studies from Bangladesh (Newman, 2013). In the case of Nepal being divorced or separated, suffering from a disability had higher odds of having depression and anxiety (Pandey et al., 2024).

## *3.2 Female Population*

Studies from different countries in South Asia show a higher prevalence of mental disorders among women as compared to males. A meta-analysis of 13 studies in India showed significantly higher prevalence rates of neuroses, affective disorders, and organic psychoses in women as compared to men (Reddy & Chandrashekar, 1998). Factors like patriarchal society, violence against women, and subordinate position of women socially and economically, and stereotypical gender roles have contributed to the higher prevalence of mental disorders among women in South Asia (Niaz & Hassan, 2006). The social structure at different stages of life places South Asian women at increased risk of mental health challenges, and the social barriers prevent them from accessing mental healthcare services (Khan et al., 2020). A meta-analysis of 34 studies among 27,379 women in South Asia showed that factors like unplanned pregnancy, intimate partner violence, male gender preference, and poor relationships with in-laws were significantly associated with antenatal anxiety or depression (Insan et al., 2022). A stakeholder perspective using open-ended, in-depth interviews in Nepal identified inadequate social support, lack of availability and accessibility of maternal health services, and restricted socioeconomic and cultural context as determinants of poor mental health among pregnant women that caused immense distress (Sah et al., 2024). A systematic review of women living in slums from different countries in India, Bangladesh, and Nepal South Asia also showed that socioeconomic level and gender had the highest correlation with poor mental health status. Apart from that, living conditions, food insecurity, social capital, and social support were associated with mental health status (Abdi et al., 2021). In a meta-analysis of 47 studies of six South Asian countries, it was found that being married remained a risk factor for suicide and other suicidal behavior (Arafat et al., 2023).

## 3.3 Adolescents

Data from global school-based student health surveys show that bullying is highly prevalent and is associated with higher reporting of mental health problems like worry, loneliness and attempting suicide attempt, and substance use problems among both boys and girls (*Mental Health Status of Adolescents in South-East Asia: Evidence for Action*, n.d.). It has also been seen that social support in terms of parental involvement and close friendship is a determinant of depression among adolescents in South Asia (Murshid, 2017). A cross-sectional analysis from the global school-based student health survey (GSHS) in Bangladesh ($n = 2989$) and in Nepal ($n = 6529$) showed that there was an association of bullying victimization with loneliness, sleeping difficulty, and suicidal behaviors among adolescents in going children (Rahman et al., 2020). A systematic review has pointed to violent victimization, poor family/home/school environment and peer relationships, history of mental health problems, and substance use to be associated factors for mental health problems in adolescents of South Asia (Mudunna et al., 2023).

## 3.4 Substance Use

Data from Demographic and Health Surveys completed in nine countries of the East Asian region showed that tobacco use in both forms (smoking and smokeless) was associated with higher age, lower education, and poverty. Smoking prevalence was much lower in women than men in all countries (Sreeramareddy et al., 2014). A multicentre cross-sectional study from 15 states of India showed that socio-demographic determinants for participants with substance use disorder were higher age, male gender, urban residence, positive family history of substance use, and lower socioeconomic class (Venkatesh et al., 2024). A systematic review from South Asia showed that male gender, age greater than 14 years, having depression, parental/family alcohol use reduced parental attention, peer-drinking/pressure/approval, and urban neighborhood were associated factors for risks of adolescent alcohol use (Athauda et al., 2020). A qualitative study from Nepal stated that family relationships, ethnic identity, and psychoactive substance use, lack of social acceptance, peer pressure, stress relief, and coping with financial challenges, accessibility, and availability of psychoactive substances in the community and lack of monitoring and reinforcement of rules/ law and regulations were major drivers for substance use (Bhandari et al., 2021).

The substance use trends in South Asia have shown certain very important trends. Though there has been a consistent decline in the rates of tobacco use, the rates of alcohol use has not shown any such trends, unlike the western countries. Additionally, these countries have a higher rate of smokeless tobacco use and newer drugs due to poor regulation of pharmaceutical products and also situation of this area in the midst of important drug-trafficking routes (Bhad & Shukla, 2024; Choudhury et al.,

2024). Though the relationship of religion and substance use requires more intensive research, there are certain indicators such as decreased prevalence of alcohol use in Islamic countries like Afghanistan and Pakistan to suggest that they may have a role (Bhad & Shukla, 2024). The rates of substance use were also found to be higher in certain sections of the society like the tribal population (Sadath et al., 2022). There is some evidence that banning alcohol in certain Indian states has led to population level health benefits like decreased prevalence and indirect benefits like the decline in the rate of intimate partner violence (Chakrabarti et al., 2024).

## *3.5 Life Adversities*

Lifetime adversities in various forms tend to play a very important role in the manifestation of various psychiatric disorders. Adverse childhood experiences tend to be one of the most important factors among them. The evidence says that adverse childhood experiences can have a positive dose–response relationship with the chances of developing various mental health conditions (Trivedi et al., 2021). The studies from the South Asian countries in this context have mostly focused on the following aspects: physical abuse, childhood sexual abuse, emotional abuse, neglect, and household substance use. The problem is made more complex by the fact that, in addition to increasing the risk of developing mental disorders, the adverse situations also increase the risk of developing physical disorders, and also increase the risk of development of mental disorders in the subsequent generations (Mudunna et al., 2025). It is also important to mention that these findings seem to be universal across other social-demographic settings as well.

## *3.6 Socio-Economic Disadvantages*

In the initial section of this chapter, we have illustrated that South Asian countries remain at higher odds of disproportionate distribution of wealth and a significant amount of the population remaining in an economically disadvantaged position. The evidence in this regard seems to convey that poverty is associated with worse mental health outcomes (Lund et al., 2010). However, other studies examining this conundrum seem to suggest that the relationship is more complex. It suggests that it is actually the changes in the life setting brought on by socio-economic deprivation rather than poverty itself that lead to poor mental health outcomes (Das et al., 2007). Though such findings direct towards further examination of this problem, they do reduce the notion that poor mental health is a disease of affluence and commit us to taking a more steadfast research approach to it.

### 3.7 Migration

The South Asian population consists of a sizeable population that has suffered direct or indirect effects of inter-country or intra-country migration. Migration often occurs as a release to an unmodifiable situation, and expectedly, that has an enormous effect on the mental health of both the migrant population and the population that is left behind. Studies that have been conducted on this topic have found that mental health issues dominate the results. Though there have been various sections of populations who have been disrupted by migration, the mental health plight of Afghan migrants and Rohingya migrants has been well documented (Sifat et al., 2024; Tay et al., 2019). The findings from these studies have been homogenous and state that these people face difficulty in various aspects of their lives including language, employment, education, and legal support that puts them in a precarious position. Various stress-inducing factors and inadequate coping resources often lead to diminished mental well-being in this population (Ahmad et al., 2005). This often leads to a higher prevalence of various psychiatric disorders in the migrated population (Islam et al., 2014). Moreover, the mental health of the close family members who have been left back prior to migration was also found to be at a higher vulnerability to developing psychiatric disorders (Graham et al., 2015).

### 3.8 Racial-Caste-Based Discrimination

The South Asian society has been a spectator of stratification of the society based on caste or racial affiliation that has also tended to intersect with other forms of differences (Gorringe et al., 2017). A systematic review conducted on this theme among studies published in South Asia found that caste-based exclusion was related to differential opportunities to access education, employment, and healthcare (Thapa et al., 2021). The current evidence posits that persons affiliated to more vulnerable caste systems tend to suffer from worse mental health outcomes. They also remain more vulnerable to being exposed to systematic failures and deprived of organizational remedial measures (Komanapalli & Rao, 2020).

### 3.9 Socio-Political Issues

South Asian countries have been plagued with different kinds of protracted conflicts in the region. Some examples of such issues in the region include the Taliban takeover in Afghanistan, India-Pakistan political tensions, the revolution in Sri Lanka by the Liberation Tigers of Tamil Eelam (LTTE), and the Monsoon Revolution in Bangladesh in 2024. There has been a steady rise in the prevalence of various psychiatric disorders in the afflicted zones. Various factors that tend to play a role in the severity of the presentations include the reason for conflict (religious or political), duration (acute or protracted), and probability of displacement (David et al., 2017). The conflict also tends to have an indirect effect on mental health. Conflict leads to a rise in health costs in a bidirectional manner. On one hand, it increases the volume of healthcare seekers; on the other hand, it hinders the healthcare delivery process. It also leads to the diversion of the public exchequer towards defence expenditures. Conflicts also lead to a higher volume of displaced population, that creates further pressure on the public health systems of the country.

## 3.10 Minority Population

The mental health implications in people belonging to minority groups has been under research focus. It has been seen that persons identifying with the lesbian, gay, bisexual, transgender, and queer (LGBTQ) tended to have a higher prevalence of various psychiatric disorders than persons with heterosexual orientation (Tan & Saw, 2023). The non-binary orientation is linked with several psychological and socio-political challenges that make them highly vulnerable to negative mental health outcomes, including suicides (Bhatia et al., 2024). Belonging to other minority groups, like religious minorities, also predisposes to higher chances of developing psychiatric morbidity (Karasz et al., 2019). There is some rudimentary evidence that religious participation translated into positive mental health outcomes in certain well-controlled models of the South Asian population (Stroope et al., 2022).

## 3.11 Suicidal Behavior

The South Asian region has shown the highest regional suicide rate among the various regions (Arafat et al., 2025). This matter is made more complex considering that this area also has one of the highest population densities. Thus, in terms of numbers, this area has been witnessing an unparalleled amount of suicide. However, there have been some noticeable differences in the trends of suicide from the Western countries. The male to female ratio of suicide is lower this region, which is unlike the Western data. Suicide in this region also tended to have a lower rate of association with psychiatric disorders and a higher association with stigma and is likely to be governed by religious affiliations (Arafat et al., 2022). The suicides in this region were likely to be more associated with psycho-social stressors (migration, loneliness, unemployment, indebtedness.

### 3.12 Culture-Specific Ways of Coping

There has been observable difference in how a person's socio-ethnic background governs how a stressful situation is responded to (Luong et al., 2020). In the South Asian context, the response has been found to be associated with social situation, living conditions, family dynamics, support system, and religion (Younas et al., 2024). Additionally, the patient's socio-cultural background seems to modify how they verbalize their complaints (Weaver & Karasz, 2022). This is an important factor to be kept in mind while interviewing a patient, and also appropriate skill needs to be exercised while interpreting the complaints of the patient for effective interventions.

## 4 Framework for Prevention for Public Mental Health Aspects

In this section, we discussed the preventive measures in universal, selected, indicated category (Table 1).

### 4.1 Measures from Global Evidence

In this section, we intend to summarize the relevant approaches from the global studies that can be implemented in the South Asian context.

**Table 1** Preventive interventions to target the social determinants of mental health

| Strategy | Examples |
|---|---|
| Universal prevention strategies | 1. School-based mental health programs<br>2. Interventions directed at parents<br>3. Anti-stigma campaigns<br>4. Community based mental health literacy programs/camps |
| Selective prevention strategies | 1. Economic interventions<br>2. Neighborhood interventions<br>3. Home visit programs<br>4. Interventions targeted at specific populations such as refugees, women facing domestic violence, and conflict affected areas |
| Indicated prevention strategies | 1. Early detection services<br>2. Peer support programs<br>3. Family support interventions<br>4. School-based interventions for at-risk students |

### 4.1.1 Interventions Directed at the Parents

Parenting is one of the most crucial aspects of a child's development. Parenting interventions that aim to enhance positive parenting techniques have been developed and studied extensively, with primarily positive findings on child mental health. The studies have consistently reported improvement in child development, behavior, and child-parent interaction after such parenting interventions (Kirkbride et al., 2024). These programs are commonly conducted in groups, with around 8–12 sessions conducted weekly. Such interventions are found to be remarkably cost-effective in terms of anxiety reduction in children. One reassuring aspect of parenting interventions is that the programs are found to be equally effective in LMICs.

### 4.1.2 School-Based Interventions

School-based mental health programs are designed to provide mental health promotion and prevention. Numerous such programs exist that focus on various aspects of mental health, such as (1) mental health literacy, (2) prevention of depression and anxiety, (3) prevention or reduction of disruptive behaviors, (4) suicide prevention, (5) substance use prevention, and (6) mindfulness-based programs. School-based programs are found to be effective in reducing disruptive behaviors, reducing anxiety and depression symptoms, and reducing stigma. They are equally effective in terms of suicide prevention, especially when they are multi-faceted (Ma et al., 2023; Weare & Nind, 2011; Werner-Seidler et al., 2017). Other benefits, such as increased prosocial behaviors and reduced aggression, were also noted (Jordans et al., 2010). School-based interpersonal therapy intervention has been found to be feasible and acceptable in the LMICs (Rose-Clarke et al., 2022).

### 4.1.3 Economic Interventions

As previously discussed, there is a strong link between socioeconomic disadvantage, poverty, and poor mental health. Thus, the interventions that focus on improving such disadvantage may not only reduce poverty and inequality but also improve mental health at the population level. A recent systematic review and meta-analysis that included 136 RCTs reported that income changes impact mental health, especially if they are associated with people moving out of poverty (Thomson et al., 2022). These effects are more robust in the LMICs. Hence, many guaranteed income and cash transfer programs have been implemented globally and have shown consistent findings of improvement in mental health. Most of these studies focus on child and adolescent mental health outcomes. For example, a recent systematic review that included 14 papers reported a significant improvement in adolescent mental health (primarily in internalizing problems) after monetary poverty alleviation programs (Zaneva et al., 2022). However, some reviews also found similar positive effects of such schemes in adults (McGuire et al., 2022).

## 4.2 *Evidence from South Asia*

As compared to the volume of literature across other countries, the evidence generated from the South Asian countries have been modest. However, in this subsequent section, we will try to provide a summary of the status of evidence emerging from the South Asian countries.

### 4.2.1 Interventions Directed at the Parents

A Cochrane review that looked into the effect of group-based parenting interventions on emotional and behavioral symptoms in children identified 24 RCTs and quasi-RCTs, with none being from South Asia. A recent scoping review that assessed the implementation of parenting programs in real-world settings included 145 original studies and only found one study from a South Asian country (India). A parenting program, *Parvarish*, was adapted in India from a similar program in South Africa, "Parenting for Lifelong Health". The study reported that the program was engaging, feasible and acceptable in India (Mathias et al., 2022). Parenting interventions have been found to reduce parental stress and overall psychosocial health of the parents as well (Janardhana & Manjula, 2020; Rishi & John, 2024). Parenting interventions that address inter-generational conflicts and anxieties have also been piloted in India (de Wit et al., 2018). A combined school and family-based intervention in Nepal for child behavior health problems was found to be acceptable and feasible by parents (Adhikari et al., 2018).

### 4.2.2 School-Based Interventions

Many school-based mental health programs are implemented in South Asian countries. For example in India, Sarva Shiksha Abhiyan trained the teachers to identify psychological issues and to provide counseling. The National Institute of Mental Health and Neurosciences (NIMHANS), Bengaluru, initiated a Life Skills Training Program. Under the program, the secondary school teachers were trained to provide life skills training to students as "life skills facilitators". Various other school-based programs, such as Zippy's Friends program in Goa, the SHAPE program in Goa, and the SEHER program in Bihar, have also been implemented with varying success rates due to reasons such as stigma, reluctance of teachers, and school management non-cooperation (Raman & Thomas, 2023).

Similarly, a cluster randomized controlled trial evaluated classroom-based psychosocial intervention in conflict-affected rural Nepal. The intervention was effective in improving the socio-behavioral and resilience indicators among the participating students. However, another study that assessed the effects of training for school teachers on psychosocial support in earthquake-affected areas of Nepal did not find any positive effect of the intervention on adolescents' mental health during the six-month follow-up period (Dhital et al., 2019). A combined school- and family-based intervention, delivered by psychosocial counselors is also found to be effective in terms of improving disruptive behaviors in children (Adhikari et al., 2018).

In Sri Lanka, a 12-session structured school-based program, "ERASE Stress Sri Lanka", was studied in a quasi-randomized setting among Tsunami-exposed children. The study reported significant improvement in depression (Berger & Gelkopf, 2009), PTSD, and other outcomes (such as stress scores, functional problems, and somatic symptoms). The study reported no new cases of PTSD in the intervention arm. Another cluster randomized trial that attempted to investigate the effects of 15 sessions of school-based cognitive behavioral techniques implemented by paraprofessionals in a war-affected area reported a positive impact on conduct problems, especially among younger children. Among boys, the intervention showed significant benefits in terms of PTSD and anxiety symptoms (Tol et al., 2012).

An early study conducted in Rawalpindi, Pakistan, supported the effectiveness of school mental health programs in improving mental health awareness in school children (Rahman et al., 1998). The children were receptive to the intervention. Another RCT was conducted to assess teachers' mental health literacy and self-efficacy after a standardized WHO School Mental Health Manual-Based Intervention (Imran et al., 2022). The study found preliminary evidence of significant improvement in the teacher's outcome (in terms of mental health literacy and self-efficacy), which was sustained over time.

In Bangladesh, UNICEF collaborated with the Ministry of Education to introduce a School-based "Mental Health and Psychosocial Support Program". Mental health and well-being is among the 10 learning areas in the national curriculum framework (*Adolescent Development and Participation | UNICEF*, n.d.). The program was implemented in January 2023, and around 5 million students have benefited.

### 4.2.3 Family Interventions

LMICs, like South Asian countries, are at a higher risk of poor mental health due to socio-economic disadvantage. Families work as a buffer to the negative impacts of community stressors on children and adolescents. Thus, strengthening the families with family interventions may give their offspring the necessary support and resources for better mental health. Extensive evidence exists for their effectiveness in reducing the relapse of psychosis, depression, suicidal ideations, and other mental health outcomes. Similar effectiveness is noted in studies conducted in LMICs using a non-specialist workforce for intervention delivery (Healy et al., 2018). Like other interventions, very few studies have been conducted in South Asian countries. A recent systematic review only found 10 studies from LMICs, of which one each were from India and Pakistan. In this combined RCT from India and Pakistan, a parent-mediated intervention was tested for children with ASD and replicated the positive findings of parenting interventions from elsewhere (Thomson et al., 2022).

#### 4.2.4 Economic Interventions

Literature accrued from the South Asian countries, though limited, supports these findings. For example, a study from Bangladesh reported that providing rural women with cash and food transfers, with nutritional BCC, may lead to improvement in terms of reduced interpersonal violence. The effect is sustained over 4 years after the program ends (Roy et al., 2019). Economic interventions such as cash transfers have improved social inclusion in Nepal (Drucza, 2016). A study from India analyzed the effects of cash transfer through the *Janani Suraksha Yojana* on maternal depression in the Indian state of Uttar Pradesh. The study reported an 8.5% reduction in maternal depression due to the cash transfer, with 68% less likelihood of being in delivery care-related debt (Powell-Jackson et al., 2016). A study in Tamil Nadu, India, assessed the effect of one-time cash transfer of 1000 INR (approx. 11.5 USD) among 1120 older people living alone and found improvement in functional impairment with a slight reduction in depression (McKelway et al., 2023). Thus, South Asian studies also consistently report the mental health benefits of cash transfer programs, which are aligned with global evidence.

#### 4.2.5 Vocational Interventions

Employment rates for patients with MSUD, especially severe mental illnesses like schizophrenia and bipolar disorders, are low. This is attributed to multiple reasons, including educational disadvantage, stigma, as well as the chronic nature of many MSUD conditions. However, the benefits of employment on MSUD conditions are well documented. Vocational interventions are associated with improved functioning, well-being, self-esteem, and social connection, besides providing financial benefits. A vocational intervention, Individual Placement and Support (IPS), is effective across HICs and LMICs (Modini et al., 2016).

Studies on the effectiveness and implementation of vocational interventions are limited in South Asian countries. A very recent scoping review from India reported a total of 12 studies (all quasi-experimental or case-based). Various vocational rehabilitation methods are employed in India, including skill training, case management, and supported employment (Thekkumkara et al., 2024). In Bangladesh, occupational therapists have introduced a new paradigm in occupational therapy. They provide mental health day treatment services to MSUD patients to transit from the mental hospitals to the community. The activities focus on skill training and engagement in meaningful activities (Alve et al., 2024).

#### 4.2.6 Interventions to Address Trauma

Trauma is consistently associated with poor mental health. It is important to consider that trauma, as assessed using standard questionnaires like the Adverse Childhood Experience (ACE) questionnaire, may not be applicable in the South Asian context.

For example, an ontological study from India reported that interpersonal events are primary sources of trauma or traumatic experience, unlike Western countries, where environmental disasters or political conflicts are major sources (Smith et al., 2024). Thus, trauma-focused interventions need to be adapted to the South Asian context. Two interventions that focus on trauma-informed care and are found to be most effective across the globe to date are trauma-focused CBT and EMDR. Such interventions are moderately effective in reducing depression, anxiety, and PTSD symptoms, even in LMICs. However, the evidence from South Asian countries is somewhat limited (Khubsing et al., 2020). A brief psychological trauma intervention was developed in India and was found to be feasible and effective for children surviving sexual abuse (Choudhary et al., 2023, 2024).

### 4.2.7 *Home* Visit Interventions by Paraprofessionals

It is a well-known fact that perinatal stress impacts brain development. Because of this, early life home visit programs are developed to support healthy development during early life years. These interventions usually target marginalized groups to foster healthy home environments. Research, including RCTs, suggests that such interventions, which include strategies like parental education, providing social support, enhancing mother–child interaction, and positive parenting, improve the home environment and parenting behaviors (Kendrick et al., 2000; Masud et al., 2019). Similar interventions have been developed and implemented in South Asian countries like India, Pakistan, and Bangladesh with varying success (Bhopal et al., 2019; Hossain et al., 2024; Mehrin et al., 2021; Shah et al., 2020).

### 4.2.8 Culture-Specific Interventions

Management of various mental health-related issues in the South Asian scenario has seen the inculcation of cultural and socio-religious practices into the practice of evidence-based medicine. The rates of seeking help from traditional healers have been found to substantial in this region. Treatment from the faith healers is well-appreciated in the region and is instrumental in addressing the culture-specific distress arising of faith healers is well-appreciated in the region and is instrumental in addressing the culture-specific distress arising from mental disorders. It has been found that the formulation of the faith healers is more culturally tuned, which is not only therapeutic for the patient, but also for the attenders. Traditional healers also remain in a position of advocacy by being aware of the patients' belief system and that can be beneficial in the management of the patients (Dein, 2020; Sharma et al., 2020).

## 5 Conclusion

The social determinants of mental health in the South Asian countries remain a paradox. The countries are bound by geographical proximity and socio-cultural similarities. On the other hand, the mutual geo-political relationships among the countries are complex and not essentially beneficial for positive health outcomes, including mental health outcomes. In our review, we could identify a number of exclusive social determinants that are rather unique for this geographical region. Other than directly influencing mental health outcomes, we could also observe the complex and intense interplay of those factors in governing the consequences. The review could identify a number of steps that have been instituted by the countries. However, there is still a need for a better appreciation of the situation and the introduction of newer strategies with more intersectoral collaboration backed by political will.

## References

Abdi, F., Rahnemaei, F. A., Shojaei, P., Afsahi, F., & Mahmoodi, Z. (2021). Social determinants of mental health of women living in slum: A systematic review. *Obstetrics & Gynecology Science, 64*(2), 143–155. https://doi.org/10.5468/OGS.20264

Adhikari, R. P., Upadhaya, N., Satinsky, E. N., Burkey, M. D., Kohrt, B. A., & Jordans, M. J. D. (2018). Feasibility study of a family- and school-based intervention for child behavior problems in Nepal. *Child and Adolescent Psychiatry and Mental Health, 12*(1), 1–11. https://doi.org/10.1186/S13034-018-0226-3/TABLES/3

*Adolescent Development and Participation | UNICEF*. (n.d.). Retrieved February 3, 2025, from https://www.unicef.org/adolescence

Ahmad, F., Shik, A., Vanza, R., Cheung, A. M., George, U., & Stewart, D. E. (2005). Voices of South Asian women: Immigration and mental health. *Women & Health, 40*(4), 113–130. https://doi.org/10.1300/J013V40N04_07

Alve, Y. A., Hasan, M. R., Sultana, R., Hossain, M. S., Koly, K., & Mahaffey, L. (2024). Introducing a new paradigm in occupational therapy for mental health in Bangladesh. *Occupational Therapy in Mental Health*. https://doi.org/10.1080/0164212X.2024.2398476

Arafat, S. M. Y., Rajkumar, R. P., & Kar, S. K. (2025). Trend of suicide research in South Asia: A bibliometric analysis of the last three decades. *Omega*, 302228251323991. Advance online publication. https://doi.org/10.1177/00302228251323991

Arafat, S. M. Y., & Kar, S. K. (2024). Epidemiology of psychiatric disorders and overview of access to mental health care in South Asia. In S. M. Y. Arafat & S. K. Kar (Eds.), Access to mental health care in South Asia. Springer, Singapore. https://doi.org/10.1007/978-981-99-9153-2_1

Arafat, S. M. Y., Menon, V., Khan, M. A. S., Htay, M. N. N., Singh, R., Biyyala, D., Krishnamoorthy, Y., & Mynampally, K. (2023). Marital status and suicidal behavior in South Asia: A systematic review and meta-analysis. *Health Science Reports, 6*(12), Article e1781. https://doi.org/10.1002/hsr2.1781

Arafat, S. M. Y., Menon, V., Varadharajan, N., & Kar, S. K. (2022). Psychological autopsy studies of suicide in South East Asia. *Indian Journal of Psychological Medicine, 44*(1), 4–9. https://doi.org/10.1177/02537176211033643

Athauda, L. K., Peiris-John, R., Ameratunga, S., McCool, J., & Wickremasinghe, R. (2020). Factors influencing alcohol use among adolescents in South Asia: A systematic review. *Journal of Studies on Alcohol and Drugs, 81*(5), 529–542. https://doi.org/10.15288/JSAD.2020.81.529

Barrass, L., Joshi, E., Dawe, J., Rubbo, B., Redaniel, M. T., Riglin, L., Lee, N. R., Howe, L. D., & Knipe, D. (2024). The association between socioeconomic position and depression or suicidal ideation in low- and middle-income countries in Southeast Asia: A systematic review and meta-analysis. *BMC Public Health, 24*(1), 1–15. https://doi.org/10.1186/S12889-024-20986-9/TABLES/3

Berger, R., & Gelkopf, M. (2009). School-based intervention for the treatment of tsunami-related distress in children: A quasi-randomized controlled trial. *Psychotherapy and Psychosomatics, 78*(6), 364–371. https://doi.org/10.1159/000235976

Bhad, R., & Shukla, S. (2024). Understanding substance use disorder and comorbidities: Insights from South Asia. *Current Perspectives on Substance Use Disorders in South Asia, 225–244*,. https://doi.org/10.1007/978-981-97-6619-2_12

Bhandari, T. R., Khatiwada, B., Rajbhandari, B., Bestman, A., Mistry, S. K., Rayamajhee, B., Rawal, L. B., & Yadavid, N. (2021). A qualitative study to understand drivers of psychoactive substance use among Nepalese youth. *PLoS ONE, 16*(11 November). https://doi.org/10.1371/journal.pone.0259021

Bhatia, G., Pal, A., Parmar, A., & Sharma, P. (2024). Suicides among sexual minority populations in Asia: A battle in the shadows. *International Review of Psychiatry*. https://doi.org/10.1080/09540261.2024.2327388

Bhattacharya, G., & Schoppelrey, S. L. (2004). Preimmigration beliefs of life success, post immigration experiences, and acculturative stress: South Asian immigrants in the United States. *Journal of Immigrant Health, 6*(2), 83–92. https://doi.org/10.1023/B:JOIH.0000019168.75062.36/METRICS

Bhopal, S., Roy, R., Verma, D., Kumar, D., Avan, B., Khan, B., Gram, L., Sharma, K., Amenga-Etego, S., Panchal, S. N., Soremekun, S., Divan, G., & Kirkwood, B. R. (2019). Impact of adversity on early childhood growth & development in rural India: Findings from the early life stress sub-study of the SPRING cluster randomised controlled trial (SPRING-ELS). *PLoS ONE, 14*(1), Article e0209122. https://doi.org/10.1371/JOURNAL.PONE.0209122

Chakrabarti, S., Christopher, A., Scott, S., Kishore, A., & Nguyen, P. H. (2024). Effects of a large-scale alcohol ban on population-level alcohol intake, weight, blood pressure, blood glucose, and domestic violence in India: A quasi-experimental population-based study. *The Lancet Regional Health - Southeast Asia, 26*. https://doi.org/10.1016/j.lansea.2024.100427

Chiu, M., Lebenbaum, M., Newman, A. M., Zaheer, J., & Kurdyak, P. (2016). Ethnic differences in mental illness severity: A population-based study of Chinese and South Asian patients in Ontario, Canada. *The Journal of Clinical Psychiatry, 77*(9), 6699. https://doi.org/10.4088/JCP.15M10086

Choudhury, S., Joshi, T., & Ghosh, A. (2024). Overview of substance use disorder in South Asia. *Current Perspectives on Substance Use Disorders in South Asia, 1–18*. https://doi.org/10.1007/978-981-97-6619-2_1

Choudhary, V., Satapathy, S., & Sagar, R. (2023). Development of a brief psychological trauma intervention for child sexual abuse in India. *Journal of Child Sexual Abuse, 32*(7), 879–903. https://doi.org/10.1080/10538712.2023.2249873

Choudhary, V., Satapathy, S., & Sagar, R. (2024). Feasibility trial of a newly developed brief psychological trauma intervention for children surviving sexual abuse in India. *Journal of Child Sexual Abuse, 33*(2), 204–228. https://doi.org/10.1080/10538712.2024.2319668

Coker, R. J., Hunter, B. M., Rudge, J. W., Liverani, M., & Hanvoravongchai, P. (2011). Emerging infectious diseases in Southeast Asia: Regional challenges to control. *The Lancet, 377*(9765), 599–609. https://doi.org/10.1016/S0140-6736(10)62004-1/ATTACHMENT/628B896E-BCA5-4907-9459-58B02141D333/MMC1.PDF

*Commission on Social Determinants of Health*. (n.d.). Retrieved December 21, 2024, from https://www.who.int/initiatives/action-on-the-social-determinants-of-health-for-advancing-equity/world-report-on-social-determinants-of-health-equity/commission-on-social-determinants-of-health

Csikar, J., Aravani, A., Godson, J., Day, M., & Wilkinson, J. (2013). Incidence of oral cancer among South Asians and those of other ethnic groups by sex in West Yorkshire and England, 2001–2006. *The British Journal of Oral & Maxillofacial Surgery, 51*(1), 25–29. https://doi.org/10.1016/J.BJOMS.2012.03.008

Das, J., Do, Q. T., Friedman, J., McKenzie, D., & Scott, K. (2007). Mental health and poverty in developing countries: Revisiting the relationship. *Social Science & Medicine, 65*(3), 467–480. https://doi.org/10.1016/J.SOCSCIMED.2007.02.037

David, S., Gazi, R., Mirzazada, M. S., Siriwardhana, C., Soofi, S., & Roy, N. (2017). Conflict in South Asia and its impact on health. *BMJ, 357*. https://doi.org/10.1136/BMJ.J1537

de Wit, E. E., Adithy, Chakranarayan, C., Bunders-Aelen, J. F. G., & Regeer, B. J. (2018). Learning about parenting together: A programme to support parents with inter-generational concerns in Pune, India. *Contemporary Family Therapy, 40*(1), 68–83. https://doi.org/10.1007/S10591-017-9429-7/TABLES/5

Dein, S. (2020). Religious healing and mental health. *Mental Health, Religion & Culture, 23*(8), 657–665. https://doi.org/10.1080/13674676.2020.1834220

Dhillon, P. K., Jeemon, P., Arora, N. K., Mathur, P., Maskey, M., Sukirna, R. D., & Prabhakaran, D. (2012). Status of epidemiology in the WHO South-East Asia region: Burden of disease, determinants of health and epidemiological research, workforce and training capacity. *International Journal of Epidemiology, 41*(3), 847–860. https://doi.org/10.1093/IJE/DYS046

Dhital, R., Shibanuma, A., Miyaguchi, M., Kiriya, J., & Jimba, M. (2019). Effect of psycho-social support by teachers on improving mental health and hope of adolescents in an earthquake-affected district in Nepal: A cluster randomized controlled trial. *PLoS ONE, 14*(10), Article e0223046. https://doi.org/10.1371/JOURNAL.PONE.0223046

Diwan, S. (2008). Limited English proficiency, social network characteristics, and depressive symptoms among older immigrants. *The Journals of Gerontology: Series B, 63*(3), S184–S191. https://doi.org/10.1093/GERONB/63.3.S184

Drucza, K. (2016). Cash transfers in Nepal: Do they contribute to social inclusion? *Oxford Development Studies, 44*(1), 49–69. https://doi.org/10.1080/13600818.2015.1065313

Ekanayake, S., Ahmad, F., & McKenzie, K. (2012). Qualitative cross-sectional study of the perceived causes of depression in South Asian origin women in Toronto. *British Medical Journal Open, 2*(1), Article e000641. https://doi.org/10.1136/BMJOPEN-2011-000641

Gorringe, H., Jodhka, S. S., & Takhar, O. K. (2017). Caste: Experiences in South Asia and beyond. *Contemporary South Asia, 25*(3), 230–237. https://doi.org/10.1080/09584935.2017.1360246

Graham, E., Jordan, L. P., & Yeoh, B. S. A. (2015). Parental migration and the mental health of those who stay behind to care for children in South-East Asia. *Social Science & Medicine, 132*, 225–235. https://doi.org/10.1016/J.SOCSCIMED.2014.10.060

Grover, S., Dutt, A., & Avasthi, A. (2010). An overview of Indian research in depression. *Indian Journal of Psychiatry, 52*(7), 178. https://doi.org/10.4103/0019-5545.69231

Healy, E. A., Kaiser, B. N., & Puffer, E. S. (2018). Family-based youth mental health interventions delivered by nonspecialist providers in low- and middle-income countries: A systematic review. *Families, Systems & Health: the Journal of Collaborative Family Healthcare, 36*(2), 182–197. https://doi.org/10.1037/FSH0000334

Hossain, S. J., Rahman, S. M., Fisher, J., Rahman, A., Tofail, F., & Hamadani, J. D. (2024). Effect of a parenting and nutrition education programme on development and growth of children using a social safety net platform in urban Bangladesh: A cluster randomized controlled trial. *The Lancet Regional Health - Southeast Asia, 25*. https://doi.org/10.1016/j.lansea.2024.100388

Imran, N., Rahman, A., Chaudhry, N., & Asif, A. (2022). Effectiveness of a school-based mental health intervention for school teachers in urban Pakistan: A randomized controlled trial. *Child and Adolescent Psychiatry and Mental Health, 16*(1). https://doi.org/10.1186/S13034-022-00470-1

Insan, N., Weke, A., Forrest, S., & Rankin, J. (2022). Social determinants of antenatal depression and anxiety among women in South Asia: A systematic review & meta-analysis. *PLoS ONE, 17*(2), Article e0263760. https://doi.org/10.1371/JOURNAL.PONE.0263760

Irwin, A., Valentine, N., Brown, C., Loewenson, R., Solar, O., Brown, H., Koller, T., & Vega, J. (2006). The commission on social determinants of health: Tackling the social roots of health inequities. *PLOS Medicine, 3*(6), Article e106. https://doi.org/10.1371/JOURNAL.PMED.0030106

Islam, F., Khanlou, N., & Tamim, H. (2014). South Asian populations in Canada: Migration and mental health. *BMC Psychiatry, 14*(1), 1–13. https://doi.org/10.1186/1471-244X-14-154/TABLES/3

Janardhana, N., & Manjula, B. (2020). Parental-group interventions for parents of children with mental health problems admitted in a tertiary care center: An experience from India. *Indian Journal of Community Medicine, 45*(1), 48–53. https://doi.org/10.4103/IJCM.IJCM_192_19

Jordans, M. J. D., Komproe, I. H., Tol, W. A., Kohrt, B. A., Luitel, N. P., MacY, R. D., & De Jong, J. T. V. M. (2010). Evaluation of a classroom-based psychosocial intervention in conflict-affected Nepal: A cluster randomized controlled trial. *Journal of Child Psychology and Psychiatry, 51*(7), 818–826. https://doi.org/10.1111/J.1469-7610.2010.02209.X

Karasz, A., Gany, F., Escobar, J., Flores, C., Prasad, L., Inman, A., Kalasapudi, V., Kosi, R., Murthy, M., Leng, J., & Diwan, S. (2019). Mental health and stress among South Asians. *Journal of Immigrant and Minority Health, 21*(Suppl 1), 7. https://doi.org/10.1007/S10903-016-0501-4

Kendrick, D., Elkan, R., Hewitt, M., Dewey, M., Blair, M., Robinson, J., Williams, D., & Brummell, K. (2000). Does home visiting improve parenting and the quality of the home environment? A systematic review and meta analysis. *Archives of Disease in Childhood, 82*(6), 443. https://doi.org/10.1136/ADC.82.6.443

Khan, M. A., Jafree, S. R., & Jibeen, T. (2020). Social barriers to mental well-being in women of South Asia. *The Sociology of South Asian Women's Health, 129–150.* https://doi.org/10.1007/978-3-030-50204-1_7

Kirkbride, J. B., Anglin, D. M., Colman, I., Dykxhoorn, J., Jones, P. B., Patalay, P., Pitman, A., Soneson, E., Steare, T., Wright, T., & Griffiths, S. L. (2024). The social determinants of mental health and disorder: Evidence, prevention and recommendations. *World Psychiatry, 23*(1), 58. https://doi.org/10.1002/WPS.21160

Knipe, D. W., Carroll, R., Thomas, K. H., Pease, A., Gunnell, D., & Metcalfe, C. (2015). Association of socio-economic position and suicide/attempted suicide in low and middle income countries in South and South-East Asia—A systematic review. *BMC Public Health, 15*(1), 1–18. https://doi.org/10.1186/S12889-015-2301-5/FIGURES/11

Komanapalli, V., & Rao, D. (2020). The mental health impact of caste and structural inequalities in higher education in India. *58*(3), 392–403. https://doi.org/10.1177/1363461520963862

Leung, J. G. (2023). Ethnopsychopharmacology: Clinical and scientific writing pearls. *The Mental Health Clinician, 13*(6), 276. https://doi.org/10.9740/MHC.2023.12.276

Lund, C., Breen, A., Flisher, A. J., Kakuma, R., Corrigall, J., Joska, J. A., Swartz, L., & Patel, V. (2010). Poverty and common mental disorders in low and middle income countries: A systematic review. *Social Science & Medicine, 71*(3), 517–528. https://doi.org/10.1016/J.SOCSCIMED.2010.04.027

Luong, G., Arredondo, C. M., & Charles, S. T. (2020). Cultural differences in coping with interpersonal tensions lead to divergent shorter- and longer-term affective consequences. *Cognition & Emotion, 34*(7), 1499. https://doi.org/10.1080/02699931.2020.1752153

Ma, K. K. Y., Anderson, J. K., & Burn, A. M. (2023). Review: School-based interventions to improve mental health literacy and reduce mental health stigma—A systematic review. *Child and Adolescent Mental Health, 28*(2), 230–240. https://doi.org/10.1111/CAMH.12543

Masud, H., Ahmad, M. S., Cho, K. W., & Fakhr, Z. (2019). Parenting styles and aggression among young adolescents: A systematic review of literature. *Community Mental Health Journal, 55*(6), 1015–1030. https://doi.org/10.1007/S10597-019-00400-0

Mathias, K., Nayak, P., Singh, P., Pillai, P., & Goicolea, I. (2022). Is the Parwarish parenting intervention feasible and relevant for young people and parents in diverse settings in India? A mixed methods process evaluation. *British Medical Journal Open, 12*(2), Article e054553. https://doi.org/10.1136/BMJOPEN-2021-054553

McGuire, J., Kaiser, C., & Bach-Mortensen, A. M. (2022). A systematic review and meta-analysis of the impact of cash transfers on subjective well-being and mental health in low- and middle-income countries. *Nature Human Behaviour, 6*(3), 359–370. https://doi.org/10.1038/s41562-021-01252-z

McKelway, M., Banerjee, A., Grela, E., Schilbach, F., Sequeira, M., Sharma, G., Vaidyanathan, G., & Duflo, E. (2023). Effects of cognitive behavioral therapy and cash transfers on older persons living alone in India. *Annals of Internal Medicine, 176*(5), 632–642. https://doi.org/10.7326/M22-2496/SUPPL_FILE/M22-2496_SUPPLEMENT-STUDYPROTOCOL.PDF

Mehrin, S. F., Hamadani, J. D., Salveen, N. E., Hasan, M. I., Hossain, S. J., & Baker-Henningham, H. (2021). Adapting an evidence-based, early childhood parenting programme for integration into government primary health care services in rural Bangladesh. *Frontiers in Public Health, 8*, Article 608173. https://doi.org/10.3389/FPUBH.2020.608173/BIBTEX

*Mental Health.* (n.d.). Retrieved December 21, 2024, from https://www.who.int/news-room/fact-sheets/detail/mental-health-strengthening-our-response/?gad_source=1&gclid=CjwKCAiA65m7BhAwEiwAAgu4JDYXtNXy4aHxpbQ1EJxkNdimCxT3GgBymsyWWJXNlXcGWUMCBKI5UxoCkAUQAvD_BwE

*Mental Health Status of Adolescents in South-East Asia: Evidence for Action.* (n.d.). Retrieved January 19, 2025, from https://www.who.int/publications/i/item/9789290225737

Mirza, A., Birtel, M. D., Pyle, M., & Morrison, A. P. (2019). Cultural differences in psychosis: The role of causal beliefs and stigma in White British and South Asians. *Journal of Cross-Cultural Psychology, 50*(3), 441–459. https://doi.org/10.1177/0022022118820168

Modini, M., Tan, L., Brinchmann, B., Wang, M. J., Killackey, E., Glozier, N., Mykletun, A., & Harvey, S. B. (2016). Supported employment for people with severe mental illness: Systematic review and meta-analysis of the international evidence. *The British Journal of Psychiatry, 209*(1), 14–22. https://doi.org/10.1192/BJP.BP.115.165092

Monawar Hosain, G. M., Chatterjee, N., Ara, N., & Islam, T. (2007). Prevalence, pattern and determinants of mental disorders in rural Bangladesh. *Public Health, 121*(1), 18–24. https://doi.org/10.1016/J.PUHE.2006.06.018

Mudunna, C., Weerasinghe, M., Tran, T., Antoniades, J., Romero, L., Chandradasa, M., & Fisher, J. (2023). *Nature, prevalence and determinants of mental health problems experienced by adolescents in South Asia: A systematic review of the evidence.* https://doi.org/10.2139/SSRN.4555280

Mudunna, C., Weerasinghe, M., Tran, T., Antoniades, J., Romero, L., Chandradasa, M., & Fisher, J. (2025). Nature, prevalence and determinants of mental health problems experienced by adolescents in south Asia: A systematic review. *The Lancet Regional Health - Southeast Asia, 33*, Article 100532. https://doi.org/10.1016/J.LANSEA.2025.100532

Murshid, N. S. (2017). Parents, friends, and depression: A multi-country study of adolescents in South Asia. *Children and Youth Services Review, 79*, 160–165. https://doi.org/10.1016/J.CHILDYOUTH.2017.06.018

Nath, Y., Paris, J., Thombs, B., & Kirmayer, L. (2011). Prevalence and social determinants of suicidal behaviours among college youth in India. *International Journal of Social Psychiatry, 58*(4), 393–399. https://doi.org/10.1177/0020764011401164

Newman, M. S. (2013). Review of studies of mental health in Bangladesh, with a focus on depression. *International Journal of Mental Health, 42*(4), 48–77. https://doi.org/10.2753/IMH0020-7411420403

Niaz, U., & Hassan, S. (2006). Culture and mental health of women in South-East Asia. *World Psychiatry, 5*(2), 118. https://pmc.ncbi.nlm.nih.gov/articles/PMC1525125/

Pal, A., Saxena, V., & Avinash, P. (2021). Stigma in bipolar affective disorder: A systematic quantitative literature review of Indian studies: *Indian Journal of Psychological Medicine, 43*(3), 187–194. https://doi.org/10.1177/0253717621996618

Pandey, A. R., Adhikari, B., Bista, B., Lamichhane, B., Joshi, D., KC, S. P., Sharma, S., & Baral, S. (2024). Prevalence, determinants and care-seeking behaviour for anxiety and depression in

Nepalese population: A secondary analysis of data from Nepal Demographic and Health Survey. *BMJ Open, 14*(8), e078582. https://doi.org/10.1136/BMJOPEN-2023-078582

Powell-Jackson, T., Pereira, S. K., Dutt, V., Tougher, S., Haldar, K., & Kumar, P. (2016). Cash transfers, maternal depression and emotional well-being: Quasi-experimental evidence from India's Janani Suraksha Yojana programme. *Social Science & Medicine, 162*, 210–218. https://doi.org/10.1016/J.SOCSCIMED.2016.06.034

Rahman, A., Mubbashar, M. H., Gater, R., & Goldberg, D. (1998). Randomised trial of impact of school mental-health programme in rural Rawalpindi, Pakistan. *Lancet, 352*(9133), 1022–1025. https://doi.org/10.1016/S0140-6736(98)02381-2

Rahman, M. M., Rahman, M. M., Khan, M. M. A., Hasan, M., & Choudhury, K. N. (2020). Bullying victimization and adverse health behaviors among school-going adolescents in South Asia: Findings from the global school-based student health survey. *Depression and Anxiety, 37*(10), 995–1006. https://doi.org/10.1002/DA.23033

Rajan, S. I. (2023). Migration in South Asia: Old and new mobilities. *IMISCOE Research Series, Part F802,* 3–15. https://doi.org/10.1007/978-3-031-34194-6_1/FIGURES/2

Raman, V., & Thomas, S. (2023). School mental health program in India—Issues and possible practical solutions. *Indian Journal of Psychological Medicine, 45*(3), 283. https://doi.org/10.1177/02537176231165033

Reddy, V. M., & Chandrashekar, C. (1998). Prevalence of mental and behavioural disorders in India: A meta-analysis. *Indian Journal of Psychiatry, 40*(2), 149. https://pmc.ncbi.nlm.nih.gov/articles/PMC2965838/

Rishi, P., & John, H. (2024). Efficacy of positive parenting programme in addressing ADHD symptomatology and parental stress in Southern India. *Psychological Studies, 69*(2), 186–193. https://doi.org/10.1007/S12646-024-00785-3/METRICS

Khubsing, R. S. I., Daemen, I. K. S., Hendriks, L., van Emmerik, A. A. P., Shapiro, E., & Dekker, J. J. M. (2020). An EMDR group therapy for traumatized former child slaves in India: A pilot randomized controlled trial. *The International Journal of Indian Psychology* https://doi.org/10.25215/0803.082

Rose-Clarke, K., Prakash, B. K., Magar, J., Pradhan, I., Shrestha, P., Hassan, E., Jaoude, G. J. A., Haghparast-Bidgoli, H., Devakumar, D., Carrino, L., Floridi, G., Kohrt, B. A., Verdeli, H., Clougherty, K., Rafaeli, A. K., Jordans, M., & Luitel, N. P. (2022). School-based group interpersonal therapy for adolescents with depression in rural Nepal: A mixed methods study exploring feasibility, acceptability, and cost. *Global Mental Health, 9*, 416–428. https://doi.org/10.1017/GMH.2022.46

Roy, S., Hidrobo, M., Hoddinott, J. F., Koch, B., & Ahmed, A. (2019). Can transfers and behavior change communication reduce intimate partner violence four years post-program? *Experimental Evidence from Bangladesh.* https://doi.org/10.2499/P15738COLL2.133421

Sadath, A., Jose, K., Jiji, K., Mercy, V., Ragesh, G., & Arensman, E. (2022). Prevalence and determinants of substance use among indigenous tribes in South India: Findings from a tribal household survey. *Journal of Racial and Ethnic Health Disparities, 9*(1), 356–366. https://doi.org/10.1007/S40615-021-00964-2/TABLES/6

Sah, L. K., Hatzidimitriadou, E., Wier, J., & Sah, R. K. (2024). Social determinants of the mental health of pregnant women in Nepal: Stakeholder perspectives. *PLoS ONE, 19*(12), Article e0314736. https://doi.org/10.1371/JOURNAL.PONE.0314736

Shah, R., Gustafson, E., Dhaded, S., Herekar, V., Metgud, D., Mastiholi, S., Kim, H., Goudar, S., & Atkins, M. (2020). Integrating an adapted, low-intensity program to promote early childhood development in routine health visits in rural India: A feasibility study. *Journal of Developmental and Behavioral Pediatrics, 41*(4), 281–288. https://doi.org/10.1097/DBP.0000000000000763

Sharma, D. B., Gupta, V., Saxena, K., Shah, U. M., & Singh, U. S. (2020). Role of faith healers: A barrier or a support system to medical care- a cross sectional study. *Journal of Family Medicine and Primary Care, 9*(8), 4298. https://doi.org/10.4103/JFMPC.JFMPC_868_20

Sifat, M. S., Kenney, S., Bekteshi, V., Chiang, S. C., Ogunsanya, M., Boozary, L. K., Alexander, A. C., & Kendzor, D. E. (2024). The association of migration-related stress with poor mental health among recently resettled Afghan refugees. *Journal of Migration and Health, 10*, Article 100282. https://doi.org/10.1016/J.JMH.2024.100282

Silva, M., Loureiro, A., & Cardoso, G. (2016). Social determinants of mental health: A review of the evidence. *The European Journal of Psychiatry, 30*(4), 259–292. https://scielo.isciii.es/scielo.php?script=sci_arttext&pid=S0213-61632016000400004&lng=es&nrm=iso&tlng=en

Smith, J. L., Lipsky, S., Joyce Green, C., & Lora Erickson, M. (2024). *Traumatic stress in India 1 social construct of traumatic stress in India.*

Sreeramareddy, C. T., Pradhan, P. M. S., Mir, I. A., & Sin, S. (2014). Smoking and smokeless tobacco use in nine South and Southeast Asian countries: Prevalence estimates and social determinants from demographic and health surveys. *Population Health Metrics, 12*(1), 1–16. https://doi.org/10.1186/S12963-014-0022-0/TABLES/5

Stroope, S., Kent, B. V., Zhang, Y., Spiegelman, D., Kandula, N. R., Schachter, A. B., Kanaya, A., & Shields, A. E. (2022). Mental health and self-rated health among U.S. South Asians: The role of religious group involvement. *Ethnicity & Health, 27*(2), 388–406. https://doi.org/10.1080/13557858.2019.1661358

Tan, K. K. H., & Saw, A. T. W. (2023). Prevalence and correlates of mental health difficulties amongst LGBTQ people in Southeast Asia: A systematic review. *Journal of Gay & Lesbian Mental Health, 27*(4), 401–420. https://doi.org/10.1080/19359705.2022.2089427

Tay, A. K., Riley, A., Islam, R., Welton-Mitchell, C., Duchesne, B., Waters, V., Varner, A., Moussa, B., Mahmudul Alam, A. N. M., Elshazly, M. A., Silove, D., & Ventevogel, P. (2019). The culture, mental health and psychosocial wellbeing of Rohingya refugees: A systematic review. *Epidemiology and Psychiatric Sciences, 28*(5), 489. https://doi.org/10.1017/S2045796019000192

Thapa, R., van Teijlingen, E., Regmi, P. R., & Heaslip, V. (2021). Caste exclusion and health discrimination in South Asia: A systematic review. *Asia-Pacific Journal of Public Health, 33*(8), 828–838. https://doi.org/10.1177/10105395211014648/ASSET/IMAGES/LARGE/10.1177_10105395211014648-FIG1.JPEG

*The South Asian Paradox*. (n.d.). Retrieved December 22, 2024, from https://www.worldbank.org/en/news/feature/2012/10/25/south-asian-paradox

Thekkumkara, S., Rawat, V. S., Jagannathan, A., & Muliyala, K. P. (2024). Vocational rehabilitation in persons with mental illness in India: A scoping review. *The International Journal of Social Psychiatry, 70*(1), 13–22. https://doi.org/10.1177/00207640231183920

Thomson, R. M., Igelström, E., Purba, A. K., Shimonovich, M., Thomson, H., McCartney, G., Reeves, A., Leyland, A., Pearce, A., & Katikireddi, S. V. (2022). How do income changes impact on mental health and wellbeing for working-age adults? A systematic review and meta-analysis. *The Lancet. Public Health, 7*(6), e515–e528. https://doi.org/10.1016/S2468-2667(22)00058-5

Tol, W. A., Komproe, I. H., Jordans, M. J. D., Vallipuram, A., Sipsma, H., Sivayokan, S., MacY, R. D., & De Jong, J. T. (2012). Outcomes and moderators of a preventive school based mental health intervention for children affected by war in Sri Lanka: A cluster randomized trial. *World Psychiatry, 11*(2), 114–122. https://doi.org/10.1016/J.WPSYC.2012.05.008

Trivedi, G. Y., Pillai, N., & Trivedi, R. G. (2021). Adverse childhood experiences & mental health—The urgent need for public health intervention in India. *Journal of Preventive Medicine and Hygiene, 62*(3), E728. https://doi.org/10.15167/2421-4248/JPMH2021.62.3.1785

Venkatesh, U., Aparnavi, P., Mogan, K. A., Durga, R., Pearson, J., Kishore, S., Joshi, H. S., Nair, N. S., Nisha, B., Agrawal, R., Vidusha, K., Chenkual, C. V., Nath, B., Epari, V. R., Kumari, R., Goyal, P., Ahamed, F., Baruah, M., Anil, R., … Group, F. S. (2024). Determinants of substance use among young people attending primary health centers in India. *Cambridge Prisms: Global Mental Health, 11*, e23. https://doi.org/10.1017/GMH.2024.13

Vora, A. R., Yeoman, C. M., & Hayter, J. P. (2000). Alcohol, tobacco and paan use and understanding of oral cancer risk among Asian males in Leicester. *British Dental Journal, 188*(8), 444–451. https://doi.org/10.1038/sj.bdj.4800506

Weare, K., & Nind, M. (2011). Mental health promotion and problem prevention in schools: What does the evidence say? *Health Promotion International, 26*(suppl_1), i29–i69. https://doi.org/10.1093/HEAPRO/DAR075

Weaver, L. J., & Karasz, A. (2022). "Tension" and distress in South Asia: A systematic literature review. *SSM - Mental Health, 2*, Article 100092. https://doi.org/10.1016/J.SSMMH.2022.100092

Werner-Seidler, A., Perry, Y., Calear, A. L., Newby, J. M., & Christensen, H. (2017). School-based depression and anxiety prevention programs for young people: A systematic review and meta-analysis. *Clinical Psychology Review, 51*, 30–47. https://doi.org/10.1016/J.CPR.2016.10.005

World Report on Social Determinants of Health Equity. (2025). https://www.who.int/teams/social-determinants-of-health/equity-and-health/world-report-on-social-determinants-of-healthy-equity. Accessed on 27 July 2025.

Younas, A., Zeb, H., Arif, I., Khan, A., Ali, A., Ali, A., & Aziz, F. (2024). Sociocultural determinants of psychological distress and coping among South Asian individuals with chronic illness. *Discover Psychology, 4*(1), 1–18. https://doi.org/10.1007/S44202-024-00148-Z/TABLES/8

Zaneva, M., Guzman-Holst, C., Reeves, A., & Bowes, L. (2022). The impact of monetary poverty alleviation programs on children's and adolescents' mental health: A systematic review and meta-analysis across low-, middle-, and high-income countries. *Journal of Adolescent Health, 71*(2), 147–156. https://doi.org/10.1016/J.JADOHEALTH.2022.02.011

# Chapter 10
# Psychosocial Interventions for Mental Illness in South Asia

**Bheemsain Tekkalaki and Ekta Yadav**

**Abstract** Mental illness poses a significant disease burden in South Asia, affecting millions and contributing to substantial disability, economic loss, and social marginalization. The region faces high prevalence rates of depression, anxiety, schizophrenia, and substance use disorders, compounded by stigma, lack of mental health infrastructure, and socio-economic disparities. Limited access to psychiatric services, inadequate mental health policies, and cultural beliefs further exacerbate the crisis. Psychosocial interventions play a critical role in addressing mental health needs in South Asia which is affected by increase treatment gap due to scarcity of Mental health professionals. Community-based care, family interventions, peer support programs, and digital mental health solutions have shown promise in bridging the treatment gap. These interventions help improve patient outcomes by fostering social support, enhancing coping mechanisms, and reducing stigma. This chapter aims to explore the regional challenges and opportunities in mental healthcare, examine the existing psychosocial intervention models in the region, and to discuss the strategies to overcome barriers such as stigma, resource constraints, and policy gaps. The chapter also provides recommendations and future directions for strengthening mental health systems in South Asia through policy reforms, community engagement, and integration of psychosocial interventions into primary healthcare.

**Keywords** Psychosocial intervention · South Asia · Mental health · Evidence-based practices · Task sharing · Community-based practices · Mental health gap

## 1 Introduction

Mental illness is increasingly recognized as a leading contributor to the global disease burden, primarily in terms of disability rather than mortality (Global Burden of Disease Collaborative Network, 2022; Walker et al., 2015). Historically, mental

B. Tekkalaki (✉) · E. Yadav
Department of Psychiatry, KAHER's J.N Medical College, Belagavi, Karnataka, India
e-mail: drbheemsainvtekkalaki@jnmc.edu



S. M. Y. Arafat et al. (eds.), *Social Psychiatry in South Asia*, South Asian Perspectives in Mental Health and Psychology , https://doi.org/10.1007/978-981-96-8078-8_10

health has been overlooked in global health priorities, with services often neglected (Whiteford et al., 2013). The Lancet Commission on Global Mental Health and Sustainable Development underscores that mental health is a fundamental human right, critical to the growth and progress of all nations (Patel et al., 2018). In 2019, an estimated 1 in 8 people worldwide—around 970 million individuals—were affected by mental disorders, highlighting the urgent need to expand services and ensure equitable access to care (Institute of Health Metrics and Evaluation, 2022). This issue is particularly pronounced in South Asia, where mental illness impacts approximately 14.2% (12.9% to 15.7%) for Common Mental Disorder (Naveed et al., 2020). This is slightly higher compared to the worldwide-pooled prevalence of mental disorders which is 13.4% (Polanczyk et al., 2015).

The South Asian region, comprising eight countries (Afghanistan, Bangladesh, Bhutan, India, Maldives, Nepal, Pakistan and Sri Lanka., is home to approximately 24% of the world's population. Seven of the eight south Asian countries are mostly comprised of low- and middle-income countries (LMIC) as classified by the World Bank (Arafat & Kar, 2024; Mudunna et al., 2025). The region presents a complex tapestry of mental health challenges due to its distinct cultural, social, and economic profiles. With a population of over 1.8 billion people from diverse linguistic, ethnic, and religious backgrounds, a tailored approach is essential to address mental health disorders in each region.

Mental health disorders have multiple underlying etiological factors: biological factors, such as genetics and neurochemistry, psychological factors, including trauma, stress, and coping mechanisms, and socio-environmental factors, such as social support, education, and socio-economic status, can either exacerbate or mitigate mental health problems (Porter, 2020).

While pharmacotherapy and psychotherapy are widely practiced treatment modalities for mental illness in the Western world, their usefulness can be limited in diverse cultural contexts. Medication may alleviate symptoms globally, but it doesn't address the unique social, economic, and cultural needs of individuals from different regions, including South Asia. Given the region's distinct socio-cultural landscape, a more holistic approach is necessary.

The balanced care model recommends that mental health systems incorporate both community-based and hospital-based care (Thornicroft & Tansella, 2013). Since the aetiology of mental health disorder is complex, involving biological, psychological, and social factors. To achieve mental well-being, it is essential to address these factors and foster balance across all domains. Psychosocial interventions are hence crucial component of this approach, playing a vital role in preventing and managing mental health disorders, as they align with the principles of personal recovery, emphasizing the attainment of a fulfilling and valued life (Asher et al., 2017). By combining medication with psychosocial interventions, mental healthcare can address the complex needs of individuals, promoting holistic recovery and well-being.

The term "psychosocial" is derived from two distinct disciplines: psychology and sociology. Psychology is the scientific study of human behaviour and mental processes, encompassing thoughts, behaviours, and emotions. Sociology, on the other hand, examines how humans interact with one another within their social environments, which can have positive, neutral, or negative impacts. The integration of these two fields gives rise to the concept "psychosocial", which recognizes the dynamic interplay between individual psychological processes and social environmental factors.

In the context of mental health, interventions aim to prevent harm, improve functioning, or intentionally influence a situation to achieve a desired outcome (Institute of Medicine, 2015). Psychosocial interventions, in particular, involve targeted psychological or social actions designed to produce positive changes in various outcomes, including: Psychological outcomes (e.g., reduced symptoms, improved mood), Social outcomes (e.g., enhanced relationships, increased social support), Biological outcomes (e.g., improved sleep, reduced stress), and Functional outcomes (e.g., improved daily functioning, increased productivity) (Institute of Medicine, 2015). Hence, Psychosocial interventions are defined as, *"interpersonal or informational activities, techniques, or strategies that target biological, behavioural, cognitive, emotional, interpersonal, social, or environmental factors with the aim of improving health functioning and well-being*" (Institute of Medicine, 2015). Psychosocial interventions can be broken down into three primary components: action, mediators, and outcomes as shown in Table 1.

Psychosocial interventions can be delivered by a diverse range of trained and supervised professionals like mental health specialists (psychologists, psychiatrists, social workers, counsellors/therapists), primary care and other nonpsychiatric physicians, nurses, allied health professionals (physical and occupational therapists), community-based providers (religious leaders, lay and peer providers, paraprofessionals and caregivers), and automated providers (e.g., Internet/audio/video-delivered interventions).

Psychosocial interventions can benefit a wide range of individuals, including—those at risk of or experiencing prodromal symptoms of an illness, individuals with acute disorders, individuals in remission, maintenance, or recovery phases of mental health disorders, and individuals who are not ill but are challenged by daily functioning, relationship problems, life events, or psychological adjustment (Institute of Medicine, 2015). This diverse range of providers and target populations highlights the flexibility and adaptability of psychosocial interventions in addressing various mental health needs.

While there is no universally accepted categorization of psychosocial interventions, the term encompasses a broad spectrum of intervention types, including: psychotherapies (e.g., psychodynamic therapy, cognitive-behavioural therapy (CBT), interpersonal psychotherapy (IPT), problem-solving therapy, community-based treatment (e.g., assertive community treatment, first episode psychosis interventions); vocational rehabilitation, peer support services, and integrated care interventions. These interventions are rooted in diverse theoretical models, including: psychodynamic, behavioural, social justice, attachment, recovery, and strength-based theories. Each theoretical orientation encompasses a range of intervention approaches, reflecting the complexity and nuance of psychosocial interventions (Institute of Medicine, 2015). While the core principles remain the same, the implementation and emphasis can vary significantly across different regions and cultures.

**Table 1** Three primary components of psychosocial interventions

| Action | Mediators | Outcomes |
|---|---|---|
| Specific activities, techniques, or strategies are employed to deliver the intervention. These actions can be:<br>a. Interpersonal: delivered through a relationship between a practitioner and a client,<br>b. Informational: presented through various media, such as bibliotherapy, internet-based therapies, or biofeedback | Mediators explain how the action of psychosocial interventions leads to specific outcomes. These mediators can involve changes in biological, behavioural, cognitive, emotional, interpersonal, social, or environmental factors (Kraemer et al., 2002) | The outcomes of psychosocial interventions encompass desired changes in three key areas:<br>a. Symptoms: reduction or alleviation of physical and mental health symptoms<br>b. Functioning: improvement in performing daily activities, such as: physical activity, activities of daily living, assigned tasks in school and work, maintaining intimate and peer relationships, raising a family, and Community involvement<br>c. Well-being: enhancement of: spirituality life satisfaction, quality of life, recovery, and self-directed living. By understanding these components, practitioners can design and deliver effective psychosocial interventions that promote positive change and improve overall well-being |

Such interventions can be integrated into health, protection, community, and other settings and used together with other forms of mental health support.

South Asia has a long history of traditional medicine systems that have been employed to promote mental well-being. Have been adapted and modified over time to address the unique mental health needs of the region. For centuries, traditional practices and religious customs have played a significant role in managing mental illness in South Asia. Communities have employed various methods and treatment by ancient systems of medicine, to care for individuals with mental health conditions Asylums or mental hospitals came with the British rule in India and colonization in other South Asian countries (Thara & Padmavati, 2013). Even today, people with mental illness often seek traditional, alternative, and complementary medicine, either before or after consulting biomedicine providers (Kleinman, 1980). In India, the Ministry of AYUSH recognizes seven systems of medicine, including Ayurveda, yoga, and naturopathy (Institute of Medicine, 2015). While these traditional approaches have are widely accepted in this region, the research to establish their effectiveness is still in preliminary stage. In contrast, the modern psychosocial interventions offer structured and evidence-based strategies but—lack the wider reach in the region, contrary to the western world. The influence of Western psychiatric models has grown in South Asia since colonial times, with modern mental healthcare systems increasingly adopting Western approaches. However, cultural adaptation and integration of western approaches with traditional practices remain essential for effective mental healthcare in the region. The development of effective and accessible mental health systems in Southeast Asia will thus require evidence-based culturally appropriate psychological and social interventions (Maramis et al., 2011). This chapter provides an in depth exploration of:

- **Regional Challenges and Opportunities:** Unique considerations and prospects for psychosocial interventions in Southeast Asia.
- **Social Intervention Models:** Examining prevention, promotion, and rehabilitation/recovery strategies that are experimented or delivered in South Asia.
- **Overcoming Barriers:** Identifying and addressing obstacles to implementing effective psychosocial interventions.
- **Recommendations and Future Directions:** Expert guidance on optimizing psychosocial interventions for mental health in South Asia.

## 2 Unique Challenges and Opportunities of Psychosocial Interventions in South Asia

Psychosocial factors, including positive social connections, safe communities, and quality education, play a crucial role in protecting against mental ill health, as highlighted in the WHO's 2022 report. (World Health Organization, 2022) Furthermore, a wealth of evidence from randomized controlled trials and meta-analyses has established the efficacy of psychosocial interventions in mitigating mental health issues (Barth et al., 2013; Cuijpers et al., 2010a, 2010b, 2011, 2013; Institute of Medicine, 2006). In high-income countries, community-based psychosocial interventions are commonly utilized for managing psychiatric disorders, yielding positive outcomes such as reduced symptoms, relapse rates, and hospital admissions, as well as improved overall functioning (McDonagh et al., 2021; Ventriglio et al., 2020).

Despite the proven efficacy of psychosocial interventions, their implementation in real-world settings is often fraught with challenges. One of the most pressing grand challenges for global mental health is to provide effective and affordable community-based care and rehabilitation. However, this goal remains elusive for the vast majority of people living with mental illness in LMICs, which includes South Asian countries (Collins et al., 2011).

This section will delve into the specific barriers and facilitators that impede the effective implementation of psychosocial interventions in South Asian countries. By examining these challenges, we can better understand the complexities of integrating psychosocial interventions into mental healthcare systems in this region.

South Asia faces unique challenges due to the region's diverse cultural, social, and economic landscape. These Barriers and facilitators operate at different levels, from the individual patient level, through to organizational difficulties (Bird et al., 2022).

## *2.1 Challenges*

### 2.1.1 Treatment Gap

The treatment gap (difference between the number of people that need care and receive care) for mental health disorders is starkly evident when comparing low-income countries to their high-income counterparts (World Health Organization, 2023). A staggering 76–85% of individuals with mental disorders in low-income countries receive no treatment, whereas this number is significantly lower in high-income countries, ranging from 35–50%. (World Health Organization, 2020a, 2020b) This disparity is particularly pronounced in South Asia, where approximately 150–200 million people live with diagnosed psychiatric disorders, yet face severe limitations in accessing mental health services (Arafat & Kar, 2024; Thara & Padmavati, 2013) The treatment gap in this region is estimated to be as high as 90% (Gururaj et al., 2016; World Health Organization, 2016) Chronic underinvestment and a severe shortage of mental health facilities and specialists further perpetuate this crisis, denying millions of people access to evidence-based treatments (Kakuma et al., 2011).

### 2.1.2 Limited Research

One of the significant challenges in implementing psychosocial interventions in South Asia is the limited research and data on mental health prevalence. The rates of mental health disorders in this region are typically under-reported due to data scarcity, and there is a significantly more limited focus on the treatment of mental health disorders in these countries (World Health Organization, 2016). Furthermore, the available data are often skewed, with most studies originating from India, while evidence from countries such as Afghanistan, Bhutan, and Maldives is particularly limited (Vidyasagaran et al., 2023). This scarcity of data is particularly pronounced among adolescents, with many South Asian countries lacking prevalence data on mental health issues in this age group (Mudunna et al., 2025). As a result, the available data often provide only a partial picture, limited to adult populations, specific communities, or aggregated at the country level. This lack of representative data hinders accurate assessment of mental health needs.

### 2.1.3 Insufficient Budget Allocation

A critical challenge in implementing psychosocial interventions in South Asia is the grossly inadequate allocation of government health funding to mental health. Alarmingly, as per Mental Health Atlas 2020 of SAARC countries less than 1% of the total national budgets in South Asian Association for Regional Cooperation (SAARC) countries, except Afghanistan (4.2%), is dedicated to mental health (Grover, 2023; World Health Organization, 2016, 2017, 2020a, 2020b). This severe budget constraint hinders the development and implementation of effective psychosocial interventions.

### 2.1.4 Severe Shortage of Mental Health Professionals

The implementation of psychosocial interventions in South Asia is severely hindered by a crippling shortage of trained mental health professionals (Issac, 2013). A staggering reality is that all SAARC countries, except Maldives (3.2 per 100,000), have less than one psychiatrist per 100,000 population, as revealed by the World Health Organization's Mental Health Atlas 2020 (Grover, 2023). This scarcity is compounded by a dire shortage of clinical psychologists, social workers, and other specialized professionals (Trivedi et al., 2007).

Furthermore, the health systems in these countries are constrained by chronic shortages of motivated and adequately trained staff, inadequate budgets, and insufficient resources, including irregular supply of drugs, lack of transportation, non-functioning equipment, and poor organization and management (Issac, 2013). This perfect storm of shortages and systemic weaknesses poses a significant challenge to delivering effective psychosocial interventions, leaving a vast treatment gap, and exacerbating the mental health crisis in the region.

### 2.1.5 Policies

Another challenge is the lack of prioritization of mental health disorders in national policies. Despite the existence of national mental health policies in most South Asian countries, their effective implementation remains a substantial hurdle (Sharan et al., 2017). The region's policies aim to promote community-based care, integrate mental health into primary care, ensure access to medication, and uphold human rights. However, the implementation of these policies varies widely across countries. While some nations, such as Bangladesh, Bhutan, Pakistan, India, and Sri Lanka, have made progress in implementing these components, others, like Nepal, focus on providing minimal care, and Maldives lacks a policy altogether (Thara & Padmavati, 2013). This inconsistent policy landscape and implementation gap pose significant challenges to delivering effective psychosocial interventions in the region.

South Asia's mental health landscape is marked by a stark contradiction: despite the existence of national mental health policies in most South Asian countries, the available services remain grossly under-utilized (Issac, 2013; Sharan et al., 2017).

The presence of policies alone is insufficient; their successful execution is crucial to ensuring that mental health services are accessible and utilized by those in need. Unfortunately, the gap between policy and practice remains a substantial hurdle in South Asia's mental healthcare system. Possible reasons contributing to this disparity include: difficult to access mental healthcare by people living in rural areas, stigma, lack of awareness and education, superstitious belief and high reliance on faith healers, hence South Asians frequently suffer in silence. In the subsequent sections, we review these hurdles in detail:

Stigma, culture influence, and preference for faith healers **are important reasons for under-utilization of the Policies.** The concept of stigma has its roots in ancient Greece, where it originally referred to a tattoo that marked slaves or criminals, signifying their diminished value in society (Arboleda-Flórez & Stuart, 2012). According to Erving Goffman, stigma can be broadly categorized into three types: physical deformities, blemishes of character such as mental health conditions or criminality, and tribal origin, which encompasses factors like race, nationality, caste, or religion (Goffman, 1963). Mental health stigma is a pervasive issue globally, severely impacting the quality of life for person with mental illnesses (PwMIs). In many Asian societies, mental health issues are stigmatized, perceived as a personal weakness or failure of self-control, bringing shame to the family, often attributed to karma, or poor upbringing, leading to social isolation and discrimination (Ahad et al., 2023). Experiments in the fields of cognitive and social psychology show that the use of such stereotypes is highly automatic, based on dominant cultural beliefs of the person or family in society or the workplace (Kohrt et al., 2018). Cultural factors in South Asia significantly contribute to the perpetuation of stigma, with varying beliefs and myths surrounding mental illness across different countries (Vaishnav et al., 2023). For instance: In Nepal and India, mental illness is often attributed to spiritual incompetency or sin and faith healing and religious coping are more prevalent, leading to greater stigma vs the Western world, where the medical model of illness is more acceptable (Gupta et al., 2013; Vaishnav et al., 2023). A recent qualitative study conducted in Pakistan shed light on the perceptions of caregivers of individuals with psychosis, revealing that many attributed their condition to spiritual and social factors, such as relationship breakdowns. Thus, significantly impacted help-seeking behaviours, with a preference for non-medical interventions (Rathod et al., 2023). Mental illness illiteracy which leads to a huge number of people avoiding bio-medical therapy and instead seeking aid from traditional and religious healers (Aswini & Deb, 2020). In many cultures, mental illness is attributed to paranormal activities, magic, and religious beliefs, rather than being recognized as a medical condition. This misconception leads to a decreased perceived need for medical treatment, exacerbating the mental health crisis. Alarmingly, these attitudes and myths are not limited to the general public, but can also be found among well-educated individuals, including medical students, who may be unaware of or misunderstand the medical model of mental illnesses (Vaishnav et al., 2023). The widespread stigma surrounding mental illness hinders the effective implementation of psychosocial interventions, exacerbating the mental health crisis in South Asian countries and leads to devastating consequences, including:

- Delayed treatment-seeking behaviour, allowing conditions to worsen (Grover, 2023; Vaishnav et al., 2023).
- Social isolation and discrimination, exacerbating feelings of loneliness, and rejection.
- Reduced treatment adherence, hindering recovery and worsening prognosis.
- Perpetuation of misconceptions, reinforcing harmful stereotypes and myths.
- Influence of gender on stigma, with gender-specific stereotypes and expectations exacerbating the stigma experienced by individuals.

These detrimental effects not only harm individuals but also perpetuate a cycle of stigma, making it even more challenging to address mental health issues and promote overall well-being (Ahad et al., 2023; Javed et al., 2021; Thornicroft et al., 2022). Unfortunately, research on mental health stigma in SAARC countries is limited, highlighting the need for further study and awareness (Javed et al., 2021; Kohrt et al., 2018).

**Another important issue is** Lack of awareness and education which is a significant contributor to misconceptions and stigma surrounding mental health. A study conducted in India and Pakistan highlighted the devastating consequences of ignorance and misconceptions. The study reported two alarming cases: one patient was forcibly confined for 18 years due to their family's lack of understanding about mental health issues, while another patient was coerced into stopping their medication by their attendant. These stories emphasize the urgent need for awareness, education, and empathy to break down the barriers surrounding mental health and promote better treatment adherence and overall well-being (Bird et al., 2022).

### 2.1.6 Urban–rural Disparities and Difficulty in Accessing Appropriate Care

India's mental health infrastructure is woefully inadequate, with only 42 mental hospitals catering to a mere 20% of the population, primarily in urban areas (Thara & Padmavati, 2013). This leaves the vast rural areas without access to any mental health services. Despite efforts to expand mental health services, several districts remain uncovered by the District Mental Health Program (DMHP), resulting in limited access to community-level mental healthcare (Kirpekar V et al., 2024). The poorly financed mental health services are inaccessible to the most deprived sections of society, creating a vulnerable population that is more susceptible to mental illness and stigma (Vaishnav et al., 2023).

### 2.1.7 Insurance

The Mental Health Care Act of 2017 (MHCA 2017) aims to provide a legal framework for improving mental healthcare services and promoting mental health equity in India. A key aspect of this legislation is providing mental health insurance coverage to reduce financial barriers to mental healthcare. Section 21, Clause 4 of the Act mandates insurers to provide medical insurance for mental illness treatment on the same basis as physical illness treatment. Additionally, the Insurance Regulatory and Development Authority of India (IRDAI) has issued circulars instructing insurers to comply with MHCA 2017 and provide mental health insurance coverage, and to disclose their underwriting philosophy and approach on their websites. Insurance Regulatory and Development Authority of India (2018). A review by Avula et al., (2024) of 235 health insurance policies in India found that 37.5% covered mental illnesses, 11.5% covered persons with disabilities, but 51% did not offer mental health coverage. Significant gaps were identified, including the exclusion of suicide and substance use disorders, disparities in outpatient care, and extended waiting periods for mental health coverage. The review recommends aligning insurance practices with the Mental Health Care Act 2017 to promote mental health equity in India. Despite the policy provisions outlined in the Mental Healthcare Act (MHCA) 2017, the current status of insurance coverage for mental health issues remains unclear. Furthermore, the extent to which these policy changes benefit marginalized populations and the actual impact on mental healthcare outcomes are unknown, warranting further investigation and assessment.

Poor coverage by insurance and government institutes. Mental health services mainly rely on private NGOs and organizations. There is often a poor organization, distribution, and utilization of services/resources for delivering mental health services (Vaishnav et al., 2023). Additionally, logistical difficulties such as long distances and high costs of services hinder access to mental healthcare, further exacerbating the existing gaps in the system (Bird et al., 2022).

### 2.1.8 World vs South Asia

South Asia lack clarity on which mental health interventions are most effective in this region. Furthermore, many international services have been criticized for being culturally insensitive and failing to integrate with local communities (Seponski et al., 2014). The majority of psychological and social mental health interventions, such as CBT, were developed in high-income countries with Western cultures, which may limit their effectiveness in South Asia. This is because emotional distress is experienced and communicated differently in various social contexts, highlighting the need for culturally adapted interventions that take into account the unique cultural nuances of Southeast Asia (Maddock et al., 2021).

### 2.1.9 Buy in or Acceptance of the Interventions

Clinician attitudes play a crucial role in the successful implementation of new interventions, and can either facilitate or hinder progress. Older psychiatrists may be hesitant to adopt new approaches due to their existing experiences.

Furthermore, creating awareness about non-pharmacological approaches is essential, not only among clinicians but also among patients and their families (Bird et al., 2022).

#### 2.1.10 Case Load and Time Constraints

High caseloads and time constraints were major barriers to implementing psychosocial interventions, according to the majority of clinicians. With limited time during routine consultations, clinicians felt that delivering structured psychosocial interventions was impractical, especially in acute presentations or busy outpatient departments (OPDs). The time required to deliver these interventions was a significant concern, as it would impact the rest of the caseload. This challenge was particularly pronounced in large government-run hospitals and OPDs, where staffs were expected to see a high volume of patients daily, with typically only 10 min allocated per patient. As a result, pharmacological approaches tended to dominate, overshadowing psychosocial interventions. Structural factors at the facilities: privacy was noted to be a challenge, and one that occurred across all facilities (Bird et al., 2022).

### *2.2 Opportunities*

As described in previous sections, numerous barriers hinder the effective implementation of psychosocial interventions in South Asia. At the organizational level, challenges include inadequate research, poor infrastructure, ineffective policies, a shortage of psychiatrists, lack of insurance coverage for psychiatric disorders, and limited budget allocations. Furthermore, individual-level barriers such as lack of awareness, stigma, and reliance on faith healers or traditional practices also exist. Rural populations face significant difficulties in accessing care, while psychiatrists struggle with heavy caseloads and time constraints. Having acknowledged these challenges, we can now shift our focus to exploring the various opportunities present in South Asia for the effective implementation of psychosocial interventions.

#### 2.2.1 A Task-Shifting Model

The scarcity of specialist mental health workers in South Asia presents a significant challenge, but also offers an opportunity for innovation. A task-shifting model, which leverages non-specialist workers such as lay health workers, peer support workers, and nursing staff without psychiatric training, can help bridge this gap (Maddock et al., 2021; Nimgaonkar & Menon, 2015). By delegating specific tasks to these workers, the burden on specialist mental health professionals can be alleviated, and the reach of mental health services can be expanded. This approach not only addresses the shortage of mental health specialists but also presents a unique opportunity for psychosocial interventions to make a meaningful impact in South Asia (Lyles et al., 2023; van Ginneken et al., 2013). By harnessing the potential of task-shifting, psychosocial interventions can be delivered more widely, increasing access to care and ultimately reducing the treatment gap in the region.

Psychosocial interventions offer a vital alternative for individuals who cannot undergo medication treatment, such as pregnant women, young children, and those with complex medical conditions. Additionally, these interventions can play a crucial role in enhancing medication compliance, addressing social and interpersonal issues, and facilitating comprehensive recovery from mental health and substance use disorders.

### 2.2.2 Community-Based Care: Establishing a Specialized Cadre of Community Health Workers (CHWs) to Address the Growing Burden Mental Health Conditions in SAARC Countries

South Asia has a long history of leveraging community health workers (CHWs) to bring healthcare services closer to communities (Riaz & Jindal, 2024; Shrestha et al., 2023) According to Scott et al., (2017) CHWs are health workers based in communities, conducting outreach from their homes or peripheral health posts, who are not professionals, and have received fewer than two years of training. Today, all South Asian countries have active cadres of CHWs, constituting a substantial proportion of the healthcare workforce: nearly half of the total health workforce in Pakistan, India, and Bangladesh (Aye et al., 2018; Mubin et al., 2021). In Nepal, there are almost three times as many Female Community Health Volunteers (FCHVs) as physicians, nurses, and midwives combined. CHWs play a vital role in bridging the gap between the community and the formal health system, they are engaged in various roles, including health promotion, disease prevention, surveillance, and providing limited curative care (Shrestha et al., 2023). With high-quality training, CHWs can effectively provide psychosocial interventions, addressing the mental health needs of their communities. Studies have shown that high-quality training can achieve a high level of knowledge among CHWs, regardless of their level of education (Mubin et al., 2021). With over two million CHWs deployed in South Asia, their potential impact on healthcare outcomes is significant. South Asian countries utilize distinct terminology for CHWs, as shown in Table 2 (Modified from Shrestha et al., 2023).

**Specialist community health workers:** In response to the COVID-19 pandemic, specialist community health workers (CHWs) were introduced, marking a significant milestone in India's healthcare landscape. Notably, India has pioneered two innovative CHW models: SEVAK (Sanitation and Health, Education in Village communities through improved Awareness and Knowledge of Prevention/Management of Diseases and Health Promotion) and SATHI (Surgical Accredited and Trained Healthcare Initiative). While SEVAK focuses on preventing diabetes and hypertension, SATHI has demonstrated remarkable success in addressing unmet surgical needs, with CHWs converting 60% of unmet surgical needs through culturally sensitive, low-cost training (Riaz & Jindal, 2024). Furthermore, a community-based

**Table 2** Community health worker terminology across South Asian countries

| S. No | Country | Terms |
|---|---|---|
| 1 | Bangladesh | • Family Welfare Assistant<br>• Health Assistant<br>• Community Healthcare Provider<br>• Shasthya Shebika<br>• Shasthya Karmi |
| 2 | India | • Accredited Social Health Activist<br>• Multi-Purpose Health Worker- Female (Auxiliary Nurse Midwife)<br>• Anganwadi Worker |
| 3 | Nepal | • Female Community Health Volunteer<br>• Auxiliary Nurse Midwife<br>• Auxiliary Health Worker<br>• Health Assistant |
| 4 | Pakistan | • Lady Health Worker<br>• Marvi Worker<br>• Community Midwives<br>• Traditional Birth Attendant<br>• Reproductive Health Volunteer |
| 5 | Sri Lanka | • Public Health Midwife<br>• Public Health Inspector<br>• Public Health Nursing Sister<br>• Health Volunteer<br>• Health Assistant |

program in rural India has shown substantial improvements in equitable contact coverage for depression and enhanced mental health literacy (Shidhaye et al., 2017). Currently, India is the only SAARC country to have implemented specialist CHWs as depicted in Table 3 (Modified from Riaz & Jindal, 2024).

A community-initiated approach to care offers a promising solution to connect with individuals who may be hesitant to seek help due to fear, stigma, financial constraints, or distrust of the formal healthcare system (Siddiqui et al., 2022).

**Table 3** Specialist community health workers in South Asian countries

| Sr. no | Country | Child and maternal CHWs | Surgical CHWs | Mental CHWs | NCD CHWs |
|---|---|---|---|---|---|
| 1 | Pakistan | Yes (LHWs) | No | No | No |
| 2 | Nepal | Yes (FCHVs) | No | No | No |
| 3 | Bangladesh | Yes (SS) | No | No | No |
| 4 | India | Yes (ASHAs) | Yes (SATHIs) | Yes | Yes (SEVAKs) |

ASHA, Accredited Social Health Activists; FCHV, Female Community Health Volunteers ; LHW, Lady Health Worker; SATHI, Surgical Accredited and Trained Healthcare Initiative; SEVAK, Sanitation and Health, Education in Village communities through improved Awareness and Knowledge of Prevention/Management of Diseases and Health Promotion; SS, Shashthya Shebikas

### 2.2.3 Traditional Healers

In developing countries, like South Asia traditional healers play a significant role in addressing mental health concerns, often in conjunction with conventional psychiatric services (Familiar et al., 2013; Kapur, 1979; Razali, 2000; Varghese et al., 2011; Wig et al., 1980). Their appeal lies in their shared cultural perspective, which enables them to tap into indigenous knowledge, beliefs, and practices (World Health Organization, 2000). This cultural resonance is particularly important in areas where formal psychiatric services are scarce or unaffordable. Traditional healers' understanding of spiritual and religious models of illness causation, which are deeply rooted in local cultures, allows them to provide psychosocial interventions that are contextually relevant and effective. The "Dava-Dua" (Medicine-Prayer) intervention, launched in 2008 by the Government of Gujarat in India, combines psychiatric treatment with faith healing at the Mira Datar Dargah, implemented in partnership with Altruist, an Ahmedabad-based organization. A study (Saha et al., 2021) in Gujarat, India, found this model to be beneficial, particularly for patients with limited access to mental healthcare. It complements primary healthcare services and protects patients' human rights. The WHO defines traditional medicine as a practice that is deeply rooted in the cultural heritage of indigenous communities, "based on experiences indigenous to different cultures" and typically having a "long history" (World Health Organization, 2013). Additionally, Nortje et al., (2016) provide a nuanced operational definition of traditional healers, characterizing them as practitioners who "explicitly appeal to spiritual, magical, or religious explanations for disease and distress"· These definitions collectively highlight the distinctive cultural and philosophical underpinnings of traditional healing practices.

Cultural variations significantly influence the perception and experience of mental illness. In many cultures, wellness is intricately linked to social and spiritual harmony, rather than solely focused on psychopathology. Traditional healers' rituals of symbolic healing can have a profound impact on individuals and communities, promoting catharsis, cognitive restructuring, and restoration of social cohesion (Kirmayer, 2004; Nortje et al., 2016).

These healers often possess a unique understanding of their patients' experiences, identifying individuals with mental health conditions, albeit with different terminology and explanations. This suggests that traditional healers are, in fact, treating patients with psychiatric disorders similar to those diagnosed in conventional medicine. By acknowledging the value of traditional healing practices, we can foster a more inclusive and culturally sensitive approach to mental healthcare (Sorsdahl et al., 2010). By leveraging their unique position within the community, traditional healers can facilitate help-seeking behaviours, provide emotional support, and offer culturally sensitive care that addresses the complex interplay between psychological, social, and spiritual factors. As such, traditional healers represent a valuable resource for mental healthcare, particularly in resource-constrained settings. Research indicates that traditional healing methods have limited impact on chronic illnesses like schizophrenia and obsessive–compulsive disorder. However, they may be effective in addressing common mental disorders such as depression, anxiety, and somatisation, with outcomes comparable to primary psychiatric care. This aligns with modern psychiatric guidelines, which recommend psychosocial interventions as first-line treatment for common mental disorders (Nortje et al., 2016).

### 2.2.4 Yoga

Yoga has its roots in ancient India, dating back over 3000 years. This holistic system was designed to promote harmony within oneself, integrating the physical, emotional, and intellectual aspects, while also fostering a harmonious relationship with nature (Satyananda, 2002). Patanjali's sutras describe yoga's main objective is to 'calm down the agitations of the mind' (Bhargav et al., 2023). Yoga, traditionally a spiritual discipline, has evolved into a promising complementary therapy for managing and preventing mental disorders over the past two decades. Free from stigma, yoga therapy has gained global popularity, offering numerous advantages. These include easy access to trained professionals, cost-effectiveness, and the flexibility of group sessions. Moreover, yoga can serve as a valuable community-based intervention, providing holistic mental healthcare, promoting mental well-being, and preventing mental illness (Varambally et al., 2020). Adopting a yoga-based lifestyle has been shown to effectively reduce psychological stress, as demonstrated by various studies (Cocchiara et al., 2019). A systematic review and meta-analysis of 19 studies (1080 participants) examined the effectiveness of physically active yoga in reducing depressive symptoms in people with diagnosed mental disorders. Results showed that yoga significantly reduced depressive symptoms compared to control groups. The frequency of yoga sessions per week was also found to be associated with greater reductions in depressive symptoms (Brinsley et al., 2021). A meta-analysis of 6 studies (405 pregnant women) found that yoga-based interventions significantly reduced symptoms of maternal depression during pregnancy (Ng et al., 2019). A systematic review and meta-analysis of 15 studies (1081 patients) found that mind-body therapies like yoga, tai-chi, qi-gong, and mindfulness may help reduce negative symptoms of schizophrenia. Mindfulness-based and yoga interventions showed the most promise, but the evidence is still limited and more research is needed to confirm these findings (Sabe et al., 2019). The growing popularity of yoga, coupled with the rise of tele-yoga, has increased its accessibility and acceptability, freeing it from stigma. Despite its potential, research on yoga's role in preventive psychiatry remains limited, highlighting the need for further investigation. Bhargav et al. (2023) discussed the rationale and latest evidence base for the use of yoga in psychiatric practice, including the neurobiological mechanisms and indications, and contraindications for yoga therapy. Hence reflecting the importance of yoga in implementation of psychosocial intervention.

### 2.2.5 Family-Centric Approach for Psychosocial Intervention in South Asia

In South Asia, where family ties are strong and collectivist values prevail, a family-centric approach to psychosocial intervention is particularly effective. This approach recognizes the family as a vital support system for individuals with mental health issues, rather than just focusing on the individual. By involving family members in the intervention process, this approach fosters a supportive environment, promotes emotional expression, and encourages collaborative problem-solving. Studies have shown that family-centric interventions can lead to improved treatment outcomes, increased family cohesion, and enhanced overall well-being. In India and neighbouring countries, the collective society plays a vital role in supporting individuals with mental illness. Family members serve as primary caregivers, fostering an environment of interdependence and mutual concern. The unique aspect of the Indian family system, as noted by Chadda et al. significantly contributes to the recovery of persons with mental illness (PMI), distinguishing it from Western approaches (Chadda & Deb, 2013).

Maladaptive family dynamics and high expressed emotions can significantly increase the perceived burden on caregivers, ultimately impacting their ability to provide effective care. In such cases, family interventions and psychoeducational approaches can be highly beneficial. By addressing unhealthy communication patterns, reducing stress, and promoting a supportive environment, these interventions can help alleviate caregiver burden and enhance overall family functioning (Chadda & Deb, 2013).

### 2.2.6 Family Structures and Family-Based Interventions

Complex family dynamics can be both supportive and obstructive to mental healthcare. Due to strong family ties, Family therapy: Addressing intergenerational dynamics. Parent-child interventions: Enhancing communication. Couples therapy: Strengthening marital relationships. Multigenerational support: Involving grandparents. Family education helps reduce stigma. Engaging family members in mental healthcare, addressing complex family dynamics (Chadda & Deb, 2013).

### 2.2.7 Person-Centric Approach

Person-centred planning is a vital psychosocial intervention in South Asia, offering a holistic approach to addressing mental health needs. This approach prioritizes the individual's unique circumstances, needs, and strengths, fostering a collaborative partnership between the client and clinician. Unlike conventional management, which focuses solely on symptom reduction, person-centred planning considers the broader context of the individual's life, including co-morbidities, psychosocial aspects, and personal dignity. A study by Trivedi et al., (2012) investigated client satisfaction with person-centred management approaches in individuals with schizophrenia. The findings revealed significantly higher levels of client satisfaction with person-centred management compared to conventional approaches, underscoring the effectiveness of this holistic and client-centred strategy. In South Asia, where mental health resources are scarce, person-centred planning provides a valuable framework for delivering comprehensive, client-centred care. By acknowledging the individual's autonomy and agency, this approach empowers clients to take an active role in their recovery, promoting resilience and overall well-being.

### 2.2.8 Digital Mental Health

The widespread adoption of mobile devices in Asia, with approximately 75% of the population using smartphones, presents a significant opportunity for implementing psychosocial interventions through digital health technologies (DHTs) (Groupe Speciale Mobile Association, 2022). Despite challenges such as unreliable internet access, limited digital literacy, and regulatory concerns, leveraging DHTs can enhance the reach and accessibility of mental health services in South Asia. For instance, telepsychiatry guidelines and tele-mental health centres of excellence are being established in countries like India, demonstrating the potential for digital technology to support and regulate service development (Issac, 2013; Thornicroft et al., 2022; Vaishnav et al., 2023). Moreover, digital platforms can facilitate training and supervision for healthcare professionals, improve documentation and data collection, and enable remote access to specialized care. By harnessing the power of digital technology, it is possible to overcome traditional barriers to mental healthcare, such as stigma and geographical constraints, and improve the implementation of psychosocial interventions in the region. However, research on using digital health technologies (DHT) for mental health in Asia, particularly in countries in the south and east is limited (Trivedi et al., 2007).

## 3 Where Do We Stand?

Having examined the prevalence of mental health disorders in South Asia and the complex challenges and opportunities that surround the implementation of psychosocial interventions in the region, this section aims to provide an overview of the current status of the research and applicability of these interventions across various South Asian countries. By shedding light on the existing landscape of psychosocial interventions, we can better understand the progress made, identify areas that require strengthening, and inform future efforts to promote mental health and well-being in the region.

The expression of mental illness symptoms, coping mechanisms, social support utilization, and help-seeking behaviours are all profoundly influenced by cultural factors. However, mainstream psychotherapies, developed in Western societies, often reflect individualistic values that may not resonate with collectivistic cultures, such as those found in South Asia (Sue et al., 2009). These cultures emphasize interdependence and cooperation, rendering the "one-size-fits-all" approach ineffective (Kleinman & Good, 1985). To be relevant and effective, psychotherapy must be adapted to incorporate the unique cultural values, beliefs, and aspirations of the society it serves (Tseng, 2001).

While most evidence for psychological treatments comes from high-income countries, its applicability to low- and middle-income countries is limited due to contextual factors like varying explanatory models, coping mechanisms, and socio-economic barriers (Patel, 2000). However, adapted psychological treatments delivered by trained lay health workers in primary care and community settings are showing promise (van Ginneken et al., 2013).

The awareness campaigns in SAARC nations have shown promising results in enhancing knowledge among the target population. However, the extent to which this increased awareness translates into actual behavioural change remains a topic for further research (Xu et al., 2018).

## *3.1 Bangladesh*

1. Bangladesh has made significant strides in addressing mental health concerns, with the enactment of the Mental Health Act in 2018, followed by the National Mental Health Policy in 2019, and the National Mental Health Strategic Plan for 2020–2030. These initiatives aim to integrate mental health into the country's social and economic development framework, protecting the rights of individuals with mental illnesses and ensuring access to essential mental health services. The new mental health act is a positive step towards addressing the mental health needs of the population. However, there are still challenges to be addressed, including the lack of a nationwide anti-stigma campaign and inadequate funding for mental health resources. Despite these challenges, early career psychiatrists are taking to social media to speak out against mental health stigma, helping to raise awareness and promote greater understanding (Vaishnav et al., 2023).
2. The **International Study of Discrimination and Stigma Outcomes (INDIGO)** partnership, launched in 2018, is a five-year research program funded by the UK Medical Research Council. This initiative aims to advance research on the mechanisms of stigma and reduce stigma against people with mental illnesses (PWMI) in low- and middle-income countries (LMICs). Furthermore, INDIGO seeks to establish a sustainable collaborative research consortium. By contributing to the field of stigma research in mental health, INDIGO has developed cross-cultural assessment tools, provided strategies for multi-level stigma reduction, and created culturally appropriate anti-stigma interventions. In 2019, an international summit in Dhaka highlighted the pressing need for an intervention to support autistic children struggling with anxiety. In response, the **Helping Your Anxious Child (HAC) program** was developed through a collaborative effort

between partners from Sri Lanka, Bangladesh, and the UK. The Helping Autistic Children (HAC) program is based on established frameworks from Western parent groups for anxious children, but has been adapted to meet the unique needs of parents in South Asia. Through a collaborative approach involving clinicians, researchers, and parents of autistic children, the program has been tailored to ensure its suitability and cultural relevance for the region. The program aims to increase parents' understanding of anxiety symptoms, identify helpful strategies, and promote children's ability to manage anxiety independently. As a cost-effective, parent-led approach, HAC has the potential to improve family and child outcomes by teaching coping strategies that can be applied across various settings. The program aims to increase parents' understanding of anxiety symptoms, identify helpful strategies, and promote children's ability to manage anxiety independently. As a cost-effective, parent-led approach, HAC has the potential to improve family and child outcomes by teaching coping strategies that can be applied across various settings (Kittridge et al., 2024).

## *3.2 Bhutan*

1. Ongoing Projects to Improve Psychosocial Intervention in LMIC

The PIECEs research project aims to investigate, adapt, and evaluate the effectiveness of DIALOG+, a low-cost, resource-oriented approach, in enhancing community-based care for individuals with psychosis in India and Pakistan. The study will be conducted in two urban sites: Karachi, Pakistan, and Chennai, India. DIALOG+ is an innovative intervention that leverages technology, patient-centred communication, and solution-focused therapy to improve quality of life. This psychosocial intervention is designed to enhance the therapeutic effectiveness of routine clinician–patient meetings for individuals with mental illness, delivered via a mobile app and grounded in principles of quality of life, patient-centred care, and solution-focused therapy.

The intervention involves a patient-centred assessment, where individuals rate their satisfaction across eight life domains and three treatment aspects, followed by a four-step solution-focused approach to identify resources and develop solutions. Research has consistently demonstrated DIALOG+'s efficacy in improving quality of life and reducing symptoms across various settings, including high-income countries (HICs) and low- and middle-income countries (LMICs) (Chatterjee et al., 2008; Dias et al., 2017; Divan et al., 2015). Notably, the intervention can be delivered by various clinical staff members with minimal training (approximately 90 min), making it a versatile and accessible tool for enhancing mental healthcare. While showing promise, DIALOG+ has not been extensively tested in India and Pakistan, highlighting the need for this research (Bird et al., 2023).

2. The PEMA is a nodal agency for mental health in Bhutan, established by Her Majesty The Gyaltsuen, with the goal of ensuring and promoting mental well-being for all Bhutanese. The PEMA has two wings: The PEMA Secretariat and The PEMA Center. The PEMA Center is a 60-bed hospital for psychiatry services and an apex centre for mental health services. The PEMA Secretariat oversees mental health planning, standardization, and consolidation of strategies. Guided by four core mandates, The PEMA aims to achieve good mental health for all individuals, reduce stigma and discrimination, and promote mental health services through service delivery, enabling mental health systems, multisectoral collaboration, and advocacy and prevention.

### *3.3 India*

1. Psychosocial interventions in India are making significant strides, leveraging innovative approaches to address mental health challenges. In India, initiatives like **The Systematic Medical Appraisal, Referral and Treatment (SMART) Mental Health Project** are being scaled up, having demonstrated effectiveness in low-resource settings through multimedia approaches and rigorous evaluations. The SMART Mental Health Project was implemented across 12 villages in West Godavari district of Andhra Pradesh (Tewari et al., 2021). This was a before–after study conducted between 2014 and 2019. The successful implementation of the program was facilitated by several key factors. Firstly, adequate training and supervision of field staff, ASHAs, and doctors ensured that they were equipped to effectively deliver the intervention. The use of electronic decision support systems (EDSS) also played a crucial role. Additionally, a door-to-door campaign was conducted to reach a wider audience, and culturally tailored dramas and videos were utilized to raise awareness about common mental disorders (CMDs). Furthermore, organizing health camps at the village level enabled the delivery of intervention activities, making healthcare more accessible to the community (Maulik et al., 2015).
2. The **Atmiyata program** in rural Gujrat, India has been rolled out across multiple settings, focusing on awareness, early detection, and support regarding mental health (Mental Health Innovation Network, n.d.). This program leverages community volunteers, training them as “Champions” and “Mitras” to provide support and facilitate interventions (Shields-Zeeman et al., 2017). A randomized controlled trial has demonstrated the program’s efficacy, with Champions accurately identifying individuals with emotional distress and counselling sessions leading to a significant reduction in elevated symptoms (Joag et al., 2020). Notably, the program also ensures a referral mechanism for individuals requiring higher-level care, highlighting the growing commitment to developing comprehensive and accessible psychosocial interventions in India.
3. The Program for Effective Mental Health Interventions in Under-Resourced Health Systems **PREMIUM program** aimed to develop and evaluate scalable,

culturally sensitive psychological treatments that are affordable and feasible for delivery by non-specialist health workers. Specifically, the program focused on addressing two major mental health concerns: moderately severe to severe depression through the Healthy Activity Program (HAP), and harmful drinking through Counselling for Alcohol Problems (CAP) (Chowdhary et al., 2016). A key aspect of the PREMIUM program is that both treatments are delivered by the same lay counsellors in routine primary care settings, mirroring real-world clinical practice (Vellakkal & Patel, 2015).

a. **The Healthy Activity Program (HAP)** is an adapted version of behavioural activation, it is a concise, evidence-based psychological treatment rooted in behavioural activation principles. This structured program encompasses several key components, including psychoeducation, behavioural assessment, activity monitoring, scheduling, social network activation, and problem-solving strategies. Typically delivered over a 6–8 week period, HAP sessions are flexible, lasting 30–40 min, and can be conducted weekly in the comfort of the patient's home or via telephone, offering a convenient and accessible treatment option (Patel et al., 2017).
b. **Counselling for Alcohol Problems (CAP)** is an adapted version of Motivational Enhancement Therapy (MET) is a structured, manual-based psychological treatment that consists of three phases, delivered over a maximum of four sessions, each lasting 30–45 min, spaced weekly to fortnightly. The treatment begins with a detailed assessment and personalized feedback (Phase 1), followed by skill-building (Phase 2) that focuses on drink refusal, peer pressure management, problem-solving, and emotional regulation. The final phase (Phase 3) emphasizes relapse prevention, empowering patients to apply the skills they have acquired to manage potential or actual relapses. Counselling for Alcohol Problems (CAP) has been found to been used for harmful drinking and is delivered by lay counsellors in primary care settings (Nadkarni et al., 2015).

   A randomized controlled trial was conducted to evaluate the effectiveness of Counselling for Alcohol Problems (CAP) plus Enhanced Usual Care (EUC) compared to EUC alone in reducing harmful drinking at 10 primary health-care (PHC) settings in Goa, India. In the EUC group, usual care was enhanced by providing screening results to the PHC physician and offering a customized version of WHO's Mental Health Gap Action Program guidelines for harmful drinking. The study enrolled 377 participants, Between Oct 28, 2013, and July 29, 2015, with 188 receiving CAP plus EUC and 189 receiving EUC alone. Results showed that the CAP plus EUC group had significantly higher rates of remission (36% vs 26%) and abstinence (42% vs 18%) compared to the EUC alone group. Additionally, the CAP plus EUC group had a higher percentage of days abstinent and a lower percentage of days of heavy drinking. The incremental cost per additional remission was estimated to be $217, with an 85% chance of being cost-effective. The study suggests that CAP delivered by lay counsellors plus

EUC is a promising strategy to reduce the treatment gap for alcohol use disorders (Nadkarni et al., 2017).

4. **The Thinking Health Program (THP)** is a peer-delivered intervention specifically designed to address perinatal depression. As evaluated by Fuhr et al., (2019) and Vanobberghen et al., (2020) THP incorporates several key components, including behavioural activation, active listening, family collaboration, guided discovery, and homework assignments. This flexible program can be delivered in either individual or group formats, spanning 6–14 weeks over a six-month period, offering a supportive and structured approach to managing perinatal depression. Research on the Thinking Healthy Program (THP) intervention in India and Pakistan has yielded promising results. A study in India found that THP, when combined with enhanced usual care, significantly improved depressive symptoms at six months, although remission rates were not significantly different (Fuhr et al., 2019). However, a subsequent meta-analysis pooling data from this study and another RCT in Pakistan revealed that THP was effective in reducing depression levels and achieving remission at six months (Vanobberghen et al., 2020). Notably, the delivery method differed between the two countries, with Pakistan employing a combination of group and individual sessions, highlighting the potential for flexible implementation approaches.
5. YOGA: Research has consistently shown that yoga can be a valuable adjunct therapy for various psychiatric illnesses. Studies have demonstrated its effectiveness in reducing symptoms of depression (Tolahunase et al., 2018), somatoform pain disorders (Gulati et al., 2025), obsessive–compulsive disorder (Bhat et al., 2024), and schizophrenia (Varambally et al., 2024). Yoga has been found to improve pain scores, anxiety, depression, and quality of life, with no significant adverse effects. As a low-cost and accessible intervention, yoga holds promise for improving mental health outcomes in India and South Asia, where mental health resources are often limited. Overall, yoga is emerging as a helpful complementary therapy for managing psychiatric illnesses. While these findings are encouraging, further rigorous and large-scale studies are necessary to fully establish the efficacy and generalizability of yoga as a complementary therapy for psychiatric illnesses.
6. **The Parent-mediated Autism Spectrum Disorder Intervention in South Asia (PASS)** is a culturally adapted communication intervention, based on the UK-developed PACT intervention. The PASS intervention is specifically designed for delivery in South Asian settings through a task-shifting approach, where parents are empowered to support their children with Autism Spectrum Disorders (ASD). The adapted PASS intervention retains the same theoretical foundation as PACT, employing a naturalistic approach to develop communication skills in children with ASD. However, to ensure contextual relevance and feasibility, key adaptations were made, including modifications to

content and delivery to enhance acceptability and facilitate delivery by non-specialists. Additionally, flexibility was introduced in targeting primary care-givers, acknowledging the common role of grandparents or nannies in caregiving responsibilities within the cultural context (Divan et al., 2015).

7. **The "Depression in Late Life" (DIL) trial,** funded by the US National Institute of Mental Health, aimed to develop and test a scalable intervention for preventing depression and anxiety disorders in older adults with sub-threshold depression. The intervention, delivered by lay health counsellors (LHCs), integrated evidence-based components, including Problem-Solving Therapy, Brief Behavioural Therapy for Insomnia, social casework, and education on self-management of chronic ailments. (Frame of Mind, n.d.) The DIL intervention is a significant step forward in addressing mental health concerns in India, particularly among older adults. Building on the success of the MANAS trial, which focused on promoting mental health, DIL extends the use of lay health counsellors to prevent common mental disorders like depression and anxiety in rural and urban primary care clinics. India's growing population of individuals aged 60 and older has led to an increased focus on preventing mental health issues in this demographic. DIL's emphasis on prevention is crucial, as it can help reduce the burden on healthcare systems and improve the quality of life for older adults. By leveraging lay health counsellors, DIL can increase accessibility to mental health services, especially in rural areas where specialized care may be scarce. This approach also aligns with global efforts to promote mental health and prevent mental disorders, highlighting the importance of community-based interventions (Dias et al., 2017).
8. **MANAS** The MANAS project aimed to integrate evidence-based treatments into routine public and private primary care settings in Goa, India. The term "MANAS" means "humanity" in the local Konkani language and stands for "MANAShanty Sudhar shodh" or "project to promote mental health". The intervention was based on two key principles: using treatments backed by evidence from published trials in low- and middle-income countries, and addressing the challenges of delivering mental healthcare in primary care settings. The MANAS intervention involved a collaborative, stepped care approach, where a health counsellor and primary care doctor worked together to detect and treat common mental disorders (CMDs), with support from a visiting psychiatrist. Treatments were tailored to individual patient needs, with brief psychoeducation as the first step, followed by more intensive treatments like antidepressants and interpersonal therapy (IPT) for those with more severe problems (Chatterjee et al., 2008).
9. **Community care for People with Schizophrenia in India (COPSI) trial:** The trial was conducted to compare the effectiveness of a collaborative community-based care intervention with standard facility-based care. The COPSI trial is a collaborative effort between multiple institutions and individual psychiatrists in India. Led by the Institute of Psychiatry (IoP) at King's College, London, the partner organizations include the London School of Hygiene and Tropical Medicine (LSHTM), Sangath in Goa, the Schizophrenia Research Foundation

(SCARF) in Chennai, the National Institute of Mental Health and Neuroscience (NIMHANS) in Bangalore, and Parivartan and Nirmittee in Satara. Additionally, private sector psychiatrists in Goa and Satara also contributed to the trial as individual collaborators. (Chatterjee et al., 2011) The COPSI study was a multi-centre, randomized controlled trial conducted across three sites in India (Tamil Nadu, Goa, and Maharashtra) from 2009 to 2010. The intervention, delivered in three phases over 12 months, consisted of:

a. **Intensive engagement phase (0–3 months)**: 6–8 home visits by community health workers.
b. Stabilisation phase (4–7 months): Sessions every 15 days.
c) Maintenance phase (8–12 months): Sessions once a month.

A manual was developed to guide the intervention, allowing for flexibility to accommodate individual participant needs. Research has shown that a collaborative community-based care approach, combined with facility-based care, yields moderately better outcomes compared to facility-based care alone. Specifically, this integrated approach has been found to be more effective in: Reducing disability and Alleviating symptoms of psychosis. This suggests that community-based care can play a valuable role in enhancing treatment outcomes for individuals with mental health conditions (Chatterjee et al., 2014).

10. A systematic search was conducted on MEDLINE, PsycINFO, Global Health, and Web of Science, and the review was prospectively. This comprehensive search yielded 26 papers that were carefully evaluated for quality and implementation readiness using two standardized scales. The included studies spanned nine distinct intervention types, including community-based interventions, assertive outreach, CaCBTp, FAP, psychoeducation, cognitive retraining/rehabilitation, social cognition/skills, family/caregiver intervention, telehealth intervention, and yoga-based intervention. Notably, these interventions were implemented across six South Asian countries. Upon analysis, the findings suggest that multicomponent community-based interventions (MCBI) demonstrated the highest level of implementation readiness. This was attributed to their standardization, positive clinical outcomes for both patients and caregivers, as well as rigorous training and cost evaluations (Lyles et al., 2023).
11. **The District Mental Health Program (DMHP),** The District Mental Health Program (DMHP) is part of India's National Mental Health Program (NMHP), launched in 1982. Over the years, DMHP has evolved from a pilot project to a key component of NMHP, expanding services, protecting rights, and integrating mental healthcare into primary healthcare. Recent efforts by the Government of India and state governments have improved service quality, leveraging technology to reach 738 districts. While progress is promising, there is still work to be done to address India's mental health challenges (Kirpekar et al., 2024).
12. **Tele MANAS** is a ground breaking initiative launched by the Government of India on World Mental Health Day, 2022. It's a digital arm of the National Mental Health Program (NMHP) aimed at providing free, 24/7 tele-mental health services to people across India, especially in remote and under-served

areas. The program features a toll-free helpline (14416 and 1-800-91-4416), a two-tier system with state Tele-MANAS cells and specialist resources, and online training courses for healthcare workers. As of December 2023, 34 States/UTs have set up 46 Tele MANAS Cells, handling over 5 lakh calls (Kirpekar et al., 2024).

13. The "camp approach", a novel method for treating alcoholism in rural populations. The first camp was established in Manjakkudi, a village in Tamil Nadu, India, in 1989, and three more camps were conducted over the next four years. A total of 105 patients received treatment through these camps, which were adapted from the standard program at the T.T. Ranganathan Clinical Research Foundation to suit the rural setting. The ultimate goal of this treatment program is total abstinence, and the details of the approach are discussed in this paper (Ranganathan, 1994).
14. A network of 19 **tobacco cessation clinics (TCCs)** was established in India from 2002 to study the feasibility of providing tobacco cessation services. Over five years, 34,741 subjects attended the clinics, with 92.2% being males and 74.1% married. The clients received simple quitting tips, behavioural counselling, and adjunct medication. Follow-up results showed that 14% had quit tobacco and 22% had reduced use by over 50% at six weeks. At subsequent three-monthly follow-ups, 26%, 21%, and 18% had either quit or significantly reduced tobacco use. The study demonstrates the feasibility of setting up effective tobacco cessation clinics in developing countries, but integrating these services into the healthcare system remains a challenge (Varghese et al., 2012).
15. **Non-governmental organizations (NGOs)** are playing a vital role in promoting mental health awareness and reducing stigma. For instance, the Schizophrenia Research Foundation has organized a film event called **"The Frame of Mind"**, which showcases short films on mental illness and hosts an international competition for short films on mental health and stigma. Additionally, many NGOs regularly publish newsletters and maintain websites to educate the community about their work and promote mental health awareness (Frame of Mind, n.d.).
16. The Indian Psychiatry Society, in partnership with **the Live Love Laugh Foundation**, initiated a nationwide anti-stigma campaign to promote mental health awareness. As part of this effort, renowned celebrities lent their support to dispel common myths surrounding mental health. The campaign aimed to sensitize the public about depression and mental illness, with a specific focus on tackling stigma. Titled "Together Against Depression", this initiative sought to encourage open conversations and foster a supportive environment for those affected by mental health issues (Vaishnav et al., 2023).
17. The Banyan, a 25 years old non-profit organization providing comprehensive mental health services to people experiencing poverty and homelessness in Tamil Nadu, Kerala, and Maharashtra. Founded in 1993, it offers emergency care, inclusive living options, and community mental health programs. NALAM, its community mental health program, has reached over 10,000 people, providing personalized care, social entitlements, livelihood support,

and mental health promotion. A survey of 346 women who accessed outpatient services showed significant improvements in occupational roles and paid employment. The Banyan has also partnered with the Government of Tamil Nadu to strengthen the District Mental Health Program.

## *3.4 Nepal*

Meanwhile, in Nepal, the **RESHAPE project** is pioneering the use of visual narrative techniques, such as PhotoVoice, to engage individuals with lived experiences in reducing stigma among primary healthcare providers. These advancements underscore the growing commitment to enhancing psychosocial interventions in the region. The RESHAPE (REducing Stigma among HealthcAre Providers to improvE mental health services) intervention is designed to enhance mental health training for non-specialist healthcare providers, with a focus on improving provider attitudes and competence to ultimately boost patient outcomes. Specifically tailored for primary healthcare workers, RESHAPE incorporates social contact with mental health service users into training programs, leveraging the proven effectiveness of contact-based interventions in reducing stigma and improving attitudes. By facilitating interactions between healthcare providers and mental health service users, such as sharing testimonials and participating in social activities, RESHAPE draws on a broader body of patient-centred research to promote a more compassionate and inclusive approach to mental healthcare (Kohrt et al., 2018).

## *3.5 Pakistan*

Pakistan has implemented various psychosocial interventions to address mental health concerns, including:

1. **Culturally adapted Cognitive Behaviour Therapy for psychosis (CaCBTp)**
   They followed the manual developed by Kingdon and Turkington encompassing collaborative understanding, exploring antecedents, normalizing rationale, treating co-morbid anxiety and depression and case formulation as well as specific techniques to address positive symptoms to explore and develop coping strategies. The cultural adaptations consisted of using culturally appropriate idioms to explain concepts relating to symptoms and causes. For example, referring to religious teachings, speaking in native language (Urdu), and involving carers and family. Adaptations were based on evidence from Naeem, 2004 these included involving family from the beginning of treatment, using a bio-psycho-spiritual-social model of mental health, and involving input from faith healers (Jagtap et al., 2024).
2. **Basic Needs Pakistan**, a non-profit organization established in 2011, has been working tirelessly to promote mental health awareness and reduce stigma. The

organization provides mental health training to community volunteers, educates people about common mental health symptoms, and challenges stereotypes that perpetuate stigma. Furthermore, in 2016, Basic Needs Pakistan established the Centre for Women's Enterprise and Development, aimed at creating career opportunities for women living with mental health conditions. The Pakistan Mental Health Ordinance, 2001, which replaced the outdated Lunacy Act of 1912, focuses on the treatment and management of property for people with mental illnesses (PWMI). While the ordinance addresses important issues such as derogatory terms, criminal and civil liability, human rights, and forced detention, it does not directly target stigma reduction. (Vaishnav et al., 2023)

### *3.6 Sri Lanka*

The Sri Lanka Society of Psychiatry has been leveraging social media outlets to promote mental health awareness and support. One notable initiative is the Community-Based Mental Healthcare Package for Children in Areas of Armed Conflict. This program has shown promising results, including improved case detection and enhanced accessibility to mental healthcare services. However, further development is needed to integrate treatment for severe mental disorders, foster stronger family involvement, and strengthen primary prevention approaches (Vaishnav et al., 2023).

## 4 Recommendation Future Research and Utilizing Existing Data

1. **Conduct Epidemiological Research**: Conduct well-designed epidemiological and clinical research to examine psychopathology in diverse population groups in South Asia.
2. **Public Education and Awareness**: Launch public education and awareness campaigns to promote understanding of mental health conditions and reduce stigma.
3. **Community-Based Treatment Centres**: Establish treatment centres at the community level to increase access to mental health services.
4. **Reform Mental Health Legislation**: Reform mental health legislation to emphasize human rights, community-based care, and inclusion of substance use disorders, and improve implementation of these laws.
5. **Prioritize Mental Health Policy**: Make mental health a policy priority, and conduct comprehensive evaluations of the prevalence of mental disorders and intentional self-harm in South Asia.

6. **Integrate Mental Health into Primary Care**: Train mental health professionals, improve access to evidence-based interventions, and integrate mental health services into primary healthcare to close treatment gaps and enhance health outcomes.
7. **Launch Campaign-Based Approaches:** Utilize campaign-based initiatives to:

    - Challenge stigmatizing attitudes and practices
    - Raise awareness and spark dialogue on mental health conditions
    - Condemn harmful media representations and advocate for accurate portrayals
    - Mobilize public opinion and push for policy reforms

    By doing so, create a supportive and inclusive environment for individuals with mental health conditions, facilitating the implementation of effective psychosocial interventions.
8. **Awareness creation, education, and training interventions**

    To effectively implement psychosocial interventions, it is essential to prioritize awareness creation, education, and training initiatives. These interventions should aim to provide comprehensive information about mental health conditions, including risk factors, prevalence, symptoms, and diagnosis, while also addressing misconceptions and myths. Furthermore, employing diverse delivery methods such as face-to-face interactions, social media, theatre, workshops, and didactic training can enhance the reach and impact of these initiatives. By educating and training individuals, communities, and healthcare professionals, we can promote a culture of understanding, reduce stigma, and ultimately facilitate the successful implementation of psychosocial interventions.
9. **Modernize CHW Training** Incorporate innovative methods such as remote learning, blended learning, AI-mediated learning, and social media to enhance CHW training effectiveness.
10. **Leverage CHWs for Public Awareness** Utilize CHWs as the first point of contact for promoting public knowledge and awareness on mental health and psychosocial interventions.
11. **Introduce Specialized CHWs** Introduce specialized CHWs in SAARC countries to address the burden of non-communicable diseases (NCDs), mental disorders, and unmet surgical needs.

## 5 Conclusion

Psychosocial interventions are a crucial component in addressing the mental health needs of South Asia. The region's unique cultural landscape, characterized by traditional healing practices, presents opportunities for innovative interventions. Task-shifting, community-based interventions, and collaborations with traditional healers have shown promise in enhancing the acceptability and effectiveness of these interventions. Evidence-based interventions, such as Tele MANAS, YOGA, PREMIUM project, and COPSI, are being implemented and tested in South Asia. However, their impact is hindered by limited awareness and under-utilization. To overcome these challenges, policy reforms and innovative strategies, leveraging technology and community resources, are essential.

A comprehensive approach integrating traditional practices, community-based interventions, and evidence-based psychosocial treatments is vital for reducing the mental health burden in South Asia. By prioritizing psychosocial interventions, promoting awareness, and increasing access, South Asia can make significant strides in addressing its mental health needs.

## References


Ahad, A. A., Sanchez-Gonzalez, M., & Junquera, P. (2023). Understanding and addressing mental health stigma across cultures for improving psychiatric care: A narrative review. *Cureus, 15*(5), Article e39549. https://doi.org/10.7759/cureus.39549

Arafat, S. M. Y., & Kar, S. K. (2024). Epidemiology of psychiatric disorders and overview of access to mental health care in South Asia. In *Access to mental health care in South Asia* (pp. 1–15). Springer. https://doi.org/10.1007/978-981-99-9153-2_1

Arboleda-Flórez, J., & Stuart, H. (2012). From sin to science: Fighting the stigmatization of mental illnesses. *Canadian Journal of Psychiatry, 57*(7), 457–463. https://doi.org/10.1177/070674371205700706

Asher, L., Patel, V., & De Silva, M. J. (2017). Community-based psychosocial interventions for people with schizophrenia in low and middle-income countries: Systematic review and meta-analysis. *BMC Psychiatry, 17*(1), 355. https://doi.org/10.1186/s12888-017-1516-4

Aswini, S., & Deb, A. (2020). Living well with mental illness: Findings from India. *Journal of Human Behavior and Social Environment*, 1–18.

Avula, V. C. R., Godi, S. M., Munivenkatappa, S., & Amalakanti, S. (2024). Mental health insurance in India: An examination of policy implementation post-MHCA 2017. *Indian Journal of Psychological Medicine, 47*(1), 9–16.

Aye, B., Goss, J., Lappin, K., Whaites, M., Barria, S., Montufar, V., & Islam, M. S. (2018). *Decent work for community health workers in South Asia: A path to gender equality and sustainable development.* International Labour Organization.

Barth, J., Munder, T., Gerger, H., Nuesch, E., Trelle, S., Znoj, H., Jüni, P., & Cuijpers, P. (2013). Comparative efficacy of seven psychotherapeutic interventions for patients with depression: A network meta-analysis. *PLoS Medicine, 10*(5), Article e1001454. https://doi.org/10.1371/journal.pmed.1001454

Bhargav, H., George, S., & Varambally, S. (2023). Yoga and mental health: What every psychiatrist needs to know. *Bjpsych Advances, 29*(1), 1–12. https://doi.org/10.1192/bja.2022.63

Bhat, S., Varambally, S., Jagannathan, A., & Phillip, M. (2024). Effectiveness of add-on yoga in reducing the symptoms of obsessive compulsive disorder (OCD): A randomized controlled trial. *Asian Journal of Psychiatry, 99*, Article 104156. https://doi.org/10.1016/j.ajp.2024.104156

Bird, V. J., Davis, S., Jawed, A., Qureshi, O., Ramachandran, P., Shahab, A., Venkatraman, L., & Wright, N. (2022). Implementing psychosocial interventions within low- and middle-income countries to improve community-based care for people with psychosis—A situation analysis. *Frontiers in Psychiatry, 13*, Article 807259. https://doi.org/10.3389/fpsyt.2022.807259

Bird, V. J., Sajun, S. Z., Peppl, R., Evans-Lacko, S., Priebe, S., Singh, S., L., Venkatraman, P., Ramachandran, A., Pasha, A., Malik, & Hanlon, C. (2023). Assessing the effectiveness and cost-effectiveness of a solution-focused resource-orientated approach (DIALOG+) to improving the quality of life for people with psychosis in India and Pakistan—A cluster RCT. *Trials, 24*(1), 59. https://doi.org/10.1186/s13063-023-06633-9

Brinsley, J., Schuch, F., Lederman, O., Girard, D., Smout, M., Immink, M. A., Stubbs, B., Firth, J., Davison, K., & Rosenbaum, S. (2021). Effects of yoga on depressive symptoms in people with mental disorders: A systematic review and meta-analysis. *British Journal of Sports Medicine, 55*(17), 992–1000.

Chadda, R. K., & Deb, K. S. (2013). Family burden and coping strategies in caregivers of individuals with schizophrenia. *Indian Journal of Psychiatry, 55*(3), 253–258. https://doi.org/10.4103/0019-5545.116301

Chowdhary, N., Anand, A., Dimidjian, S., Shinde, S., Weobong, B., Balaji, M., Hollon, S. D., Rahman, A., Wilson, G. T., Verdeli, H., Araya, R., & Patel, V. (2016). The healthy activity program lay counsellor delivered treatment for severe depression in India: Systematic development and randomised evaluation. *The British Journal of Psychiatry, 208*(5), 381–388. https://doi.org/10.1192/bjp.bp.114.161098

Chatterjee, S., Chowdhary, N., Pednekar, S., Cohen, A., Andrew, G., Araya, R., Simon, G., King, M., Telles, S., Verdeli, H., Clougherty, K., & Patel, V. (2008). Integrating evidence-based treatments for common mental disorders in routine primary care: Feasibility and acceptability of the MANAS intervention in Goa, India. In *World Psychiatry* (Vol. 7, pp. 39–46). https://doi.org/10.1002/j.2051-5545.2008.tb00151.x

Chatterjee, S., Leese, M., Koschorke, M., McCrone, P., Naik, S., John, S., Dabholkar, H., Goldsmith, K., Balaji, M., Varghese, M., Thara, R., Patel, V., & The Community Care for People with Schizophrenia in India (COPSI) Group. (2011). Collaborative community-based care for people and their families living with schizophrenia in India: Protocol for a randomised controlled trial. *Trials, 12*, 12. https://doi.org/10.1186/1745-6215-12-12

Chatterjee, S., Naik, S., John, S., Dabholkar, H., Balaji, M., Koschorke, M., Varghese, M., Thara, R., Weiss, H. A., Williams, P., McCrone, P., & Patel, V. (2014). Effectiveness of a community-based intervention for people with schizophrenia and their caregivers in India (COPSI): A randomised controlled trial. *The Lancet, 383*(9926), 1385–1394. https://doi.org/10.1016/S0140-6736(13)62629-6

Cocchiara, R. A., Peruzzo, M., Mannocci, A., & Villari, P. (2019). The use of Yoga to manage stress and burnout in healthcare workers: A systematic review. *Journal of Clinical Medicine, 8*(3), 284. https://doi.org/10.3390/jcm8030284

Collins, P. Y., Patel, V., Joestl, S. S., March, D., Insel, T. R., Daar, A. S., & Walport, M. (2011). Grand challenges in global mental health. *Nature, 475*(7354), 27–30. https://doi.org/10.1038/475027a

Cuijpers, P., Geraedts, A. S., van Oppen, P., Andersson, G., Markowitz, J. C., & van Straten, A. (2011). Interpersonal psychotherapy for depression: A meta-analysis. *American Journal of Psychiatry, 168*(6), 581–592. https://doi.org/10.1176/appi.ajp.2010.10101487

Cuijpers, P., Sijbrandij, M., Koole, S. L., Andersson, G., Beekman, A. T., & Reynolds, C. F. (2013). The efficacy of psychotherapy and pharmacotherapy in treating depressive and anxiety disorders: A meta-analysis of direct comparisons. *World Psychiatry, 12*(2), 137–148. https://doi.org/10.1002/wps.20038

Cuijpers, P., Smit, F., Bohlmeijer, E., Hollon, S. D., & Andersson, G. (2010a). Efficacy of cognitive-behavioural therapy and other psychological treatments for adult depression: Meta-analytic study of publication bias. *British Journal of Psychiatry, 196*(3), 173–178. https://doi.org/10.1192/bjp.bp.109.066001

Cuijpers, P., van Straten, A., Schuurmans, J., van Oppen, P., Hollon, S. D., & Andersson, G. (2010b). Psychotherapy for chronic major depression and dysthymia: A meta-analysis. *Clinical Psychology Review, 30*(1), 51–62. https://doi.org/10.1016/j.cpr.2009.09.003

Dias, A., Azariah, F., Health, P., Cohen, A., Anderson, S., Morse, J., Cuijpers, P., M., Sequeira, V., Gaude, S., Soares, V., Patel, C. F., & Reynolds III. (2017). Intervention development for the indicated prevention of depression in later life: The "DIL" protocol in Goa, India. *Contemporary Clinical Trials Communications, 6*, 131–139. https://doi.org/10.1016/j.conctc.2017.03.005

Divan, G., Hamdani, S. U., Vajartkar, V., Minhas, A., Taylor, C., Aldred, C., Leadbitter, K., Rahman, A., Green, J., & Patel, V. (2015). Adapting an evidence-based intervention for autism spectrum disorder for scaling up in resource-constrained settings: The development of the PASS intervention in South Asia. *Global Health Action, 8*, 27278. https://doi.org/10.3402/gha.v8.27278

Familiar, I., Sharma, S., Ndayisaba, H., & Bolton, P. (2013). Community perceptions of mental distress in a post-conflict setting: A qualitative study in Burundi. *Global Public Health, 8*(9–10), 943–957. https://doi.org/10.1080/17441692.2013.859721

Frame of Mind. (n.d,). https://www.frameofmind.in/. Last Accessed on 13 August 2023.

Fuhr, D. C., Weobong, B., Lazarus, A., Vanobberghen, F., Weiss, H. A., Singla, D. R., Tabana, H., Afonso, E., De Sa, A., D'Souza, E., Joshi, A., & Patel, V. (2019). Delivering the thinking healthy programme for perinatal depression through peers: An individually randomised controlled trial in India. *The Lancet Psychiatry, 6*(2), 115–127. https://doi.org/10.1016/S2215-0366(18)30280-3

Global Burden of Disease Collaborative Network. (2022). Global, regional, and national burden of 12 mental disorders in 204 countries and territories, 1990–2019: A systematic analysis for the Global Burden of Disease Study 2019. *The Lancet Psychiatry, 9*(2), 137–150. https://doi.org/10.1016/S2215-0366(21)00395-3

Goffman, E. (1963). *Stigma: Notes on the management of spoiled identity*. Penguin Books.

Groupe Speciale Mobile Association. (2022). *The mobile economy: Asia Pacific 2022.*

Grover, S. (2023). Status of mental health in South Asian countries. *Journal of SAARC Psychiatrists Federation, 1*(1), 1–5. https://doi.org/10.4103/jspf.jspf_15_23

Gulati, K., Gunasekaran, D. M., Bhargav, H., Bhaskarapillai, B., Nandakumar, D. N., Varambally, S., Gangadhar, B. N., & Desai, G. (2025). The efficacy of add-on yoga intervention in somatoform pain disorders: An open-label controlled trial. *Indian Journal of Psychiatry, 67*(3), 316–322. https://doi.org/10.4103/indianjpsychiatry.indianjpsychiatry_932_24

Gupta, A., Lohiya, A., & Kharya, P. (2013). Mental health issues and challenges in India: A review. *International Journal of Science Research and Publication, 3*(1), 2250–3153.

Gururaj, G., Varghese, M., Benegal, V., Rao, G. N., Pathak, K., Singh, L. K., et al. (2016). National mental health survey of India, 2015–16: Prevalence, patterns and outcomes. National Institute of Mental Health and Neuro Sciences.

Institute of Health Metrics and Evaluation. (2022). *Global Health Data Exchange (GHDx).*

Institute of Medicine. (2006). *Improving the quality of care for mental and substance use conditions.* The National Academies Press.

Institute of Medicine. (2015). *Psychosocial interventions for mental and substance use disorders: A framework for establishing evidence-based standards.* National Academies Press.

Insurance Regulatory and Development Authority of India. (2018). *Medical insurance for treatment of mental illness on the same basis as is available for treatment of physical illness.*

Issac, M. (2013). Mental health services in South Asia: Past, present and future. *South Asian Journal of Psychiatry, 2*, 4–11.

Jagtap, S., Zahid, A., Dere, J., Gerritsen, C., D'Arcey, J., Romanowska, S., Naeem, F., & Best, M. W. (2024). Culturally adapted cognitive behavioral therapy for psychosis (CaCBTp): A review of key features of cultural adaptation and considerations for psychologists. *Psychological Services, 21*(4), 880–892. https://doi.org/10.1037/ser0000654

Javed, A., Lee, C., Zakaria, H., Buenaventura, R. D., Cetkovich-Bakmas, M., Duailibi, K., Ng, B., Ramy, H., Saha, G., Arifeen, S., Elorza, P. M., & Zhang, Y. (2021). Reducing the stigma of mental health disorders with a focus on low- and middle-income countries. *Asian Journal of Psychiatry, 58*, Article 102601. https://doi.org/10.1016/j.ajp.2020.102601

Joag, K., Shields-Zeeman, L., Kapadia-Kundu, N., Kawade, R., Balaji, M., & Pathare, S. (2020). Feasibility and acceptability of a novel community-based mental health intervention delivered by community volunteers in Maharashtra, India: The Atmiyata programme. *BMC Psychiatry, 20*, 48. https://doi.org/10.1186/s12888-020-2464-4

Kakuma, R., Minas, H., van Ginneken, N., Dal Poz, M. R., Desiraju, K., Morris, J. E., Saxena, S., & Scheffler, R. M. (2011). Human resources for mental health care: Current situation and strategies for action. *The Lancet, 378*(9803), 1654–1663. https://doi.org/10.1016/S0140-6736(11)60893-7

Kapur, R. L. (1979). The role of traditional healers in mental health care in rural India. *Social Science & Medicine, 13B*(1), 27–31. https://doi.org/10.1016/0160-7987(79)90005-6

Kirpekar, V., Faye, A., Bhave, S., Gawande, S., & Tadke, R. (2024). District mental health program: Then and now. *Indian Journal of Psychiatry, 66*(7), 603–613. https://doi.org/10.4103/indianjpsychiatry.indianjpsychiatry_1021_22

Kittridge, C., Rob, P., Fisher-Rogers, A., Anis, T., Attygalle, U., Islam, F., Sharma, A. N., Rodgers, J., & Singla, D. R. (2024). The development of the Helping your Anxious Child programme: A parent-mediated group intervention for parents of autistic children in South Asia. *Bjpsych International, 21*(2), 26–28. https://doi.org/10.1192/bji.2023.17

Kleinman, A. (1980). *Patients and healers in the context of culture*. University of California Press.

Kleinman, A., & Good, B. (1985). *Culture and depression: Studies in the anthropology and cross-cultural psychiatry of affect and disorder*. University of California Press.

Kirmayer, L. J. (2004). The cultural diversity of healing: Meaning, metaphor and mechanism. *British Medical Bulletin, 69*, 33–48. https://doi.org/10.1093/bmb/ldh024

Kohrt, B. A., Jordans, M. J. D., Turner, E. L., Sikkema, K. J., Luitel, N. P., Rai, S., & Shrestha, P. (2018). Reducing stigma among healthcare providers to improve mental health services (RESHAPE): Protocol for a pilot cluster randomized controlled trial of a stigma reduction intervention for training primary healthcare workers in Nepal. *Pilot and Feasibility Studies, 4*, 36. https://doi.org/10.1186/s40814-018-0253-3

Kraemer, H. C., Wilson, G. T., Fairburn, C. G., & Agras, W. S. (2002). Mediators and moderators of treatment effects in randomized clinical trials. *Archives of General Psychiatry, 59*(10), 877–883. https://doi.org/10.1001/archpsyc.59.10.877

Lyles, S., Khan, Z., Qureshi, O., & Shaikh, M. (2023). A systematic review of the effectiveness and implementation readiness of psychosocial interventions for psychosis in South Asia. *PLoS ONE, 18*(11), Article e0283411. https://doi.org/10.1371/journal.pone.0283411

Maddock, A., Blair, C., Ean, N., & Dawson, L. (2021). Psychological and social interventions for mental health issues and disorders in Southeast Asia: A systematic review. *International Journal of Mental Health Systems, 15*, 56. https://doi.org/10.1186/s13033-021-00479-9

Maramis, A., Van Tuan, N., & Minas, H. (2011). Mental health in Southeast Asia. *The Lancet, 377*(9767), 700–702. https://doi.org/10.1016/S0140-6736(11)60069-3

Maulik, P. K., Devarapalli, S., Kallakuri, S., Praveen, D., Jha, V., & Patel, A. (2015). Systematic Medical Appraisal, Referral and Treatment (SMART) Mental Health Programme for providing innovative mental health care in rural communities in India. *Global Mental Health, 2*, Article e13. https://doi.org/10.1017/gmh.2015.12

McDonagh, M. S., Dana, T., Kopelovich, S. L., Monroe-DeVita, M., Blazina, I., Bougatsos, C., Grusing, S., Selph, S. S., & Buckley, D. I. (2021). Psychosocial interventions for adults with schizophrenia: An overview and update of systematic reviews. *Psychiatric Services, 72*(5), appips202000649. https://doi.org/10.1176/appi.ps.202000649

Mental Health Innovation Network. (n.d.). ATMIYATA: A community-led intervention in rural India.

Mubin, N., Bin Abdul Baten, R., Jahan, S., Zohora, F. T., Chowdhury, N. M., Faruque, G. M., & Alam, S. (2021). Cancer-related knowledge, attitude, and practice among community health care providers and health assistants in rural Bangladesh. *BMC Health Services Research, 21*(1), 191. https://doi.org/10.1186/s12913-021-06162-4

Mudunna, C., Weerasinghe, M., Tran, T., Antoniades, J., Romero, L., Chandradasa, M., Fisher, J., & Dawson, L. (2025). Nature, prevalence, and determinants of mental health problems experienced by adolescents in South Asia: A systematic review. *Lancet Regional Health - Southeast Asia, 33*, Article 100532. https://doi.org/10.1016/j.lansea.2024.100532

Nadkarni, A., Velleman, R., Dabholkar, H., Shinde, S., Bhat, B., McCambridge, J., Murthy, P., Wilson, T., Weobong, B., & Patel, V. (2015). The systematic development and pilot randomized evaluation of counselling for alcohol problems, a lay counselor-delivered psychological treatment for harmful drinking in primary care in India: The PREMIUM Study. *Alcoholism: Clinical and Experimental Research, 39*(10), 1631–1638. https://doi.org/10.1111/acer.12841

Nadkarni, A., Weobong, B., Weiss, H. A., McCambridge, J., Bhat, B., Katti, B., Murthy, P., King, M., McDaid, D., Park, A. L., Wilson, G. T., & Patel, V. (2017). Counselling for Alcohol Problems (CAP), a lay counsellor-delivered brief psychological treatment for harmful drinking in men, in primary care in India: A randomised controlled trial. *The Lancet, 389*(10065), 186–195. https://doi.org/10.1016/S0140-6736(16)32267-8

Naeem, F. (2004). Review of the book Family work for schizophrenia: A practical guide, second edition, by E. Kuipers, J. Leff, & D. Lam. *Psychiatric Bulletin, 28*, 185–186.

Naveed, S., Waqas, A., Chaudhary, A. M. D., Kumar, S., Abbas, N., Amin, R., Jamil, N., Saleem, S., & Husain, N. (2020). Prevalence of common mental disorders in South Asia: A systematic review and meta-regression analysis. *Frontiers in Psychiatry, 11*, Article 573150. https://doi.org/10.3389/fpsyt.2020.573150

Ng, Q. X., Venkatanarayanan, N., Loke, W., Yeo, W. S., Lim, D. Y., Chan, H. W., & Sim, W. S. (2019). A meta-analysis of the effectiveness of yoga-based interventions for maternal depression during pregnancy. *Complementary Therapies in Clinical Practice, 34*, 8–12.

Nimgaonkar, A. U., & Menon, S. D. (2015). A task shifting mental health program for an impoverished rural Indian community. *Asian Journal of Psychiatry, 16*, 41–47. https://doi.org/10.1016/j.ajp.2015.04.005

Nortje, G., & Sorsdahl, K. (2016). Effectiveness of traditional healers in treating mental disorders: A systematic review. *The Lancet Psychiatry, 3*(2), 154–170. https://doi.org/10.1016/S2215-0366(15)00515-5

Patel, V. (2000). The need for treatment evidence for common mental disorders in developing countries. *Psychological Medicine, 30*(4), 743–746. https://doi.org/10.1017/S0033291799002435

Patel, V., Saxena, S., Lund, C., Thornicroft, G., Baingana, F., Bolton, P., Chisholm, D., Collins, P. Y., Cooper, J. L., Eaton, J. Herrman, H., & Unützer, J. (2018). The Lancet Commission on global mental health and sustainable development. *Lancet, 392*(10157), 1553–1598. https://doi.org/10.1016/S0140-6736(18)31612-X

Patel, V., Weobong, B., Weiss, H. A., Anand, A., Bhat, B., Katti, B., Dimidjian, S., Araya, R., Hollon, S. D., King, M., & Vijayakumar, L. (2017). The Healthy Activity Program (HAP), a lay counsellor-delivered brief psychological treatment for severe depression, in primary care in India: A randomised controlled trial. *The Lancet, 389*(10065), 176–185. https://doi.org/10.1016/S0140-6736(16)32265-4

Polanczyk, G. V., Salum, G. A., Sugaya, L. S., Caye, A., & Rohde, L. A. (2015). Annual research review: A meta-analysis of the worldwide prevalence of mental disorders in children and adolescents. *Journal of Child Psychology and Psychiatry, 56*(3), 345–365. https://doi.org/10.1111/j.1469-7610.2012.02567.x

Porter, R. J. (2020). The biopsychosocial model in mental health. *Australian and New Zealand Journal of Psychiatry, 54*(7), 773–774. https://doi.org/10.1177/0004867420927183

Ranganathan, S. (1994). The Manjakkudi experience: A camp approach towards treating alcoholics. *Addiction, 89*(8), 1071–1075. https://doi.org/10.1111/j.1360-0443.1994.tb01764.x

Rathod, S., Javed, A., Iqbal, R., & Kingdon, D. (2023). Results of a qualitative study of patient, carer and clinician views on the experience of caring for individuals with psychosis in Pakistan. *Cognitive Behaviour Therapy, 16*, Article e17. https://doi.org/10.1080/16506073.2022.2150424

Razali, S. M. (2000). Complementary treatment of mental illness in Southeast Asia. *International Medical Journal, 7*(3), 189–191.

Riaz, M. M. A., & Jindal, R. M. (2024). Reimagining the role of community health workers in SAARC countries. *Annals of Medicine and Surgery, 86*(8), 4608–4612. https://doi.org/10.1016/j.amsu.2023.10.025

Sabe, M., Sentissi, O., & Kaiser, S. (2019). Meditation-based mind-body therapies for negative symptoms of schizophrenia: Systematic review of randomized controlled trials and meta-analysis. *Schizophrenia Research, 212*, 15–25.

Saha, S., Chauhan, A., Hamlai, M., Saiyad, V., Makwana, S., Shah, K., & Pandya, A. (2021). Unique collaboration of modern medicine and traditional faith-healing for the treatment of mental illness: Best practice from Gujarat. *Journal of Family Medicine and Primary Care, 10*(1), 521–526. https://doi.org/10.1016/j.schres.2019.07.030

Satyananda, S. (2002). *Four chapters on freedom: Commentary on the yoga sutras of Patanjali.* Nesma Books.

Scott, K., Beckham, S., Gross, M., & Pearson, L. (2017). What do we know about community health workers? A systematic review of existing reviews. *Human Resources for Health Observer, 19*, 1–35. https://doi.org/10.1186/s12960-017-0206-3

Seponski, D. M., Lewis, D. C., & Megginson, M. C. (2014). A responsive evaluation of mental health treatment in Cambodia: Intentionally addressing poverty to increase cultural responsiveness in therapy. *Global Public Health, 9*(10), 1211–1224. https://doi.org/10.1080/17441692.2014.934255

Sharan, P., Sagar, R., & Kumar, S. (2017). Mental health policies in South-East Asia and the public health role of screening instruments for depression. *WHO South-East Asia Journal of Public Health, 6*(1), 5.

Shields-Zeeman, L., Pathare, S., Walters, B. H., Kapadia-Kundu, N., & Joag, K. (2017). Promoting wellbeing and improving access to mental health care through community champions in rural India: The Atmiyata intervention approach. *International Journal of Mental Health Systems, 11*, 6. https://doi.org/10.1186/s13033-016-0114-6

Shidhaye, R., Murhar, V., Gangale, S., Aldridge, L., Shastri, R., Parikh, R., Shrivastava, R., Damle, S., Raja, T., Nadkarni, A. & Patel, V. (2017). The effect of VISHRAM, a grass-roots community-based mental health programme, on the treatment gap for depression in rural communities in India: A population-based study. *The Lancet Psychiatry, 4*(2), 128–135. https://doi.org/10.1016/S2215-0366(16)30342-4

Shrestha, P., & Dawson, L. (2023). Strengthening primary health care through community health workers in South Asia. *The Lancet Regional Health - Southeast Asia, 28*, Article 100463. https://doi.org/10.1016/j.lansea.2023.100463

Siddiqui, S., Morris, A., Ikeda, D. J., Balsari, S., Blanke, L., Pearsall, M., Rodriguez, R., Saxena, S., Miller, B. F., Patel, V., & Naslund, J. A. (2022). Scaling up community-delivered mental health support and care: A landscape analysis. *Frontiers in Public Health, 10*, Article 992222. https://doi.org/10.3389/fpubh.2022.992222

Sorsdahl, K., Stein, D. J., & Flisher, A. J. (2010). Traditional healer attitudes and beliefs regarding referral of the mentally ill to Western doctors in South Africa. *Transcultural Psychiatry, 47*(5), 591–609. https://doi.org/10.1177/1363461510382154

Sue, S., Zane, N., Nagayama Hall, G. C., & Berger, L. K. (2009). The case for cultural competency in psychotherapeutic interventions. *Annual Review of Psychology, 60*, 525–548. https://doi.org/10.1146/annurev.psych.60.110707.163651

Thornicroft, G., & Tansella, M. (2013). The balanced care model: The case for both hospital- and community-based mental healthcare. *British Journal of Psychiatry, 202*(4), 246–248. https://doi.org/10.1192/bjp.bp.112.114829

Thornicroft, G., Sunkel, C., Aliev, A.A., Baker, S., Brohan, E., El Chammay, R., Davies, K., Demissie, M., Duncan, J., Fekadu, W., Gronholm, P.C., & Yeeles, K. (2022). The Lancet Commission on ending stigma and discrimination in mental health. *The Lancet, 400*(10363), 1438–1448. https://doi.org/10.1016/S0140-6736(22)01532-4

Tewari, A., Kallakuri, S., Devarapalli, S., Peiris, D., Patel, A., & Maulik, P. K. (2021). SMART Mental Health Project: Process evaluation to understand the barriers and facilitators for implementation of multifaceted intervention in rural India. *International Journal of Mental Health Systems, 15*, 15. https://doi.org/10.1186/s13033-021-00431-8

Thara, R., & Padmavati, R. (2013). Community mental health care in South Asia. *World Psychiatry, 12*(2), 176–177. https://doi.org/10.1002/wps.20042

Tolahunase, M. R., Sagar, R., Faiq, M., & Dada, R. (2018). Yoga- and meditation-based lifestyle intervention increases neuroplasticity and reduces severity of major depressive disorder: A randomized controlled trial. *Restorative Neurology and Neuroscience, 36*(3), 423–442. https://doi.org/10.3233/RNN-170810

Trivedi, J. K., Goel, D., Kallivayalil, R. A., Isaac, M., Shrestha, D. M., Gambheera, H. C., & Gupta, S. (2007). Regional cooperation in South Asia in the field of mental health. *World Psychiatry, 6*(1), 57–59.

Trivedi, J. K., Jilani, A. Q., & Kar, S. K. (2012). Levels of client satisfaction following the application of a person-centered management approach in persons suffering with schizophrenia. *The International Journal of Person Centered Medicine, 2*(1), 234–239.

Tseng, W. S. (2001). *Handbook of cultural psychiatry*. Elsevier Science.

Vaishnav, M., Javed, A., Gupta, S., Kumar, V., Vaishnav, P., Kumar, A., Salih, H., NG, B., Alkhoori, S., Luguercho, C., Soghoyan, A., & Singh, S. (2023). Stigma towards mental illness in Asian nations and low-and-middle-income countries, and comparison with high-income countries: A literature review and practice implications. *Indian Journal of Psychiatry, 65*(10), 995–1011. https://doi.org/10.4103/psychiatry.indpsychiatry_1561_22

van Ginneken, N., Tharyan, P., Lewin, S., Rao, G. N., Meera, S. M., Pian, J., Chandrashekar, S., & Patel, V. (2013). Non-specialist health worker interventions for the care of mental, neurological and substance-abuse disorders in low- and middle-income countries. *Cochrane Database of Systematic Reviews, 2013*(11), CD009149. https://doi.org/10.1002/14651858.CD009149.pub2

Vanobberghen, F., Weiss, H. A., Fuhr, D. C., Sikander, S., Afonso, E., Ahmad, I., Atif, N., Bibi, A., Bibi, T., Bilal, S. De Sa, A., & Patel, V. (2020). Effectiveness of the Thinking Healthy Programme for perinatal depression delivered through peers: Pooled analysis of two randomized controlled trials in India and Pakistan. *Journal of Affective Disorders, 265*, 660–668. https://doi.org/10.1016/j.jad.2019.11.121

Varghese, C., Kaur, J., Desai, N. G., Murthy, P., Malhotra, S., Subbakrishna, D. K., Prasad, V. M., Munish, V. G., & Jain, R. (2012). Initiating tobacco cessation services in India: Challenges and opportunities. *WHO South-East Asia Journal of Public Health, 1*(2), 159–168. https://doi.org/10.4103/2224-3151.207037

Varghese, K. J., Gopal, B., & Thomas, T. M. (2011). Revisiting psychotherapeutic practices in Karnataka, India: Lessons from indigenous healing methods. *International Journal of Health Promotion and Education, 49*(2), 128–136. https://doi.org/10.1080/14635240.2011.10708185

Varambally, S., George, S., & Gangadhar, B. N. (2020). Yoga for psychiatric disorders: From fad to evidence-based intervention? *The British Journal of Psychiatry, 216*(4), 291–293. https://doi.org/10.1192/bjp.2020.36

Varambally, S., Holla, B., Venkatasubramanian, G., Mullapudi, T., Raj, P., Shivakumar, V., Christopher, R., Debnath, M., Philip, M., Bharath, R. D., & Gangadhar, B. N. (2024). Clinical effects of a yoga-based intervention for patients with schizophrenia: A six-month randomized controlled trial. *Schizophrenia Research, 269*, 144–151. https://doi.org/10.1016/j.schres.2024.05.007

Vellakkal, S., & Patel, V. (2015). Designing psychological treatments for scalability: The PREMIUM approach. *PLoS ONE, 10*(10), Article e0134189. https://doi.org/10.1371/journal.pone.0134189

Ventriglio, A., Ricci, F., Magnifico, G., Chumakov, E., Torales, J., Watson, C., & Bhugra, D. (2020). Psychosocial interventions in schizophrenia: Focus on guidelines. *International Journal of Social Psychiatry, 66*(7–8), 735–747. https://doi.org/10.1177/0020764020929935

Vidyasagaran, A. L., McDaid, D., Faisal, M. R., Nasir, M., Muliyala, K. P., Thekkumkara, S., Wright, J., Huque R., Benkalkar, S., Siddiqi, N., & Prince, M. (2023). Prevalence of mental disorders in South Asia: A systematic review of reviews. *Global Mental Health, 10*, Article e78. https://doi.org/10.1017/gmh.2022.28

Walker, E. R., McGee, R. E., & Druss, B. G. (2015). Mortality in mental disorders and global disease burden implications: A systematic review and meta-analysis. *JAMA Psychiatry, 72*(4), 334–341. https://doi.org/10.1001/jamapsychiatry.2014.2502

Whiteford, H. A., Degenhardt, L., Rehm, J., Baxter, A. J., Ferrari, A. J., Erskine, H. E., Charlson, F. J., Norman, R. E., Flaxman, A. D., Johns, N., Burstein, R., Murray, C. J. L., & Vos, T. (2013). Global burden of disease attributable to mental and substance use disorders: Findings from the Global Burden of Disease Study 2010. *Lancet, 382*(9904), 1575–1586. https://doi.org/10.1016/S0140-6736(13)61611-6

Wig, N. N., Suleiman, M. A., Routledge, R., Srinivasa Murthy, R., Ladrido-Ignacio, L., Ibrahim, H. H. A., & Harding, T. W. (1980). Community reactions to mental disorders: A key informant study in three developing countries. *Acta Psychiatrica Scandinavica, 61*(1), 111–126. https://doi.org/10.1111/j.1600-0447.1980.tb04571.x

World Health Organization. (2000). *General guidelines for methodologies on research and evaluation of traditional medicine*. World Health Organization.

World Health Organization. (2013). *WHO traditional medicine strategy: 2014–2023*. World Health Organization.

World Health Organization. (2016). *mhGAP Intervention Guide—Version 2.0 for mental, neurological and substance use disorders in non-specialized health settings*. World Health Organization.

World Health Organization. (2017). *Mental health atlas*. World Health Organization.

World Health Organization. (2020a). *Mental health atlas*. World Health Organization.

World Health Organization. (2020b). *WHO mental health gap action programme (mhGAP)*. World Health Organization.

World Health Organization. (2022). *Mental health fact sheets*. World Health Organization.

World Health Organization. (2023). *Mental health action plan for the WHO South-East Asia region 2023–2033*. World Health Organization Regional Office for South-East Asia.

Xu, Z., Müller, M., Lay, B., Oexle, N., Drack, T., Bleiker, M., Lengler, S., Blank, C., Vetter, S., Rössler, W., Rüsch, N., & Kawohl, W. (2018). Involuntary hospitalization, stigma stress and suicidality: A longitudinal study. *Social Psychiatry and Psychiatric Epidemiology, 53*(4), 309–312. https://doi.org/10.1007/s00127-018-1494-9

# Chapter 11
# Traditional Approaches to Mental Illness in South Asia

**Syeda Ayat-e-Zainab Ali, Tamkeen Saleem, and S. M. Yasir Arafat**

**Abstract** The traditional methods of treating mental illness in South Asia have their roots in indigenous healing techniques as well as cultural, religious, and spiritual practices. Due to cultural beliefs, stigma, accessibility, and religious understanding, South Asians continue to seek alternative treatments for mental illness even as evidence-based treatments for mental health issues have grown in popularity. When it comes to coping with mental health issues, individuals in South Asia frequently exhibit a stronger propensity to rely on religion and spirituality than those in other countries. Ayurvedic medicine, Tibb, aromatherapy, breathing techniques, yoga, and meditation are frequently utilized by South Asians in managing mental health issues. But there are also concerns about the lack of scientific support and possible harm from unauthorized practices. It is possible to bridge treatment gaps and improve mental health outcomes by combining evidence-based mental health care with traditional approaches. Further, research is required to assess the effectiveness and safety of traditional methods in order to ensure comprehensive and efficient mental health treatment outcomes. Therefore, a religiously integrated, community-driven, culturally sensitive strategy is needed that recognizes traditional healing while implementing contemporary psychiatric interventions that could enhance access to mental health care in South Asia.

**Keywords** Traditional approaches · Mental illness · South Asia

S. A.-Z. Ali (✉) · T. Saleem
Department of Clinical Psychology, Shifa Tameer-E-Millat University, Islamabad, Pakistan
e-mail: ayat.dcp@stmu.edu.pk

S. M. Y. Arafat
Department of Psychiatry, Bangladesh Specialized Hospital, Dhaka, Bangladesh



S. M. Y. Arafat et al. (eds.), *Social Psychiatry in South Asia*, South Asian Perspectives in Mental Health and Psychology , https://doi.org/10.1007/978-981-96-8078-8_11

## 1 Introduction

South Asia, composed of Afghanistan, Bangladesh, Bhutan, India, Nepal, Pakistan, and Sri Lanka, is home to about 24% of the world's population. Seven of the eight South Asian nations are categorized as LMICs by the World Bank (Arafat & Kar, 2024; Mudunna et al., 2025) and it is reported that more than 80% of those with mental health issues reside in low- and middle-income nations (LMICs) (Naveed et al., 2020). There are a lot of disparities in South Asia. Over the past few decades, this region has seen significant social and economic changes. Mental, substance use, and neurological problems account for most of the disease burden in South Asian countries. South Asia's population is diverse in terms of religion, socioeconomic status, and culture, and it is expanding too quickly (Tripathi, 2023). Research indicates that compared to many other parts of the world, South Asia has a higher prevalence of mental health issues (Tripathi, 2023). Affected by high rates of poverty, between 150 and 200 million people in this area have a diagnosed mental disorder and have restricted access to mental health care (Thara & Padmavati, 2013). Additionally, there is a dearth of thorough research on the epidemiological and psychological burden of mental diseases, which has a significant impact on the development and application of mental health policies and services (Hossain & Purohit, 2019; Hossain et al., 2020; Naveed et al., 2020; Shidhaye et al., 2015).

Because of the high population density in the region, all of the South Asian countries struggle with a lack of suitable medical facilities. Additionally, as there are few resources and a lack of qualified specialists, mental health services are sometimes insufficient or difficult to access (Arafat & Kar, 2024; Tripathi, 2023). The burden of mental disorders at the population level is increased by a number of sociocultural barriers, such as the stigma associated with mental illnesses and a lack of awareness, which frequently result in underreporting or delayed reporting of mental illnesses (Hossain et al., 2020; Naveed et al., 2020). South Asians often endure mental illness in silence because of the stigma attached to it (Tripathi, 2023).

Furthermore, mental health is not well acknowledged in those countries as a priority for health policy. A large number of South Asian nations lack strategic plans, programs, laws, regulations, and other instrumental measures necessary to effectively address mental health issues in their populations (Hossain & Purohit, 2019; Hossain et al., 2020). Also, the social, cultural, religious, spiritual, historical, and holistic facets of human existence are also strongly intertwined with mental health (Gopalkrishnan, 2018). Since South Asians share all of these psychosocial categories to varied degrees (Hossain et al., 2020), research on mental health in this region also needs to take a cross-cultural and multi-national approach. Hence, a comprehensive assessment of the incidence of mental diseases in South Asian countries is necessary to address these problems and enhance the body of knowledge for improved decision-making and future research.

## 2 Traditional Healers in the Treatment of Mental Disorders in South Asia

Historically, mental illness has been viewed and handled differently across cultures. In South Asia, beliefs pertaining to culture, religion, spirituality, and community-based practices have long served as the foundation for traditional approaches to mental health treatment. In nations like India, Pakistan, Bangladesh, Afghanistan, Maldives, Bhutan, Nepal, and Sri Lanka, perspectives and approaches to mental health illnesses are still shaped by these practices, which are frequently inspired by Hinduism, Islam, Buddhism, and indigenous traditions.

A significant portion of the worldwide mental health workforce consists of traditional healers (Nortje et al., 2016). By applying indigenous knowledge systems that are firmly anchored in cultural and spiritual practices, traditional healers in South Asia play a vital role in treating mental health illnesses. Particularly in impoverished and rural areas, these traditional healing techniques sometimes supplement or even replace conventional mental health treatments. Many people in developing nations seek out traditional healers for mental health issues, often in addition to accessing professional psychiatric services, according to a substantial body of published literature covering the last 50 years (Familiar et al., 2013; Marques et al., 2021; Nortje et al., 2016). The attractiveness of traditional healers lies in their shared viewpoint with clients and their application of local culturally specific information, beliefs, and practices (Nortje et al., 2016). Spiritual and religious explanations of illness aetiology are common among these shared beliefs, especially in developing nations, and they influence help-seeking behaviors (Bhikha et al., 2012). Traditional healers are particularly popular and offer a potentially beneficial source of mental health care in places where conventional psychiatric facilities are limited or prohibitively expensive (Farooqi, 2006; Gureje et al., 2015; Nortje et al., 2016). In South Asian countries, traditional healing practices involve not only natural medical substances but also objects such as amulets, religious phrases, incantations, charms, magic (sorcery), sacrifices, ceremonies, and even intrusive physical and mental suffering. This approach is referred to as "traditional" since it has been used for many generations to treat a variety of physical and mental illnesses (Haque et al., 2018).

### *2.1 Religious and Spiritual Healing Practices in Mental Health Treatment*

Healing, which seeks to relieve suffering and restore health and wholeness, is generally a key element of all religious systems. It encompasses the physical, psychological, social, and spiritual facets of human existence and is typically strongly ingrained in religion. Religious healing can take many different forms, such as social and interpersonal reorganization, metaphysical energy manipulation, and miraculous supernatural interventions (Dein, 2020). Religious healing, according to Vellenga (2008), is a therapeutic approach that "assumes the presence of a supernatural power which can restore the natural order." In numerous religious traditions across a range of historical and geographic contexts, there exist accounts of the therapeutic effects of religious rituals or practices. With roots in Buddhism, Islam, Hinduism, and indigenous traditions, these approaches link mental diseases to karma, supernatural forces, or divine intervention. Reading religious materials, praying, and doing rituals are frequent techniques. Religions vary in the kinds of religious healers they employ, such as shamans or "miraculous" healers, as well as in how they employ self-help techniques (Dein, 2020).

Over the last twenty years, there has been a growing emphasis on religion as a coping mechanism. While negative religious coping typically has the opposite effect, positive religious coping has favorable correlations with mental health (Ali & Saleem, 2024; Skalski-Bednarz et al., 2022). Individuals in South Asia are more likely than people in other regions to turn to religion and spirituality as coping strategies when they are experiencing mental health issues. The existing and quickly growing body of research on religion and mental health supports the positive impacts of religious participation on mental health and overall well-being (Ali et al., 2024). For instance, higher levels of mental health are typically associated with increased religious activity or attendance and believe in God (Aggarwal et al., 2023; Ali & Saleem, 2024; Ali et al., 2024; Estrada et al., 2019). Moreover, a fundamental aspect of religions is prayer (Dein, 2020). Being a multifaceted phenomenon, it can help people find meaning, purpose, and coping mechanisms in their lives as well as promote social bonding (Aggarwal et al., 2023). These elements may enhance mental health. Although it would seem that prayer would benefit mental health (Levin, 2020), there is inconsistent empirical evidence in this area (Bartkowski et al., 2017).

South Asian societies are intricately woven with religion and spirituality, which influence daily practices, values, and beliefs. They are therefore well-known and easily accessible sources of assistance. Accessible and cost-effective mental health services are frequently a problem in many South Asian nations, especially in rural areas. Because of this, religious institutions are often the first place people turn to when they need help with mental health issues. Unfortunately, in many South Asian cultures, stigma around mental illness is still quite strong. This may deter people from getting professional assistance and instead lead them to look for spiritual or religious solutions. The utilization of rituals, ceremonies, and the engagement of spiritual healers to address mental health issues are some of the common features of religious and spiritual healing practices in South Asian nations. Following are key religious and spiritual healing practices integrated for mental health care across South Asian countries:

### 2.1.1 Faith Healing Practices in India and Nepal

Hinduism in India provides a number of rituals that many people find useful in managing mental health issues, such as reciting mantras, engaging in puja (worship), and asking priests for blessings (Dein, 2020). Residential stays at temples, daily prayers and meditations at religious shrines devoted to healing particular mental diseases, music and drums, and in some extreme situations, the patient was shackled to the walls to help them focus on their recovery (Dein et al., 2020). According to Raguram and colleagues (2002), temple healing traditions and other traditional community resources are frequently employed in India to treat mental diseases. Their research showed that objective assessments of clinical psychopathology were better after a short visit to a healing temple in South India.

The majority of people in Nepal are spiritualists, as the country is primarily Hindu. Many practices associated with spiritualism are therefore in use. Early morning prayer, pilgrimage, intermittent fasting, meditation, music, and bhajan are some of the behavioral practices that help improve mental health and provide comfort by fostering hope and optimistic thinking (Nadi & Ghahremani, 2014; Poudel, 2020). The benefits of fasting for fostering mental wellness are explained by numerous studies. Fasting is said to have a larger favorable impact on self-esteem, which helps people maintain a healthy mental state (Poudel, 2020). Additionally, it has been demonstrated that fasting enhances social functioning and lessens the symptoms of despair and anxiety (Nair & Khawale, 2016). As part of mental health, listening to bhajan and yoga music significantly enhances focus and attention (Dey et al., 2013).

### 2.1.2 Healing Through Quran, and Sunnah in Pakistan, Bangladesh, Afghanistan and Maldives

Muslims embrace religion in times of adversity, increasing the frequency and intensity of their religious practices such as reading the Qur'an, praying, confessing their sins, and surrendering to God's will. The holiest book of Islam, the Qur'an, introduces God as "The most compassionate, most merciful" (Al-Fatihah, 1:1). It then goes on to describe God as an entity to turn to for guidance and assistance. By submitting to and depending on God, these opening lays the groundwork for the Islamic religion (Ghuloum et al., 2024). Therefore, Islamic traditions like as reciting the Quran, engaging in Sufi zikr (remembrance), and consulting imams are frequently employed for mental health in Muslim nations like Bangladesh, Afghanistan, Pakistan, and the Maldives. People often seek Ruqya as a treatment that involves recitation of Quranic verses for protection and healing from spiritual or emotional problems. Remembering the Almighty and praying every day are also seen as effective therapies (Dein et al., 2020). According to Dein et al. (2020), these therapy techniques are believed to help people regain their belief, which is a crucial component of healing or recovery.

A particular component of how mental illness is conceptualized in Muslim culture is governed by supernatural forces. According to an Islamic perspective, mental health issues are caused by black magic, the Jinn (genie), and the evil eye (Rassool, 2018). It implies that those who have lost faith and place greater significance on the material world will be particularly impacted by these factors (Haque, 2004). For instance, according to a study by Rassool (2018), most Muslim patients believe that their symptoms are signs of spiritual distress, divine retribution, or supernatural powers like black magic or the evil eye (Ghuloum et al., 2024). The Muslim community frequently attributes symptoms including anxiety, hyperactivity, altered consciousness, and psychotic disorders to the evil eye, sorcery, or jinn possession, according to research by Al-Ashqar (2003) and Al-Habeeb (2003). In case of possession, evil eye and black magic, Ruqya and dhikar is performed to ward off bad spirits and jinn.

According to an extensive review by Koenig and Al-Shohaib (2019), practicing Islam by reading and reciting the Qur'an, praying frequently, adhering strictly to its teachings, and having a committed belief system can reduce stress and improve mental health, general well-being, and happiness. Quran recitation ceremonies (khatam) are held to bring emotional and spiritual healing to individuals or families. Incense (Lauban) is burned for purification and to ward off negative energies believed to cause distress. Similarly, use of Amulets (Taweez) where Quranic verses written on paper, wrapped in leather are worn for protection against negative influences. People visit Sufi shrines for spiritual solace, healing, and emotional relief through rituals such as dhamaal (spiritual dance). Vows or offerings are made at shrines or sacred places to seek divine intervention for mental health issues (Khan & Kalhoro, 2016). In the context of faith or belief system, these interpretations are crucial to take into account because religiosity frequently leads patients to turn to faith healers, religious leaders, or traditional healers for assistance in addition to or instead of professional mental health care (Ghuloum et al., 2024).

#### 2.1.3 Religious Factors and Mental Health in Bhutan and Sri Lanka

Both Bhutan and Sri Lanka are primarily Buddhist nations, with over 90% and 70% of their respective populations reporting to be spiritual (Sithey et al., 2018). Participating in religious activities has been linked to improved coping mechanisms for stress, depression, substance misuse, anxiety, and suicide (Koenig, 2009). The law of karma, acceptance, and forgiveness are all part of Buddhist principles that may promote tolerance and ease social tensions while improving mental health individually (Sithey et al., 2018). Buddhists can participate in their religion by chanting, prayers, sermons, Bodhipuja, and other rituals, or through mental exercises like meditation (De Zoysa & Wickrama, 2011). People engage in religious activities for an average of 51 min per day (Sithey et al., 2018).

### 2.2 *Use of Traditional Remedies*

In South Asian region, traditional remedies for mental health issues often integrate spiritual rituals, herbal, and holistic treatments to address mental well-being. Following are some key traditional healing remedies:

### 2.2.1 Ayurvedic Medicine

Indian practices include Ayurvedic medicine, which offers some dietary adjustments, herbal remedies, and lifestyle tailored to individual needs and problems. The fundamental principle of Ayurveda revolves around the equilibrium of the three doshas; Vata (air and space), Pitta (fire and water), and Kapha (Earth and water), a disequilibrium among these may cause a disease. It addresses physical as well as mental health problems through practices like Panchakarma detoxification (cleansing on the mind and body) and the use of calming herbs. Shirodhara is a distinctive Ayurvedic therapy that involves a steady stream of warm oil or medicated liquid being poured onto the forehead. It is thought to calm the mind, alleviate stress and anxiety, and encourage profound relaxation (Gupta, 2024; Verma et al., 2024).

### 2.2.2 Siddha Medicine

One of the oldest traditional healing systems is Siddha medicine, which is mostly practiced in Tamil Nadu, India. By emphasizing the equilibrium of the body's basic components and energy, it addresses mental wellness. Among the treatments include lifestyle modifications, mineral supplements, and herbal formulations. In order to address imbalances considered to be the source of mental disorders, detoxification treatments and specialized diets are recommended. It is noteworthy, nonetheless, that despite the cultural significance of these techniques, there are still obstacles to their scientific confirmation and incorporation into mainstream treatment (Ottilingam et al., 2015).

### 2.2.3 The Unani Tibb System

In Pakistan, the Unani Tibb system is fundamental to traditional healing. Hellenistic Greece is where this Greco-Arabic medical system first emerged. The notion of humors is central to Unani Tibb—balancing the four vital body fluids (blood, phlegm, yellow bile, and black bile) to maintain health. In order to restore equilibrium, practitioners combine dietary changes, lifestyle alterations, and herbal therapies (Arooj, 2023).

### 2.2.4 Aromatherapy

In South Asia, aromatherapy is being used more and more as an adjunct to mental health treatment. Because of their potential relaxing benefits, essential oils like lavender, chamomile, and rosemary are frequently used (Ringu & Ranjan, 2024). According to a review of aromatherapy's effectiveness in psychiatric diseases, essential oils used topically or inhaled can have quantifiable psychological effects, suggesting possible advantages in the treatment of mental health issues like anxiety and depression (Perry & Perry, 2006).

### 2.2.5 Lifestyle and Therapeutic Practices

South Asian populations, including Indians, Nepalese, Pakistanis, and Bangladeshis, also frequently engage in a holistic practice that combines physical postures, breathing exercises (pranayama), and meditation. High-intensity exercises like Pranayama are suggested to combat feelings of fatigue and encourage the release of "happy hormones" like serotonin and dopamine, which improve mental health (Barua, 2025). Yoga is widely recognized for reducing stress, anxiety, and enhancing overall mental well-being. In Bhutan, Nepal, and Sri Lanka, mindfulness exercises including meditation and consulting monks are common coping strategies. Yoga asanas and mindfulness-based practices are becoming increasingly popular for stress management in Buddhists, Indians, and Muslim regions (Barua, 2025; Khajuria et al., 2023; Sharma & Sharma, 2024). Mindfulness meditation, which has its roots in Buddhist teachings, is a framework for mental training that uses nonjudgmental observation to develop awareness of one's current feelings and senses (Black & Slavich, 2016). According to a prior study that included a systematic review of randomized controlled trials, mindfulness meditation may be linked to immune system modulation, such as a reduction in proinflammatory processes or an increase in cell-mediated defense systems (Black & Slavich, 2016). Numerous beneficial psychological outcomes of mindfulness include enhanced behavioral regulation, decreased psychological symptoms and emotional reactivity, and a rise in subjective well-being (Keng et al., 2011). Furthermore, a culturally-driven approach to health and well-being is evident in Muslim South Asian countries, where herbal remedies, cupping therapy (hijama), and spiritual healing (ruqyah) are frequently sought in addition to conventional medical care (Ghuloum et al., 2024).

## 3 Family Factors in Mental Health

For South Asians, the family environment has continuously been identified as a significant factor in psychological functioning (Roysircar et al., 2003). According to clinical research, a breakdown in the support system of both nuclear and extended families, especially for South Asians, can lead to feelings of loneliness, distress and acute anxiety (Ahmed & Lemkau, 2000). In South Asia, family systems are usually close-knit and extended, making them an ideal support system for people dealing with mental health issues (Masood et al., 2009). Family members frequently have a significant impact on the diagnosis, treatment, and recovery of people with mental illnesses and suicidal behavior (Arafat et al., 2022). Their engagement can include anything from providing emotional support and arranging access to medical specialists or traditional healers to monitoring medicine adherence. However, societal views on mental illness have an impact on how successful family-based care is. Misconceptions and stigma can cause people to underreport and be reluctant to ask for outside assistance. For supportive intentions to be translated into effective care, educational programs that raise mental health literacy within families are necessary.

## 4 Integration of Traditional and Modern Approaches

In South Asia, efforts have been made recently to combine contemporary mental health treatments with traditional healing methods (Sabki et al., 2019). Mental health practitioners understand the value of culturally sensitive methods that take into account the part that religion, spirituality, and culture play in their patients' lives. In addition to lowering stigma and increasing access to care, collaborative efforts among religious leaders, faith and traditional healers, community organizations, and mental health professionals seek to advance holistic well-being. For better therapeutic outcomes, it is vital to incorporate the cultural and religious beliefs into mental health treatment as it aligns with their worldview, thus, making the therapy more relevant and effective. For instance, a mental health professional working with a Muslim client might incorporate mindfulness practices that are supported with Islamic perspectives, like reflective meditation/grounding during prayers or using Quranic verses for comfort. Similarly, with a Hindu client yoga and meditation or mantas rooted in their cultural practices may enhance therapeutic rapport and stimulate emotional regulation.

The Dava-Dua project in Gujarat, India, is a prime example of how religious prayers and medical care can be combined to address mental health concerns. At the Mira Datar Dargah in Mehsana District, this project blends ancient faith-based therapeutic techniques (Dua) with contemporary mental medicine (Dava) (Saha et al., 2021). Patients who receive both treatments think that their recovery depends on both medicine and healing. Patients can get diagnostics, treatments, and counseling in the Dava-Dua center's outpatient department. In order to create a network of referrals between the Dava-Dua centre and priests (Mujavars), the center provides them with mental health education. This partnership promotes recovery from mental diseases and makes medical care more accessible. The Dava-Dua model enhances current basic healthcare services, despite certain implementation issues, such as outstation patients' treatment adherence and therapy cessation after patients begin to improve. It gives people access to contemporary healthcare without interfering with their spiritual and religious beliefs. Patients whose access to mental health care would otherwise be restricted benefit from this integrated approach, which upholds their human rights (Saha et al., 2021). By addressing people's cultural, religious, spiritual, and psychological needs, this approach promotes cultural resonance, trust, and therapy efficacy.

# 5 Conclusion

In the South Asian setting, it is imperative to recognize the intricate and multi-dimensional role that culture, religion, and spirituality play in the treatment of mental illness. Despite the fact that they can provide invaluable comfort and support, depending alone on them might not be enough to combat mental illness. To ensure the holistic well-being of individuals in the region, a comprehensive strategy that combines professional mental health care with traditional practices is required.

# References


Aggarwal, S., Wright, J., Morgan, A., Patton, G., & Reavley, N. (2023). Religiosity and spirituality in the prevention and management of depression and anxiety in young people: A systematic review and meta-analysis. *BMC Psychiatry, 23*(1), 729. https://doi.org/10.1186/s12888-023-05091-2

Ahmed, S. M., & Lemkau, J. P. (2000). Cultural issues in the primary care of South Asians. *Journal of Immigrant Health, 2*, 89–96. https://doi.org/10.1023/A:1009585918590

Al-Ashqar, U. S. (2003). *The world of the jinn and devils in the light of the Qur'an and Sunnah*. International Islamic Publishing House.

Al-Habeeb, T. A. (2003). A pilot study of faith healers' views on evil eye, jinn possession, and magic in the kingdom of Saudi Arabia. *Journal of Family & Community Medicine, 10*(3), 31–38.

Ali, S. A. E. Z., & Saleem, T. (2024). Psychological autopsies: Religious and spiritual factors for suicide in cases and controls. *Frontiers in Psychiatry, 15*, 1419669. https://doi.org/10.3389/fpsyt.2024.1419669

Ali, S. A. E. Z., Arafat, S. M. Y., Rezaeian, M., Khan, M. M. (2024). Suicide prevention in Muslim countries: Current status and way forward. In S. M. Y. Arafat, M. Rezaeian, & M. M. Khan (Eds.), *Suicidal behavior in Muslim majority countries*. Springer, Singapore. https://doi.org/10.1007/978-981-97-2519-9_22

Arafat, S. M. Y., Kar, S. K. (2024). Epidemiology of psychiatric disorders and overview of access to mental health care in South Asia. In S. M. Y. Arafat & S. K. Kar (Eds.), *Access to mental health care in South Asia*. Springer, Singapore. https://doi.org/10.1007/978-981-99-9153-2_1

Arafat, S. M. Y., Saleem, T., Edwards, T. M., Ali, S. A., & Khan, M. M. (2022). Suicide prevention in Bangladesh: The role of family. *Brain and Behavior, 12*(5), Article e2562. https://doi.org/10.1002/brb3.2562

Arooj, N. (2023). Understanding the role of traditional healing practices in Pakistan: Leading towards holistic healthcare. *Qlantic Journal of Social Sciences, 4*(1), 27–32. https://doi.org/10.55737/qjss.717809184

Barua, R. (2025). Harmonizing body and mind: Investigating the combined impact of yoga and mindfulness meditation on depression, anxiety, and stress. In *Global innovations in physical education and health* (pp. 203–232). IGI Global. https://doi.org/10.4018/979-8-3693-3952-7.ch008

Bartkowski, J. P., Acevedo, G. A., & Van Loggerenberg, H. (2017). Prayer, meditation, and anxiety: Durkheim revisited. *Religions, 8*(9), 191. https://doi.org/10.3390/rel8090191

Bhikha, A. G., Farooq, S., Chaudhry, N., & Husain, N. (2012). A systematic review of explanatory models of illness for psychosis in developing countries. *International Review of Psychiatry, 24*(5), 450–462. https://doi.org/10.3109/09540261.2012.711746

Black, D. S., & Slavich, G. M. (2016). Mindfulness meditation and the immune system: A systematic review of randomized controlled trials. *Annals of the New York Academy of Sciences, 1373*(1), 13–24.

Dein, S. (2020). Religious healing and mental health. *Mental Health, Religion & Culture, 23*(8), 657–665. https://doi.org/10.1080/13674676.2020.1834220

Dein, S., Persaud, A., Tribe, R., Bhugra, D., Bhui, K., Lashley, M., & ChiYing Chung, R. (2020). Moving beyond Christianity: Islam, Judaism, Hinduism and Mental Health. *World Cultural Psychiatry Research Review, 14*(1–2), 13–19.

Dey, B., Hankey, A., & Kumari, S. (2013). Listening to Bhajan improves sustained attention. *Voice of Research, 2*(2), 26–30.

De Zoysa, P., & Wickrama, T. (2011). Mental health and cultural religious coping of disabled veterans' in Sri Lanka. *Journal of Military and Veterans Health, 19*(3), 4–12.

Estrada, C. A. M., Lomboy, M. F. T. C., Gregorio, E. R., Amalia, E., Leynes, C. R., Quizon, R. R., & Kobayashi, J. (2019). Religious education can contribute to adolescent mental health in school settings. *International Journal of Mental Health Systems, 13*, 1–6. https://doi.org/10.1186/s13033-019-0286-7

Familiar, I., Sharma, S., Ndayisaba, H., Munyentwari, N., Sibomana, S., & Bass, J. K. (2013). Community perceptions of mental distress in a post-conflict setting: A qualitative study in Burundi. *Global Public Health, 8*(8), 943–957. https://doi.org/10.1080/17441692.2013.819587

Farooqi, Y. N. (2006). Traditional healing practices sought by Muslim psychiatric patients in Lahore, Pakistan. *International Journal of Disability, Development and Education, 53*(4), 401–415. https://doi.org/10.1080/10349120601008530

Ghuloum, S., Al-Thani, H. A., & Al-Amin, H. (2024). Religion and mental health: An Eastern Mediterranean region perspective. *Frontiers in Psychology, 15*, 1441560. https://doi.org/10.3389/fpsyg.2024.1441560

Gopalkrishnan, N. (2018). Cultural diversity and mental health: Considerations for policy and practice. *Frontiers in Public Health, 6*, 179. https://doi.org/10.3389/fpubh.2018.00179

Gupta, R. (2024). Integrating ayurveda with modern medicine for enhanced patient care: Analysis of realities. *The Physician, 9*(1), 1–6. https://doi.org/10.38192/1.9.1.3

Gureje, O., Nortje, G., Makanjuola, V., Oladeji, B. D., Seedat, S., & Jenkins, R. (2015). The role of global traditional and complementary systems of medicine in the treatment of mental health disorders. *The Lancet Psychiatry, 2*(2), 168–177. https://doi.org/10.1016/S2215-0366(15)00013-9

Haque, M. I., Chowdhury, A. A., Shahjahan, M., & Harun, M. G. D. (2018). Traditional healing practices in rural Bangladesh: A qualitative investigation. *BMC Complementary and Alternative Medicine, 18*, 1–15. https://doi.org/10.1186/s12906-018-2129-5

Haque, A. (2004). Psychology from Islamic perspective: Contributions of early Muslim scholars and challenges to contemporary Muslim psychologists. *Journal of Religion and Health, 43*, 357–377. https://doi.org/10.1007/s10943-004-4302-z

Hossain, M. M., Purohit, N., Sultana, A., Ma, P., McKyer, E. L. J., & Ahmed, H. U. (2020). Prevalence of mental disorders in South Asia: An umbrella review of systematic reviews and meta-analyses. *Asian Journal of Psychiatry, 51*, Article 102041. https://doi.org/10.1016/j.ajp.2020.102041

Hossain, M. M., & Purohit, N. (2019). Improving child and adolescent mental health in India: Status, services, policies, and way forward. *Indian Journal of Psychiatry, 61*(4), 415–419. https://doi.org/10.4103/psychiatry.IndianJPsychiatry_217_18

Keng, S. L., Smoski, M. J., & Robins, C. J. (2011). Effects of mindfulness on psychological health: A review of empirical studies. *Clinical Psychology Review, 31*(6), 1041–1056.

Khajuria, A., Kumar, A., Joshi, D., & Kumaran, S. S. (2023). Reducing stress with yoga: A systematic review based on multimodal biosignals. *International Journal of Yoga, 16*(3), 156–170. https://doi.org/10.4103/ijoy.ijoy_218_23

Khan, S., & Kalhoro, Z. A. (2016). The impact of international migration on spiritual Healing practices in rural Punjab. *Journal of the Pakistan Historical Society, 64*(4), 71–94.

Koenig, H. G., & Al Shohaib, S. S. (2019). Religiosity and Mental Health in Islam. In H. Moffic, J. Peteet, A. Hankir, & R. Awaad (Eds.), *Islamophobia and psychiatry*. Springer, Cham. https://doi.org/10.1007/978-3-030-00512-2_5

Koenig, H. G. (2009). Research on religion, spirituality, and mental health: A review. *The Canadian Journal of Psychiatry, 54*(5), 283–291. https://doi.org/10.1177/0706743709054005
Levin, J. (2020). Religion and medicine: A history of the encounter between humanity's two greatest institutions. *Oxford University Press.* https://doi.org/10.1093/oso/9780190867355.001.0001
Marques, B., Freeman, C., & Carter, L. (2021). Adapting traditional healing values and beliefs into therapeutic cultural environments for health and well-being. *International Journal of Environmental Research and Public Health, 19*(1), 426. https://doi.org/10.3390/ijerph19010426
Masood, N., Okazaki, S., & Takeuchi, D. T. (2009). Gender, family, and community correlates of mental health in South Asian Americans. *Cultural Diversity & Ethnic Minority Psychology, 15*(3), 265–274. https://doi.org/10.1037/a0014301
Mudunna, C., Weerasinghe, M., Tran, T., Antoniades, J., Romero, L., Chandradasa, M., & Fisher, J. (2025). Nature, prevalence and determinants of mental health problems experienced by adolescents in south Asia: A systematic review. *The Lancet Regional Health-Southeast Asia, 33*, Article 100532. https://doi.org/10.1016/j.lansea.2025.100532
Nadi, M. A., & Ghahremani, N. (2014). The relationship between dimensions of religiosity/spirituality with mental health and hope for future between staff of public hospitals in Shiraz. *Journal of Education and Health Promotion, 3*(1), 20. https://doi.org/10.4103/2277-9531.127600
Nair, P. M., & Khawale, P. G. (2016). Role of therapeutic fasting in women's health: An overview. *Journal of mid-Life Health, 7*(2), 61–64. https://doi.org/10.4103/0976-7800.185325
Naveed, S., Waqas, A., Chaudhary, A. M. D., Kumar, S., Abbas, N., Amin, R., & Saleem, S. (2020). Prevalence of common mental disorders in South Asia: A systematic review and meta-regression analysis. *Frontiers in Psychiatry, 11*, Article 573150. https://doi.org/10.3389/fpsyt.2020.573150
Nortje, G., Oladeji, B., Gureje, O., & Seedat, S. (2016). Effectiveness of traditional healers in treating mental disorders: A systematic review. *The Lancet Psychiatry, 3*(2), 154–170. https://doi.org/10.1016/S2215-0366(15)00515-5
Ottilingam, S., Murthy, T., & Raghavan, V. (2015). Mental health: Concepts and treatment in the Siddha (Tamil) system of medicine. *ASEAN Journal of Psychiatry, 16*(2).
Perry, N., & Perry, E. (2006). Aromatherapy in the management of psychiatric disorders: Clinical and neuropharmacological perspectives. *CNS Drugs, 20*(4), 257–280. https://doi.org/10.2165/00023210-200620040-00001
Poudel, A. (2020). Role of spirituality in mental health in Nepal. *JNMA; Journal of the Nepal Medical Association, 58*(226), 439–441. https://doi.org/10.31729/jnma.5110
Raguram, R., Venkateswaran, A., Ramakrishna, J., & Weiss, M. G. (2002). Traditional community resources for mental health: A report of temple healing from India. *BMJ, 325*(7354), 38–40. https://doi.org/10.1136/bmj.325.7354.38
Rassool, G. H. (2018). *Evil eye, jinn possession, and mental health issues: An Islamic perspective.* Routledge.
Ringu, K., & Ranjan, A. (2024). A Review on effectiveness of aromatherapy on mental health and well-being. *International Journal of Scientific Research in Modern Science and Technology, 3*(11), 1–13. https://doi.org/10.59828/ijsrmst.v3i11.260
Roysircar, G. E., Sandhu, D. S. E., & Bibbins Sr, V. E. (2003). *Multicultural competencies: A guidebook of practices.* Association for Multicultural Counseling & Development.
Sabki, Z. A., Sa'ari, C. Z., Muhsin, S. B. S., Kheng, G. L., Sulaiman, A. H., & Koenig, H. G. (2019). Islamic integrated cognitive behavior therapy: A Shariah-compliant intervention for Muslims with depression. *Malaysian Journal of Psychiatry,* 28(1), 29–38.
Saha, S., Chauhan, A., Hamlai, M., Saiyad, V., Makwana, S., Shah, K., & Pandya, A. (2021). Unique collaboration of modern medicine and traditional faith-healing for the treatment of mental illness: Best practice from Gujarat. *Journal of Family Medicine and Primary Care, 10*(1), 521–526. https://doi.org/10.4103/jfmpc.jfmpc_979_19
Sharma, D., & Sharma, B. R. (2024). The impact of yoga and meditation on mental and Physical well-being. *Journal of Ayurveda and Integrated Medical Sciences, 9*(5), 144–153. https://doi.org/10.21760/jaims.9.5.23

Shidhaye, R., Sikander, S., Jordans, M., De Silva, P., & Chatterjee, S. (2015). Mental health programs and policies in South Asia: Initiatives and obstacles. *In Mental health in South Asia: Ethics, resources, programs and legislation* (pp. 95–111). Springer. https://doi.org/10.1007/978-94-017-9017-8_7

Sithey, G., Li, M., Wen, L. M., Kelly, P. J., & Clarke, K. (2018). Socioeconomic, religious, spiritual and health factors associated with symptoms of common mental disorders: A cross-sectional secondary analysis of data from Bhutan's Gross National Happiness Study, 2015. *British Medical Journal Open, 8*(2), Article e018202. https://doi.org/10.1136/bmjopen-2017-018202

Skalski-Bednarz, S. B., Konaszewski, K., Toussaint, L. L., Büssing, A., & Surzykiewicz, J. (2022). Positive religious coping acts through perception of nature and silence in its association with well-being and life satisfaction among Polish Catholics. *Frontiers in Public Health, 10*, 1020007. https://doi.org/10.3389/fpubh.2022.1020007

Thara, R., & Padmavati, R. (2013). Community mental health care in South Asia. *World Psychiatry, 12*(2), 176–177. https://doi.org/10.1002/wps.20042

Tripathi, S. (2023). Mental health in South Asia: A growing cause for concern. *The round Table, 112*(2), 195–196. https://doi.org/10.1080/00358533.2023.2201071

Verma, S. K., Pandey, M., Sharma, A., & Singh, D. (2024). Exploring Ayurveda: Principles and their application in modern medicine. *Bulletin of the National Research Centre, 48*(1), 77. https://doi.org/10.1186/s42269-024-00658-9

Vellenga, S. J. (2008). Longing for health. A practice of religious healing and biomedicine compared. *Journal of Religion and Health, 47(3)*, 326–337. https://doi.org/10.1007/s10943-008-9175-0

# Chapter 12
# Culture-Bound Syndromes in South Asia

**Sujita Kumar Kar**

**Abstract** South Asia known for its cultural diversity, is recognized as the most densely populated region in the world. The majority of its countries fall into the categories of low- and middle-income, known as LAMICs. Within this richly varied cultural landscape, deeply ingrained beliefs and practices significantly influence the understanding and manifestation of psychopathology. The unique cultural nuances in South Asia give rise to specific forms of psychological distress, which may evolve in different ways across different communities. These forms of psychopathology can emerge as isolated instances or, at times, manifest in larger epidemic patterns, reflecting the intricate interplay between culture and mental health. This chapter discusses about the culture-bound syndromes that are prevalent in South Asia, exploring how these conditions are shaped by and interwoven with local customs, traditions, and societal norms.

**Keywords** Culture · Culture-bound syndrome · Cultural concepts of distress · South Asia · Dhat syndrome · Koro · Mental health

## 1 Introduction

South Asia is a heavily populated region of the globe, which harbors nearly 1.94 billion population by 2023 with a life expectancy at birth of 68 years and an annual growth rate of 1.0% (World Bank Group, 2024). The majority of the countries of South Asia are developing countries. A large number of people migrate each year out of South Asia with an estimated figure of 1,175,806 in the year 2023 (World Bank Group, 2024). Unemployment, poverty, environmental adversities, pollution, deforestation, debts, politico-religious conflicts, terrorism and war are significant other challenges of this region (World Bank Group, 2024). The culture of South Asia is highly rich and diverse. Religious beliefs and customs also vary significantly between South Asian regions (Dokuru et al., 2024).

S. K. Kar (✉)
Department of Psychiatry, King George's Medical University, Lucknow, India
e-mail: sujitakumarkar@kgmcindia.edu



S. M. Y. Arafat et al. (eds.), *Social Psychiatry in South Asia*, South Asian Perspectives in Mental Health and Psychology , https://doi.org/10.1007/978-981-96-8078-8_12

Culture has a significant influence on mental health (Aina & Morakinyo, 2011; Levine & Gaw, 1995; Ventriglio et al., 2016). Culture colors the meanings people give to illness and their attributes. People use culture-specific coping measures to deal with illness, life challenges and socio-cultural adversities (Aina & Morakinyo, 2011; Levine & Gaw, 1995; Ventriglio et al., 2016). Clinicians dealing with specific health issues in a given culture should be sensitive to cultural belief systems to accurately identify health ailments and their effective remediation. This chapter attempts to highlight the culture-bound syndromes of South Asia and the underlying culture-specific beliefs. The focus also extends to variations of the phenomenology and management of culture-bound syndromes of South Asia.

## 2 Culture-Bound Syndrome

Diversity in cultural beliefs produces diverse impacts on the mental health (Gopalkrishnan, 2018). Culture-bound syndromes commonly refer to the common mental health conditions that have a peculiar presentation in the people of a particular culture, due to the unique set of beliefs of that culture (Levine & Gaw, 1995). Various other synonyms (cultural concepts of distress, folk diagnostic categories) are used to explain them. The culture-bound syndromes were initially described around 1960s (Ventriglio et al., 2016).

It has been noticed that despite being called as "culture-bound syndrome", these conditions are also seen across other cultures. As a result, many a times researchers questioned the credibility of culture-bound syndrome (Levine & Gaw, 1995; Perez et al., 2000). Due to contradicting opinions of prominent researchers based on culture-bound syndrome, it struggled to find a place in the existing diagnostic and classificatory systems (Balhara, 2011; Perez et al., 2000).

Culture-bound syndromes are often sporadic. Sometimes culture-bound syndromes may manifest in the form of epidemics. Imitation and internalization explain, how mass behavior evolves due to cultural vulnerabilities (Carel & Cooper, 2010). Rapid globalization, industrialization, migration and socio-cultural integration in the twenty-first century resulted in changes in the prevalence and pattern of culture-bound syndromes (Kar, 2015; Ventriglio et al., 2016).

## 3 Culture-Bound Syndromes of South Asia

There are significant differences between the cultural beliefs of East and West (Gopalkrishnan, 2018).

### 3.1 Dhat Syndrome

Dhat syndrome is a prominent culture-bound syndrome of South East Asia, characterized by psychological, somatic, and sexual symptoms which is often attributed to semen loss (Bhatia et al., 1989; Chadda & Ahuja, 1990; Dhungana et al., 2017; Kar & Mishra, 2018; Kar & Sarkar, 2015; Khan, 2005, 2008; Khan et al., 2011; Maruf et al., 2024; Mullick et al., 1995; Shakya, 2019). Indian Psychiatrist Late Prof. NN Wig, has introduced the term "Dhat syndrome" in 1960s, and elaborated on it (Kar & Mishra, 2018; Malhotra & Wig, 1975; Wig, 1960). In the Indian subcontinent, semen is considered as a precious body fluid which is formed by the process of multi-step ultra-condensation of food extract in the body (Kar & Sarkar, 2015; Mishra & Roy, 2018; Prakash, 2007; Prakash et al., 2014). Ayurveda describes semen to be highly precious and as the elixir of life; hence, a lot of emphasis is given to its preservation through practice of celibacy, in the religious texts (Kar & Sarkar, 2015; Prakash et al., 2014; Sahu, 2018). Similar set of beliefs and patients presenting similar patterns of symptoms has also been reported in several parts of Europe (Janssen, 2024). Patients with Dhat syndrome often manifest with anxiety, low mood, worry, health anxiety, irritability, multiple somatic complaints, weakness, lethargy, sexual dysfunction, reduced appetite, sleep disturbances, pre-occupations related to semen loss and withdrawn behavior (Deb & Balhara, 2013; Prakash & Kar, 2019; Prakash et al., 2014; Sumathipala et al., 2004).

Similar entity has been reported in females as well, where females often show concerns to non-pathological vaginal discharge and manifest with multiple non-specific somatic symptoms and anxiety. It is popularly known as female Dhat syndrome (Chaturvedi et al., 1993; Joshi et al., 2022; Kar & Singh, 2017; Kar et al., 2021; Mehra et al., 2021; Prakash & Kar, 2019; Swami, 2018). Dhat syndrome was initially included in the International Classification of Diseases version 10 (ICD-10) and the Diagnostic and Statistical Manual of Mental Disorders, Text Revision of the fourth edition (DSM-IV-TR) (Kar, Menon, et al., 2024; Sridhar et al., 2018). In the DSM-5, it has been placed under "cultural concepts of distress". As the existing diagnostic systems do not have specific diagnostic criteria or diagnostic category to include female Dhat syndrome, these patients are often diagnosed with somatization disorder, anxiety disorder or depression (Kar & Singh, 2017; Kar, Arafat, et al., 2024; Sharma et al., 2024; Tripathi et al., 2021). Individuals with Dhat syndrome often have multiple psychiatric comorbidities; sexual dysfunction (premature ejaculation and erectile dysfunction) is the most common one (Grover et al., 2015; Grover, Avasthi, et al., 2016).

Individuals suffering from Dhat syndrome often seek care from the quacks, traditional healers, and doctors of alternative systems of medicine. They often reach the mental health professionals after seeking care from multiple non-credible sources (Grover, Gupta, et al., 2016; Singh, 2018, 2024; Singh et al., 2016). Psycho-education, addressing sexual myths, cognitive behavior therapy, supportive psychotherapy, multivitamins, anxiolytic medications and antidepressants are commonly being used in the treatment of Dhat syndrome (Kar et al., 2021; Kar, Arafat, et al., 2024; Prakash & Kar, 2019; Salam et al., 2012; Udina et al., 2013).

## 3.2 *Sorcery (Possession Syndrome)*

It is a well-known and commonly prevalent entity in several parts of India. It is known by various local names. It manifests with a dissociative phenomenon characterized by being possessed by an evil spirit, soul of a dead person or God (Rao, 1978). Affected individuals are often young females from lower educational background. It is more prevalent in tribal areas and may manifest in the form of epidemics (Rao, 1978). Such phenomenon are commonly reported in specific situations (during specific festivals or cultural rituals, in specific temples, where the religious crown reinforce such behavior positively) (Rao, 1978). In several parts of the southern India, a form of possession is prevalent which is known by the name "Bhanmati Sorcery" (Kapoor et al., 2018). It is speculated that presence of primary psychiatric illnesses like dissociative disorder, somatoform disorder, mood disorder and even schizophrenia increases the vulnerability to "Bhanmati Sorcery" (Kapoor et al., 2018). "Yakshi syndrome" is a form of possession by supernatural spirit seen in Indian culture (Jalarajan & Suresh, 2023a, 2023b). In Pakistan possession by Jinn (Jinn possession) is commonly reported culture-bound syndrome, which refers to possession by evil spirit (Ayub, 2021; Khalifa & Hardie, 2005; Khan & Sanober, 2016; Zaman, 2016).

## 3.3 *Koro*

Koro is a culture-bound syndrome characterized by the belief of progressive shrinkage of one's own penis ultimately merging with the abdomen leading to death of the individual (Chowdhury, 1996; Garg et al., 2017). It is commonly reported in Chinese and South East Asian populations. In Indian population, it is prevalent in the North-East region (Chowdhury, 1996; Garg et al., 2017). However, cases of Koro are reported from other parts of the world like—Africa (Elghazouani & Barrimi, 2018; Kar et al., 2022), Europe, Singapore (Crozier, 2012). The first published report of Koro was in the year 1895 as genital retraction syndrome in a Dutch medical journal (Chowdhury, 2021).

Koro has been included in the classificatory system of DSM-III R and ICD-10 (Chowdhury, 1996). However, the recent classificatory system DSM-5, places Koro under the category of obsessive–compulsive related disorders (Chowdhury, 2021).

Individuals suffering from Koro have cognitive distortions related to body morphology (mostly the penis) (Kar, 2023). However, Koro has also been reported in females, where the belief is centered around shrinkage of the genitalia and breast, producing significant psychological distress (Kar et al., 2022).

Koro-related psychopathology has been reported in other psychiatric disorders like schizophrenia (Garg et al., 2017), delusional disorder (Sinha et al., 2024), obsessive–compulsive disorder (Ghosh & Chowdhury, 2020), dhat syndrome (Ghosh & Chowdhury, 2020), depression (Bandinelli et al., 2011; Kennedy & Flick, 1991), anxiety (Crozier, 2012), cannabis use (Earleywine, 2001; El-Tantawy, 2017; Kalaitzi & Kalantzis, 2006; Kanwar et al., 2018), and depersonalization syndrome (Yap, 1965). The individuals affected with koro are often from low socio-economic status, poor educational level and rural background (Debbarma et al., 2016).

### 3.4 *Latah*

Latah is a culture-bound syndrome of South Asia, commonly prevalent in the Malay region and Indonesia (Lim et al., 2022; Massard-Vincent, 1996; Winzeler, 1995). It is characterized by exaggerated startle response, echo- phenomenon (echolalia, echopraxia), coprolalia, palilalia, and forced obedience. Latah is often triggered by stimulus-like sound (Bakker & Tijssen, 2010; Lim et al., 2022). It is predominantly seen among females (Bakker & Tijssen, 2010).

### 3.5 *Suchi Bai*

Suchi Bai is characterized by a morbid preoccupation with cleanliness rituals, commonly seen in Bengal (Rao, 1978). The cultural basis of this syndrome is the emphasis of the Indian system of Medicine "Ayurveda" on purity (cleanliness or hygiene), which is widely accepted in several parts of India (Kashyap et al., 2015).

The features were initially described in 1975 and had close resemblance with obsessive–compulsive disorder (than obsessive–compulsive neurosis) (Rao, 1978). An earlier literature describes the context of obsessive and compulsive phenomenon among the Bengali patients and it reveals that the most chronic cases are of Suchi bai (Chakraborty & Banerji, 1975). Often the individuals with Suchi bai syndrome indulge in excessively cleaning rituals, not allowing others to touch their things, not eating anything outside, excessive bathing and avoiding touching of anything dirty on the streets or roads (Kapoor et al., 2018).

### 3.6 *Lizard Syndrome (Squirrel or Gilhari Syndrome)*

It has been commonly reported in the western part of Rajastan (Kapoor et al., 2018). The people suffering from it often present that lizard or squirrel is present in their body underneath the skin, which moves towards the neck (Kapoor et al., 2018). It provokes a lot of anxiety in them and choking sensation (when they feel that the lizard or the squirrel is moving towards the neck) (Kapoor et al., 2018). Supportive psychotherapy and antianxiety medications are often useful. Medical evaluations are often uneventful. Patients often misinterpret the contraction of muscles (due to anxiety) as a lizard or squirrel and not convinced by alternative explanations (Kapoor et al., 2018). Often such cases meet the diagnosis of somatization disorder.

## 3.7 *Jhin-Jhinia*

It is characterized by a feeling of tingling sensation and numbness in the legs, which quickly spread to other parts of the body. This progression of symptoms result in intense anxiety and fear of death (Kapoor et al., 2018; Nandi et al., 1992). It has been reported in epidemic form during 1982 in the Arkhali village area of 24 paraganas district of west Bengal (Nandi et al., 1992). The local remedies and intervention of traditional healers often improve the condition in several hours. The spread of information of such events in general public during 1982 resulted in the development of similar episodes among other people (Nandi et al., 1992). Jhin-jhinia affected both genders and people were mostly younger adults (Kapoor et al., 2018; Nandi et al., 1992). Jhin-jhinia when occur in epidemic form or seen among people within a family, it can be explained by mean of "hysterical contagion" which is a form of social contagion (Chowdhury, 1993).

## 3.8 *Other Culture-Bound Syndromes*

### 3.8.1 Braid Cut Anxiety

Recently in 2017–2018, in several parts of north India a form of anxiety, possession and emotional dysregulation manifested in an epidemic form (Kar & Dwivedi, 2018). The episodes were triggered by cutting of hair of women by unknown persons when the women were sleeping during the nights. The affected individuals were females and mostly from rural backgrounds (Kar & Dwivedi, 2018). The individuals with braid cut anxiety mostly responded to reassurance, psycho-education, relaxation exercises and anxiolytic medications (Kar & Dwivedi, 2018).

### 3.8.2 Bachadani Syndrome

The term "Bachadani" is a phrase in Indian languages like -Hindi, which refers to the uterus (Hussain et al., 2016). The affected individuals are invariably females, who report that their uterus is either displaced or diseased and it is often accompanied with multiple non-specific somatic symptoms and anxiety (Hussain et al., 2016). It is highly prevalent in the Kashmiri women as well other parts of India (Hussain et al., 2016).

### 3.8.3 Culture-Bound Suicide

Suicide is associated with several cultural contexts. Sati and Jouhar are two prominent examples of suicidal behavior in cultural context (Chhabra et al., 2008; Thomas & Sharma, 2016). In Indian religious history, *sati* was the daughter of Daksha Prajapati, who married to Lord Shiva. She attended a religious sacrifice (popularly known as Daksha Yajna) organized by her father Daksha Pajapati, where her husband Lord Shiva was not invited (Ramos, 2015; Schmelzle & Timalsina, 2021; Wikipedia, 2025). When Daksha Prajapati disrespected and criticized Lord Shiva at the function (in his absence) before Sati, she could not tolerate it and jumped into the religious pyre as a protest against her husband's disrespect (Ramos, 2015; Wikipedia, 2025). Her sacrifice was a model of not tolerating disrespect and impending disrespect for the females. It continued for a long-time in various parts of India, particularly among the women of the upper caste. Similarly, *Jouhar* is seen mostly in Rajasthan, where females choose suicide for honor. Indian history documents the *Jouhar* of queen of Chittor (Rani Padmini) along with several other females of the Chittor fort following the conquer of Chittor by cruel invader Alauddin Khilji.

### 3.8.4 Suudu

It is a culture-bound syndrome prevalent in southern states of India characterized by feeling of heat in the pelvic region (Chhabra et al., 2008; Thomas & Sharma, 2016). People often attribute it to the manifestation of inner heat. It is reported both among males and females (Chhabra et al., 2008; Thomas & Sharma, 2016).

### 3.8.5 Ascetic Syndrome

It is characterized by strict abstinence from sexual practices, social withdrawal behavior, firm adherence to religious practices and extreme form of negligence to general wellbeing (Chhabra et al., 2008; Masson, 1976). Though Ascetic syndrome is common among followers of Vedic philosophy, it is also seen among the followers of eastern Christianity (Bradford, 2016). Asceticism is the branch that deals with development of purity, holiness and perfection in an individual's life (Cross & Thoma, 2006). Setting discipline in life is expected to bring all these virtues to life (Cross & Thoma, 2006). It is reflected in the life of the individuals with ascetic syndrome.

## 4 Impact of Culture-Bound Syndromes Mental Health Service Delivery

The culture-bound syndromes affect mental health service delivery in several ways. The important effects of culture-bound syndrome on mental health service delivery are:

I. Misdiagnosis: As the manifestations of the culture-bound syndromes occur in a typical fashion, a clinician's lack of cultural awareness may result in a misdiagnosis of the condition.
II. Reaching to mental health facilities: As people with the culture-bound syndrome often attribute their distress to a cultural belief; so they do not consider it to be a mental health issue and are reluctant to seek psychiatric consultation.
III. Resistance to therapeutic suggestions: A strong cultural belief often result in significant resistance to therapeutic suggestions.
IV. Challenges in estimating burden of culture-bound syndrome: As majority of the culture-bound syndromes are not included in diagnostic systems, often the epidemiological studies on mental health fail to estimate the burden of culture-bound syndromes in the community.
V. Challenges on mental healthcare facilities: Sometimes culture-bound syndromes occur in the form of an epidemic, which often increases the burden on mental healthcare facilities unexpectedly.

## 5 Approach and Management of Culture-Bound Syndromes of South Asia

- **Help-seeking behavior & Pathway of Care:** Access to mental healthcare is adversely affected by the cultural beliefs and stigma in South Asia (Arafat & Kar, 2024). Several factors (socio-demography of the client, availability and accessibility of the mental health services, knowledge about the condition, acceptability of the condition as a health issue, referral practice, coordination between the healthcare facilities) influence the help-seeking behavior in culture-bound syndromes (Grover, Gupta, et al., 2016; Singh, 2018, 2024; Singh et al., 2016). The majority of people with culture-bound syndrome often seek help from unqualified practitioners or traditional healers (Singh, 2024). Often the people with culture-bound syndrome follow a long pathway of care before reaching a qualified specialist mental health professional (Grover, Gupta, et al., 2016; Singh, 2024).
- **Treatment models:** Various treatment models have been proposed for managing culture-bound syndromes. The conventional treatment model emphasizes management of myths and cultural conflicts, strengthening psychosocial support, coping with stress, awareness of reality, and handling comorbid psychiatric

conditions such as depression, anxiety, and sleep disturbances through appropriate psychological and medical interventions in a culturally sensitive manner. However, the needs of every individual with a culture-bound syndrome, as well as those of different culture-bound syndromes, are unique; thus, a person-centered model of care is expected to be more effective (Kar & Singh, 2016). As several culture-bound syndromes like Dhat syndrome and Koro have multi-systemic manifestations, probably a multidisciplinary approach and integrated model of approach (involving mental health professions, traditional healers, family members and professionals of relevant allied systems of medicine) may be beneficial in providing holistic care to the individuals with culture-bound syndrome (Kar & Sarkar, 2015).

- **Treatment modalities:** Individuals suffering from culture-bound syndrome, also need detailed evaluation in a culture-sensitive manner. A detailed history taking, evaluation of comorbid medical and psychiatric conditions, and detailed physical examination help in formulating an appropriate management plan (Rekha & Mangalwedhe, 2018; Singh & Tripathi, 2018). Various psychological and pharmacological interventions are often used in the management of culture-bound syndromes (Fig. 1). Dealing the individuals with culture-bound syndrome requires a culture-sensitive approach and better understanding of the cultural nuances.

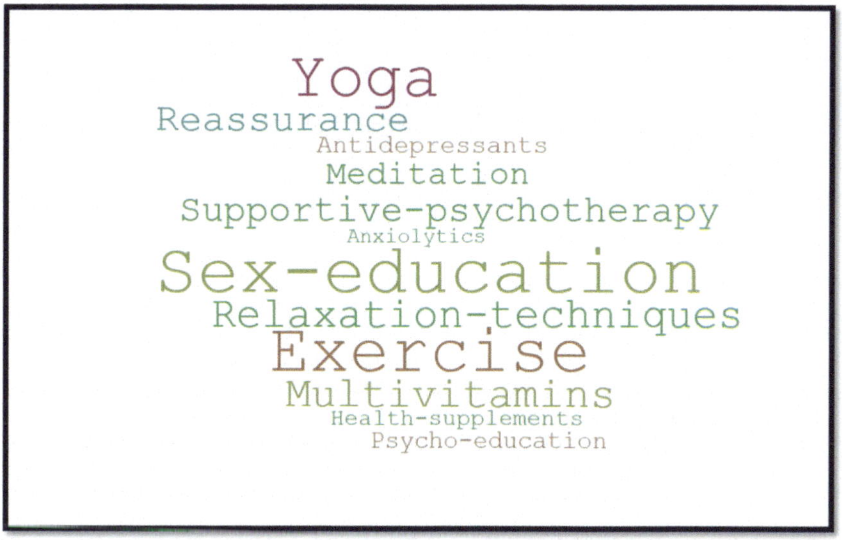


**Fig. 1** Commonly used modalities of interventions for culture-bound syndromes

## 6 Conclusion and Future Directions

Culture-bound syndromes survive on cultural beliefs. Cultures are undergoing rapid transformation, which is likely to affect the belief systems and the psychopathology based on these beliefs. It is important to carry out research to understand the change in the manifestation of the culture-bound syndrome with reference to the change in cultural beliefs and values. Also, there is a need to develop specific diagnostic criteria to distinctly identify these conditions. Also, there is a need for systematically conducted epidemiological studies and qualitative research to have an in-depth understanding of these conditions.

## References

Aina, O. F., & Morakinyo, O. (2011). Culture-bound syndromes and the neglect of cultural factors in psychopathologies among Africans. *African Journal of Psychiatry, 14*(4), 278–285. https://doi.org/10.4314/ajpsy.v14i4.4

Arafat, S. M. Y., & Kar, S. K. (Eds.). (2024). *Access to mental health care in South Asia: Current status, potential challenges, and ways out*. Springer Nature. https://doi.org/10.1007/978-981-99-9153-2

Ayub, A. (2021). *Jinn possession, black magic, or mental illness the impact of demographic factors & religion on people's perceptions*. Unpublished Undergraduate Project. Institute of Business Administration, Pakistan. https://Ir.Iba.Edu.Pk/Sslace/76. https://www.researchgate.net/profile/Aayma-Ayub/publication/355789883_Jinn_Possession_Black_Magic_Or_Mental_Illness_The_Impact_of_Demographic_Factors_Religion_on_People's_Perceptions/links/617e66333c987366c30acd6a/Jinn-Possession-Black-Magic-Or-Mental-Illness-The-Impact-of-Demographic-Factors-Religion-on-Peoples-Perceptions.pdf

Bakker, M. J., & Tijssen, M. A. J. (2010). Latah. In K. Kompoliti & L. V. Metman (Eds.), *Encyclopedia of movement disorders* (pp. 120–122). Academic Press. https://doi.org/10.1016/B978-0-12-374105-9.00477-9

Balhara, Y. P. S. (2011). Culture-bound syndrome: Has it found its right niche? *Indian Journal of Psychological Medicine, 33*(2), 210–215. https://doi.org/10.4103/0253-7176.92055

Bandinelli, P. L., Trevisi, M., Kotzalidis, G. D., Manfredi, G., Rapinesi, C., & Ducci, G. (2011). Chronic Koro-like Syndrome (KLS) in recurrent depressive disorder as a variant of Cotard's delusion in an Italian male patient. A case report and historical review. *Rivista Di Psichiatria, 46*(3), 220–226.

Bhatia, M. S., Bohra, N., & Malik, S. C. (1989). "Dhat" syndrome—A useful clinical entity. *Indian Journal of Dermatology, 34*(2), 32–41.

Bradford, D. T. 1951-. (2016). *The spiritual tradition in Eastern Christianity: Ascetic psychology, mystical experience, and physical practices*. Peeters.

Carel, H., & Cooper, R. (2010). Introduction: Culture-bound syndromes. *Studies in History and Philosophy of Biological and Biomedical Sciences, 41*(4), 307–308. https://doi.org/10.1016/j.shpsc.2010.10.004

Chadda, R. K., & Ahuja, N. (1990). Dhat syndrome. A sex neurosis of the Indian subcontinent. *The British Journal of Psychiatry: the Journal of Mental Science, 156*, 577–579. https://doi.org/10.1192/bjp.156.4.577

Chakraborty, A., & Banerji, G. (1975). Ritual, a culture specific neurosis, and obsessional states in Bengali culture. *Indian Journal of Psychiatry, 17*(4), 273.

Chaturvedi, S. K., Chandra, P. S., Isaac, M. K., Sudarshan, C. Y., & Rao, S. (1993). Is there a female Dhat syndrome. *NIMHANS Journal, 11*(2), 89–93.

Chhabra, V., Bhatia, M., & Gupta, R. (2008). Cultural bound syndromes in India. *Delhi Psychiatry Journal, 11*(1), 15–18.

Chowdhury, A. N. (1993). Jhin-Jhini—A hysterical contagion? *Indian Journal of Psychiatry, 35*(2), 141.

Chowdhury, A. N. (1996). The definition and classification of Koro. *Culture, Medicine and Psychiatry, 20*(1), 41–65. https://doi.org/10.1007/BF00118750

Chowdhury, A. N. (2021). Loss of cultural tag of Koro. In A. N. Chowdhury (Ed.), *Koro: Clinical and historical developments of the culturally defined genital retraction disorder* (pp. 93–140). Springer International Publishing. https://doi.org/10.1007/978-3-030-87962-4_5

Cross, R., & Thoma, D. (2006). The collapse of ascetical discipline and clerical misconduct: Sex and prayer. *The Linacre Quarterly, 73*(1), 1–114. https://doi.org/10.1080/20508549.2006.11877771

Crozier, I. (2012). Making up koro: Multiplicity, psychiatry, culture, and penis-shrinking anxieties. *Journal of the History of Medicine and Allied Sciences, 67*(1), 36–70. https://doi.org/10.1093/jhmas/jrr008

Deb, K. S., & Balhara, Y. P. S. (2013). Dhat syndrome: A review of the world literature. *Indian Journal of Psychological Medicine, 35*(4), 326–331. https://doi.org/10.4103/0253-7176.122219

Debbarma, S., Das, S. K., Kumar, A., Debbarma, D., Das, A., & Reang, T. (2016). Koro epidemic: A descriptive study. *Hindu, 5*(76), 5634–5638.

Dhungana, M., Ghimire, S. R., & Thapa, M. (2017). A study of Dhat syndrome-a culture bound syndrome in Nepalese context. *Journal of Psychiatrists' Association of Nepal, 6*(1), 33–37.

Dokuru, D. R., Horwitz, T. B., Freis, S. M., Stallings, M. C., & Ehringer, M. A. (2024). South Asia: The missing diverse in diversity. *Behavior Genetics, 54*(1), 51–62. https://doi.org/10.1007/s10519-023-10161-y

Earleywine, M. (2001). Cannabis-induced Koro in Americans. *Addiction, 96*(11), 1663–1666. https://doi.org/10.1046/j.1360-0443.2001.9611166312.x

Elghazouani, F., & Barrimi, M. (2018). Koro syndrome: When culture interacts with psychopathology. *Revue Medicale De Bruxelles, 39*(2), 108–110. https://doi.org/10.30637/2018.17-097

El-Tantawy, A. (2017). Chronic Koro-like syndrome co-morbid with schizophrenia and history of cannabis abuse in an Egyptian patient: Case report. *Arab Journal of Psychiatry, 28*(1), 92–96.

Garg, K., Kumar, C. N., & Sharadhi, C. (2017). Koro: Much more than just a culture bound syndrome. *Asian Journal of Psychiatry, 29*, 146–147. https://doi.org/10.1016/j.ajp.2017.05.022

Ghosh, S., & Chowdhury, A. N. (2020). A case of two culture-bound syndromes (Koro and Dhat syndrome) coexisting with obsessive-compulsive disorder. *Indian Journal of Psychiatry, 62*(2), 221–222. https://doi.org/10.4103/psychiatry.IndianJPsychiatry_298_19

Gopalkrishnan, N. (2018). Cultural diversity and mental health: Considerations for policy and practice. *Frontiers in Public Health, 6*, 179. https://doi.org/10.3389/fpubh.2018.00179

Grover, S., Avasthi, A., Gupta, S., Dan, A., Neogi, R., Behere, P. B., Lakdawala, B., Tripathi, A., Chakraborty, K., Sinha, V., Bhatia, M. S., Patjoshi, A., Rao, T. S. S., & Rozatkar, A. (2016). Phenomenology and beliefs of patients with Dhat syndrome: A nationwide multicentric study. *The International Journal of Social Psychiatry, 62*(1), 57–66. https://doi.org/10.1177/0020764015591857

Grover, S., Gupta, S., Mahajan, S., & Avasthi, A. (2016). Pathway of care among patients with Dhat syndrome attending a psychosexual clinic in tertiary care center in North India. *Industrial Psychiatry Journal, 25*(1), 72–77.

Grover, S., Gupta, S., Mehra, A., & Avasthi, A. (2015). Comorbidity, knowledge and attitude towards sex among patients with Dhat syndrome: A retrospective study. *Asian Journal of Psychiatry, 17*, 50–55. https://doi.org/10.1016/j.ajp.2015.07.002

Hussain, T., Bhat, J. A., Shamshad, M., Malik, A. A., Mir, S. A., & Shafat, M. (2016). *Bachadani (Uterine) syndrome among Kashmiri women, a culture bound syndrome? 6*(8), 78–83.

Jalarajan, R. S., & Suresh, A. K. (2023a). 5 The Yakshi syndrome in Indian popular culture. *Culture-Bound Syndromes in Popular Culture*. https://books.google.com/books?hl=en&lr=&id=Hs7bEAAAQBAJ&oi=fnd&pg=PT113&dq=Suudu+culture+bound+syndrome&ots=l4DhWeC4HO&sig=jW4iPByKS066bVYISOI2I32EFEs

Jalarajan, R. S., & Suresh, A. K. (2023b). The Yakshi syndrome in Indian popular culture: Representation of possessed female bodies in Indian cinema. In *Culture-bound syndromes in popular culture* (pp. 106–123). Routledge. https://www.taylorfrancis.com/chapters/edit/10.4324/9781003379096-8/yakshi-syndrome-indian-popular-culture-raj-sony-jalarajan-adith-suresh

Janssen, D. F. (2024). Dhat syndrome east and west: A history in two acts. *Culture, Medicine, and Psychiatry*. https://doi.org/10.1007/s11013-024-09874-4

Joshi, S., Tripathi, A., Agarwal, S., Singh, N., Gupta, B., Nischal, A., & Kar, S. K. (2022). Phenomenology, disability and sexual functioning in female Dhat syndrome: A study of tertiary care gynaecology outpatients. *General Psychiatry, 35*(5), Article e100863. https://doi.org/10.1136/gpsych-2022-100863

Kalaitzi, C. K., & Kalantzis, A. (2006). Cannabis-induced koro-like syndrome: A case report and mini review. *Urologia Internationalis, 76*(3), 278–280.

Kanwar, P., Kumar, R., & Sharma, R. C. (2018). Cannabis induced koro in a Nepali migrant. *Asian Journal of Psychiatry, 31*, 86–87.

Kapoor, A., Juneja, R., & Chand Singh, D. (2018). Cultural specific syndromes in India—An overview. *International Journal of Current Research and Review, 10*(11), 2–6.

Kar, S. K. (2015). Dhat syndrome: Will it reach a height or die soon? *Journal of Human Reproductive Sciences, 8*(4), 246. https://doi.org/10.4103/0974-1208.170421

Kar, S. K. (2023). Penis size: Body image. In T. K. Shackelford (Ed.), *Encyclopedia of sexual psychology and behavior* (pp. 1–3). Springer International Publishing. https://doi.org/10.1007/978-3-031-08956-5_1792-1

Kar, S. K., Arafat, S. M., Menon, V., Sharma, P., Das, A., Perera, S., & Shankar, A. (2022). A bibliometric analysis of Koro syndrome. *Global Psychiatry Archives, 5*(1), 36–41. https://doi.org/10.52095/gp.2022.4460.1039

Kar, S. K., Arafat, S. Y., & Menon, V. (2024). *Dhat syndrome: medical, psychological and sociocultural aspects*. Springer Nature. https://doi.org/10.1007/978-981-99-8870-9

Kar, S. K., & Dwivedi, S. (2018). Braid cut anxiety in females: A newly emerged epidemic of mass hysteria in North India. *Asian Journal of Psychiatry, 32*, 116–117. https://doi.org/10.1016/j.ajp.2017.12.003

Kar, S. K., Menon, V., & Arafat, S. M. Y. (2024). Dhat syndrome as a diagnostic category: The nosological struggle. In S. K. Kar, S. M. Y. Arafat, & V. Menon (Eds.), *Dhat syndrome: Medical, psychological and sociocultural aspects* (pp. 29–35). Springer Nature. https://doi.org/10.1007/978-981-99-8870-9_3

Kar, S. K., Menon, V., Arafat, S. Y., Singh, A., Das, A., Shankar, A., Sharma, P., & Perera, S. (2021). Dhat syndrome: Systematic review of epidemiology, nosology, clinical features, and management strategies. *Asian Journal of Psychiatry, 65*, Article 102863. https://doi.org/10.1016/j.ajp.2021.102863

Kar, S. K., & Mishra, S. R. (2018). Prof. NN Wig & his contribution to understand Dhat syndrome. *Indian Journal of Health, Sexuality, and Culture, 4*(2), 39–40.

Kar, S. K., & Sarkar, S. (2015). Dhat syndrome: Evolution of concept, current understanding, and need of an integrated approach. *Journal of Human Reproductive Sciences, 8*(3), 130–134. https://doi.org/10.4103/0974-1208.165143

Kar, S. K., & Singh, A. (2016). Person centered management approach for the Dhat syndrome. *International Journal of Person Centered Medicine, 6*(4), Article 4. https://doi.org/10.5750/ijpcm.v6i4.615

Kar, S. K., & Singh, A. (2017). Where lies the fault in diagnosing Dhat syndrome among females? Understanding through a case study. *Indian Journal of Psychological Medicine, 39*(4), 506–508. https://doi.org/10.4103/0253-7176.211742

Kashyap, H., Kumar, J. K., Kandavel, T., & Reddy, Y. C. J. (2015). The dysfunctional inner mirror: Poor insight in obsessive-compulsivedisorder, contributions to heterogeneity and outcome. *CNS Spectrums, 20*(5), 460–462. https://doi.org/10.1017/S1092852915000619

Kennedy, B., & Flick, G. R. (1991). Classification of Koro. *American Journal of Psychiatry, 148*(9), 1278-b-1279. https://doi.org/10.1176/ajp.148.9.1278-b

Khalifa, N., & Hardie, T. (2005). Possession and Jinn. *Journal of the Royal Society of Medicine, 98*(8), 351–353. https://doi.org/10.1177/014107680509800805

Khan, N. (2005). Dhat syndrome in relation to demographic characteristics. *Indian Journal of Psychiatry, 47*(1), 54–57. https://doi.org/10.4103/0019-5545.46077

Khan, N. (2008). Dhat syndrome: Physical and psychological implications. *Unpublished Doctoral Thesis Submitted to University of Health Sciences, Lahore, Pakistan.* http://www.uhs.edu.pk/downloads/dr_nashi.pdf

Khan, N., Kausar, R., & Chaudhary, H. R. (2011). Demographic characteristics and implications of Dhat syndrome in Pakistan. *Indian Journal of Clinical Psychology, 38*(1), 69–78.

Khan, Q. U. A., & Sanober, A. (2016). "Jinn possession" and delirious mania in a Pakistani woman. *American Journal of Psychiatry, 173*(3), 219–220. https://doi.org/10.1176/appi.ajp.2015.15030281

Levine, R. E., & Gaw, A. C. (1995). Culture-bound syndromes. *The Psychiatric Clinics of North America, 18*(3), 523–536.

Lim, T. T., Tan, K., Eow, G. B., & Bhidayasiri, R. (2022). A South East Asian perspective of neuropsychiatric startle syndromes of latah. *Parkinsonism & Related Disorders, 95*, 138–142. https://doi.org/10.1016/j.parkreldis.2022.01.013

Malhotra, H. K., & Wig, N. N. (1975). Dhat syndrome: A culture-bound sex neurosis of the orient. *Archives of Sexual Behavior, 4*(5), 519–528. https://doi.org/10.1007/BF01542130

Maruf, M. M., Mubassara, L., & Ahsan, M. S. (2024). Psychosexual disorders in Bangladesh: From bench to community. In S. M. Y. Arafat (Ed.), *Mental health in Bangladesh* (pp. 139–165). Springer Nature Singapore. https://doi.org/10.1007/978-981-97-0610-5_9

Massard-Vincent, J. (1996). Latah in Southeast Asia. The history and ethnography of a culture-bound syndrome. In *Publications of the society for psychological anthropology* (Vol. 7). JSTOR. https://www.jstor.org/stable/27976372

Masson, J. M. (1976). The psychology of the ascetic. *The Journal of Asian Studies, 35*(4), 611–625. https://doi.org/10.2307/2053674

Mehra, A., Kathirvel, S., Gainder, S., Avasthi, A., & Grover, S. (2021). Female Dhat syndrome in primary care setting. *Industrial Psychiatry Journal, 30*(2), 278–284.

Mishra, K. K., & Roy, P. (2018). Historical perspective of Dhat syndrome: A brief overview. *Indian Journal of Health, Sexuality, and Culture, 4*(2), 4–7.

Mullick, M. S. I., Karim, M. E., Islam, M. S., Chowdhury, S., Rahman, M., & Islam, M. R. (1995). Clinical pattern of Dhat syndrome. *Age, 16*(20), 29.

Nandi, D. N., Banerjee, G., Saha, H., Sen, B., & Bhattacharjee, A. (1992). An epidemic of "Jhin-Jhini"—A strange contagious psychogenic disorder in a village in West Bengal. *Indian Journal of Psychiatry, 34*(4), 366.

Perez, S., Junod, A., & Pilard, M. (2000). Culture-bound syndromes: Pertinence as a diagnostic category. *Medecine Tropicale: Revue Du Corps De Sante Colonial, 60*(1), 75–82.

Prakash, O. (2007). Lessons for postgraduate trainees about Dhat syndrome. *Indian Journal of Psychiatry, 49*(3), 208–210. https://doi.org/10.4103/0019-5545.37324

Prakash, O., & Kar, S. K. (2019). Dhat syndrome: A review and update. *Journal of Psychosexual Health, 1*(3–4), 241–245. https://doi.org/10.1177/2631831819894769

Prakash, O., Kar, S. K., & Sathyanarayana Rao, T. S. (2014). Indian story on semen loss and related Dhat syndrome. *Indian Journal of Psychiatry, 56*(4), 377–382. https://doi.org/10.4103/0019-5545.146532

Ramos, I. (2015). The fragmentation of Sati: Constructing Hindu identity through pilgrimage souvenirs. *Journal of Decorative and Propaganda Arts, 27*, 12–35.

Rao, A. V. (1978). Some aspects of psychiatry in India. *Transcultural Psychiatric Research Review, 15*(1), 7–27. https://doi.org/10.1177/136346157801500101

Rekha, H. G., & Mangalwedhe, S. B. (2018). Management of Dhat syndrome: An overview. *Indian Journal of Health, Sexuality and Culture, 4*(2), 25–28.

Sahu, S. K. (2018). Ayurvedic concept of semen. *Indian Journal of Health, Sexuality, and Culture, 4*(2), 32–35.

Salam, K. P. A., Sharma, M. P., & Prakash, O. (2012). Development of cognitive-behavioral therapy intervention for patients with Dhat syndrome. *Indian Journal of Psychiatry, 54*(4), 367–374. https://doi.org/10.4103/0019-5545.104826

Schmelzle, L., & Timalsina, S. (2021). *Hindu mythology: The effect of ancient Vedic myths of Lord Krishna and Lord Shiva.* https://www.academia.edu/download/67263358/Writing_on_Rel_Final_Paper.pdf

Shakya, D. R. (2019). Dhat syndrome: Study of clinical presentations in a teaching institute of Eastern Nepal. *Journal of Psychosexual Health, 1*(2), 143–148. https://doi.org/10.1177/2631831819853742

Sharma, P., Singh, S., & Pal, A. (2024). Female Dhat syndrome. In S. K. Kar, S. M. Y. Arafat, & V. Menon (Eds.), *Dhat syndrome* (pp. 127–136). Springer Nature Singapore. https://doi.org/10.1007/978-981-99-8870-9_12

Singh, A. (2018). Pathways to care for Dhat syndrome. *Indian Journal of Health, Sexuality, and Culture, 4*(2), 15–18.

Singh, A. (2024). Care-seeking, pathway to care and disease burden in Dhat syndrome. In S. K. Kar, S. M. Y. Arafat, & V. Menon (Eds.), *Dhat syndrome* (pp. 73–83). Springer Nature Singapore. https://doi.org/10.1007/978-981-99-8870-9_7

Singh, A., Tripathi, A., Gupta, B., & Agarwal, V. (2016). Pathways to care for Dhat (semen loss anxiety) syndrome: A study from North India. *International Journal of Mental Health, 45*(4), 253–261. https://doi.org/10.1080/00207411.2016.1238741

Singh, J., & Tripathi, A. (2018). Approach to a case of Dhat syndrome. *Indian Journal of Health, Sexuality, and Culture, 4*(2), 19–24.

Sinha, N., Suresh, S. B., Patil, P. S., & Unni, N. (2024). A rare presentation of delusional parasitosis with Koro-like syndrome. *Cureus, 16*(5), Article e59946. https://doi.org/10.7759/cureus.59946

Sridhar, V. K., Subramanian, K., & Menon, V. (2018). Current nosology of Dhat syndrome and state of evidence. *Indian Journal of Health, Sexuality, and Culture, 4*(2), 8–14.

Sumathipala, A., Siribaddana, S. H., & Bhugra, D. (2004). Culture-bound syndromes: The story of dhat syndrome. *The British Journal of Psychiatry: the Journal of Mental Science, 184*, 200–209. https://doi.org/10.1192/bjp.184.3.200

Swami, M. K. (2018). Dhat syndrome among females: Is there enough evidence? *Indian Journal of Health, Sexuality and Culture, 4*(2), 29–31.

Thomas, C., & Sharma, M. K. (2016). Culture-bound syndromes in India. *Journal of Psychiatric Nursing, 5*(2), 77–80.

Tripathi, A., Roy, D., & Kar, S. K. (2021). Distress due to nonpathological vaginal discharge: A new face of Dhat syndrome in females. *Journal of Psychosexual Health, 3*(4), 315–321. https://doi.org/10.1177/26318318211049547

Udina, M., Foulon, H., Valdés, M., Bhattacharyya, S., & Martín-Santos, R. (2013). Dhat syndrome: A systematic review. *Psychosomatics, 54*(3), 212–218.

Ventriglio, A., Ayonrinde, O., & Bhugra, D. (2016). Relevance of culture-bound syndromes in the 21st century. *Psychiatry and Clinical Neurosciences, 70*(1), 3–6. https://doi.org/10.1111/pcn.12359

Wig, N. N. (1960). Problems of mental health in India. *J Clin Soc Psychiatry, 17*, 48–53.

Wikipedia. (2025). Sati (Hindu goddess). In *Wikipedia*. Wikipedia. https://en.wikipedia.org/w/index.php?title=Sati_(Hindu_goddess)&oldid=1270818308

Winzeler, R. L. (1995). *Latah in South-East Asia: The history and ethnography of a culture-bound syndrome* (Vol. 7). Cambridge University Press. https://books.google.com/books?hl=en&lr=&id=cx6lttzLAGMC&oi=fnd&pg=IA6&dq=culture+bound+syndrome+south+asia&ots=3dLpy-GL1i&sig=wPzsldf_hIGJFehVRDkYcY875JQ

World Bank Group. (2024). *South Asia: World Bank open data.* World Bank Open Data. https://data.worldbank.org

Yap, P. M. (1965). Koro—A culture-bound depersonalization syndrome. *The British Journal of Psychiatry, 111*(470), 43–50.

Zaman, M. (2016). Association of delirious mania with Jinn possession phenomenon—A study from Pakistan Qurat ul Ain Khan, Aisha Sanober. *Mariam Opel, 11*(1/2), 29–37.

# Chapter 13
# Marriage and Mental Health in South Asia

**Mudita Chaturvedi, Bhavika Rai, and Snehil Gupta**

**Abstract** This chapter focuses on understanding marriage from a mental health perspective and its evolving narrative in the context of South Asia. Marriage's salutary benefit is determined by the perceived and actual social support and attachment with the partners. In this chapter, the authors have outlined critical aspects of marriage and mental health, including differences between South Asia and Western societies, experience of marriage in people with mental illness and their partners, including caregiver burden. Here, we have also discussed the impact of age on marriage and mental health outcomes, intimate partner violence, perceived social support, gender differences concerning the marriage and mental health. Towards, the later part of the chapter, tools to measure dimensions of marriage and relationships, therapeutic management of marital issues, legal aspects of marriage and mental health in South Asia, and current research gap which needs further exploration were also highlighted. Essential research has been included to give a comprehensive glimpse into marriage and mental health while underlining the areas that need more in-depth understanding and empirical evidence.

**Keywords** Marriage · Mental health · Theories · Implication · Gender differences · Cultural differences · Perceived social support · Social psychiatry · South Asia · India

## 1 Introduction: Marriage and Its Impact on Mental Health

Social scientists have generated a considerable amount of evidence showing that married individuals enjoy better mental health than never-married and previously-married individuals (Marcussen, 2005). Marriage is typically thought to increase

---

M. Chaturvedi · S. Gupta (✉)
Department of Psychiatry, All India Institute of Medical Sciences (AIIMS), Bhopal, India
e-mail: snehil2161@gmail.com

B. Rai
Department of Psychiatry, All India Institute of Medical Sciences (AIIMS), Nagpur, India

 
S. M. Y. Arafat et al. (eds.), *Social Psychiatry in South Asia*, South Asian Perspectives in Mental Health and Psychology , https://doi.org/10.1007/978-981-96-8078-8_13

psychological, social, and economic resources and help individuals avoid the stress of separation from their romantic partners (Williams & Umberson, 2004). Though marriage, on average, may confer mental health benefits, this positive association may not hold across different contexts or groups of people. The salutary mental health benefits of marriage are the result of underlying social attachment and support (Ross, 1995).

Relationships of various kinds fall along a continuum of social attachment, from singles to non-co-habiting romantic relationships to co-habiting relationships to marriage. The mental health advantages accrue as individuals move from less attachment to more attachment; thus, marriage has the most benefits.

Two hypotheses have been proposed to explain the connection between marital status and psychiatric disability, namely, premarital and postmarital disability hypotheses. *The premarital disability hypotheses* suggest that individuals with severe psychiatric impairments face difficulties in both getting married and maintaining a marriage, which accounts for the observed link between marital status and the use of mental health services. The primary hypothesis within this group is known as the *selection hypothesis* (Segraves, 1980).

The *postmarital disability hypotheses* encompass variations of the protection and stress hypotheses. The *protection hypothesis* argues that marriage offers a shield against psychiatric disorders, mainly because close emotional bonds are thought to be protective against mental health issues. On the other hand, the *stress hypothesis* proposes that divorce represents a major life stressor, potentially triggering psychiatric illness in individuals who would otherwise remain mentally healthy. The premarital disability hypotheses view human beings as having limited adaptability in response to life stressors. In contrast, the postmarital disability hypotheses, often supported by social psychiatrists and social psychologists, consider humans as highly influenced by their environment (Segraves, 1980).

Married people do not have better mental health because they are married; rather, people with better mental health are the ones who get married. The benefit of early marriage may be selective for individuals with good mental health (Marcussen, 2005).

A sense of relationship permanence often accompanies marriage. Since relationship dissolution may harm mental health, relationship stability explains marriage's positive effects on mental health. The most tested variables concerning marriages' impact on mental health are relationship stability and self-image. Ending relationships can cause psychological distress in young adults. In contrast, marriage, although not permanent, serves as a buffer and protects many young adults from such distress. Individuals' immediate social context, including structural (e.g., neighbourhood disadvantage) and cultural (e.g., local age norms) factors, may buffer or exacerbate marriage's effect on mental health (Clarke & Wheaton, 2005; Simon & Barrett, 2010). Marriage may also affect the mental health of both spouses differentially. Women's mental health seems to be especially sensitive to relationship factors, inside or outside of marriage. Women have more self-esteem bound up in the success of the relationship, which might be because they have higher affiliation needs and higher sensitivity to rejection than men; therefore, when affiliation is endangered, they tend to suffer more (Moffitt et al., 1986).

## 2 Marriage and Its Implications on Mental Health—Differences Between South Asia and the Western Societies

Research consistently shows that marital status is a powerful predictor of mental health (Horwitz et al., 1996). Eickmeyer et al. (2019) reported that marriage (not co-habitation) leads to greater income pooling, which enables the partners to cushion against idiosyncratic shocks (Eickmeyer et al., 2019). Married people are less likely to experience depression following a job loss, which amounts to 22% of the variance of experiencing a depressive episode. In this sense, although job-related income loss is still associated with a substantial increase in experiencing mental health problems, marriage nonetheless serves as a protective factor. Marriage is still associated with a stronger protective effect for males (although for females as well, to a lesser extent). Finally, although younger individuals also exhibit a protective effect, older individuals exhibit an even stronger one. A work by Tumin and Zheng (2018) shows heterogeneous effects of marriage on mental health moderated by the length of the marriage (Tumin & Zheng, 2018).

Globally, the trend of a decreasing proportion of married individuals and increasing age at marriage is observed, especially in Nordic countries. However, a rise in consensual unions has counterbalanced this. Despite the observed mental health benefits of marriage, couples are choosing to co-habit over getting married, as the notion is similar to marriage due to limited changes in their legal rights (Härkönen et al., 2021; Perelli-Harris et al., 2019).

Well-documented health and survival advantages for the married probably result partly from various protective effects of having a spouse. This includes economic benefits, widening of social network, provision of companionship and emotional support. Emotional closeness not only has practical implications (healthier lifestyle, smoother recovery from diseases), but also carries direct physiological effects, like lowering cortisol levels (Kravdal et al., 2023).

Kravdal et al. (2023) noted that, in Norway, the trend in mental health is more favourable after direct marriage than after a marriage preceded by co-habitation (Kravdal et al., 2023). Among women, the number of visits to general practitioners for mental health issues continued to decrease for a few years following direct marriage (Vs. an increase after marriage through co-habitation). Among those who have experienced dissolution earlier, there is much less evidence of mental health benefits from co-habitation and marriage.

Thc institution of marriage, its social connotations, and impact on mental health differ between Western and Asian countries. Despite the changing trends of relationships observed in the Western population and their impact on the individuals' mental health, the trend in Asian countries has not been paradigm-shifting. Hence, it is of paramount importance to discuss the relationship between marriage and mental illness in Asian countries, especially in countries like India, where marriage is perceived to be a remedy for mental illness.

In contrast to Western countries, in Asian countries, not being married is considered a stigma, particularly in the case of women, while being married translates into an elevation in social status. Marriages in India have certain distinctive features. It is usually an arranged relationship between two families with little scope for personal choices. A patriarchal ideology exists, and the husband is considered the head of the family and the breadwinner (Behere et al., 2011). Women have a social pressure to accept a position subservient to males, control their sexual impulses and to subordinate their personal preferences to the needs of the family. Women are typically the primary caregivers in the family and are responsible for ensuring the smooth functioning of the household. There is a strong social and moral compulsion to continue the relationship despite facing difficulties in the marriage. Divorce is frowned upon in the traditional Indian society (Avasthi, 2010).

Literature shows greater psychological distress among married women as compared to married men in the Indian setting. It can be attributed to psychological, social, and biological stress in women, including more responsibilities in taking care of the family, adjusting to a new family, pregnancy, childbirth and motherhood.

The protective effect of marriage, particularly when reinforced by children, significantly lessens the risks of suicide. The suicide rate is 11/100000 for married persons, almost half of the never-married/single individuals (Nambi, 2005). However, marital and family problems can be important stressors leading to suicidal behaviour, especially in married women, for whom, in the traditional Indian social fabric, separation/divorce is not a very feasible alternative. A systematic review & metanalysis (involving 47 studies from six countries) by Arafat et al. (2023) on marital status and suicidal behaviour in South – Asia revealed that the proportion of married people with suicide behaviours, completed suicide, and suicide attempts was 55.4% (95% CI: 50.1–60.5), 52.7% (95% CI: 44.5–60.7), and 43.1 (95% CI: 32.9–53.9), respectively. There was a significant difference in suicide attempts across the countries, with the highest prevalence in India (61.8%; 95% CI: 57.2–66.2), followed by Bangladesh (52.5%; 95% CI: 41.8%-62.9%) and Pakistan (45.1%; 95% CI: 30.9–59.9). This finding suggests that marital status may play a significant role in suicidal behaviour in this region. This contrasting finding from the Western literature suggests that the association between marital status and suicidal behaviour may be influenced by cultural, social, and economic factors specific to the South Asian region. Specifically, gender stereotyping, limited agency for women, and the expectation of fulfilling certain marital responsibilities may contribute to stress and psychological distress within marriages, potentially increasing the risk of suicidal behaviour among married women (Arafat et al., 2023).

Major mental health disorders have a bi-directional relationship with marital disharmony. Research shows that divorce-seeking couples have high psychiatric morbidity in comparison to well-adjusted couples with more neurotic traits (Srivastava, 2013).

Varying sociocultural practices also influence marital outcomes within the South Asian diaspora. Polygyny is a cultural practice that accepts men marrying multiple women at a time. Sueyoshi and Ohtsuka (2003) found that polygynous women tend to have significantly more children than monogamous women. Studies have posed

Islamic ideology as a main factor for increased fertility in Muslim countries. Fertility and population dynamics in Pakistan play a critical role in shaping the country's socio-economic development. While the household wealth index typically negatively affects fertility, this pattern does not apply to polygynous families, where wealthier households tend to have more children than monogamous ones (Shah et al., 2025). Thus, even though marriage confers a protective effect on mental health, both in Western as well as Asian countries, the sociocultural differences lead to an inequality in these benefits among both genders in the Asian setting.

## 3 Experience of Marriage in People with Mental Illness

The concept of marriage has been identified as a major variable predicting quality of life (QoL) in Asian countries. A study in India has found that marriage in persons with severe mental illness (SMI) can lead to poor treatment adherence, relapse, and separation or divorce (Kulhara et al., 1998). On the contrary, a study from China showed that marriage can be a source of support and prevent homelessness and suicide among persons with SMIs (Ran et al., 2006). Thus, marriage may affect the treatment and recovery of a person with SMI.

Marriage is emerging as a prominent right and cultural need among people living with SMI. A qualitative study from Chennai, India by Thara et al. (2003), involving persons with SMI and their caregivers on marriage, reported that caregivers found it difficult to get marital alliance for their patients due to ongoing symptoms. Often, patients experience rejection from prospective partners, leading to distress. Another qualitative study revealed concerns among participants in forming and maintaining romantic relationships due to their illness. Most of the caregivers are filled with apprehension as to who will take care of the patients in the future. To most of them, marriage is a solution to ensure their patients are cared for (Kumar et al., 2019; Thara et al., 2003).

Numerous studies between healthy and control groups reported that the rate of sexual dysfunction was quite high in persons with SMI, with women having a higher rate. For instance, a Chinese study on 607 persons with schizophrenia reported that 69.9% had sexual dysfunction (60% in males and 80% in females) (Hou et al., 2016). Notably, the marital rates among persons with SMI in Asian countries are high compared to Western countries; (Li et al., 2015) a 10-year follow-up study of 76 persons with the first onset of schizophrenia in South India reported that 70% of the individuals were married (Deshmukh et al., 2016). A study from Sweden, which consists of 1750 males and 1506 females in the age group of 16–64 who were diagnosed with schizophrenia and discharged from the hospital, has reported only a 27% marriage rate (Olsson et al., 2016).

Studies examining individuals with SMI across various regions of South Asia have consistently shown that factors such as the presence and duration of mental illness, employment status, and gender influence marriage prospects (Bursalioglu et al., 2013; Deshmukh et al., 2016; Drisya et al., 2019). Most studies have found that most of the females with SMIs are married, versus the males with SMIs. Most women (77.5%) are married within 5 years of the start of the illness (Elkington et al., 2013). A retrospective case-control study in India among persons with schizophrenia revealed that 42.5% of married persons with schizophrenia were divorced, and about 70% of them were divorced within two years of their marriage (Behere et al., 2020). Almost 70% of the general population would not consider a partner with mental illness. Hence, families of individuals with Schizophrenia often conceal their condition due to fear of rejection. Women, individuals with lower educational status, and employed individuals were more likely to be married (Bursalioglu et al., 2013; Deshmukh et al., 2016; Drisya et al., 2019). Factors that increased the chances of remaining in marriage included marriage before the onset of illness, state of remission from the mental illness and having children, whereas not having children and disability were associated with poor marital outcomes (Salokangas et al., 2001).

There is a common belief in Indian society that marriage can cure mental illness. Although on one hand, marriage can provide good emotional support, which can help in the physical and mental well-being of both individuals, on the other hand, adjustment issues in marriage can cause mental distress (Behere et al., 2011). Thus, marriage can have protective as well as debilitating effects on the course of mental illness. In an Indian retrospective case–control study on schizophrenia, it was found that there were more relapses (70%) in married subjects as compared to never-married subjects (57.5%) (Behere et al., 2020). Findings of this study were similar to a study done by Kulhara et al., which also suggests that married individuals with schizophrenia have more relapses (Kulhara et al., 1998).

In Nepal, family members mentioned losing prestige in society as an important cultural reason for not disclosing the diagnosis or seeking care. Another reason, especially for parents of persons with mental illness, was not being able to marry off their children, particularly for daughters. Not being able to marry off one's daughter is considered one of the biggest cultural burdens for parents in Nepal, which is further amplified by the myth that marriage will heal mental disorders (Brenman et al., 2014). Persons with mental illness are also considered ineligible for work or marriage, and even if they do get married, mental disorders are considered to be acceptable grounds for divorce. High levels of perceived stigma are reported among persons with mental illness in the context of marriage, where they experience that their opinions are taken less seriously, they are looked down upon and they often feel that they are being treated as less intelligent or as a failure. This leads them to not seek help or adhere to treatments (Gurung et al., 2022).

Similar to Nepal and India, in Pakistan, people frequently share their privacy concerns about receiving mental health care due to perceptions of others in their communities, and fear that others would not marry into their families (Shafiq, 2020). In a study based in Pakistan, over half of the sample population indicated that it would be better not to marry someone with a mental illness, and over one-third suggested that being around those with mental illness can cause mental illness in oneself. Societal stigma against those with mental illness is high in many Pakistani individuals, and such fears increase the negative impacts of mental illness on those who are affected by it (Ahmad & Koncsol, 2022).

## 4 Caregiver Burden of Partners of Persons with Mental Illness (PwMI)

Mental illness brings with it a range of adverse consequences not only for the individual suffering from the disorder, but also for their families, particularly the primary caregiver. Caregiver burden refers to the '*significant amount of strain and difficulties experienced by the caregiver or family member of mentally ill people and includes a range of psychological, emotional, social, physical, and financial problems*' (Stanley et al., 2016). This includes subjective and objective burdens like perceived psychological distress such as feelings of loss, embarrassment in social situations, and depression, and issues such as reduced social and family activities and financial difficulties, respectively. Increased symptom severity also leads to increased family burden (Ohaeri, 2003).

In the Indian context, the caregiving function is usually discharged by the family, parents, or spouse. In marital relationships, the burden of care usually falls on the spouse, and a woman is perceived as a natural caregiver, and one is morally bound owing to religious and cultural expectations. A comparative study found that caregiver burden scores in the caregivers of psychiatric patients were significantly higher than that of chronic medical illness (Ampalam et al., 2012). Similar to Western world, higher levels of caregiver stress, anxiety, and depression have also been reported in Indian literature (Dalui et al., 2014; Idstad et al., 2010). A study from India that observed the perceived burden in spouses of persons with psychotic illnesses, using the Burden Assessment Schedule, remarked that the caregivers' age differentiates them in terms of the perceived severity of illness, and this was highest for young caregivers (Vs relatively older ones) (Stanley et al., 2016). Furthermore, a study from India involving primary caregivers of persons with schizophrenia observed that as compared to respondents with low stigma (score below the mean of the study population), participants with high stigma reported being depressed or in sorrow, are of young age, with their patients being younger and of female gender (Thara & Srinivasan, 2000).

A study from Nepal showed that the sex-wise distribution of burden in different dimensions of the Burden Assessment Schedule had female caregivers report more spouse-related burden than that of male. The psychotic symptoms occurring for the first time are more frightening for the spouse of the person affected as the illnesses occur unexpectedly. Mean score burden was found to be high among caregivers of patients with more than five years of illness ($75.45 \pm 14.007$), with mood disorders ($79.12 \pm 10.176$), with first hospitalization ($75.96 + 12.833$) and cared for by the spouse ($82.67 \pm 9.642$) (Bhandari et al., 2017).

In a study from Pakistan, caregivers who were married ($t = -2.98$, $p < 0.01$), and provided longer hours of caregiving ($F = 19.12$, $p < 0.001$) reported significantly higher caregiver burden than caregivers who were unmarried. A Bangladeshi study reported that most of the caregivers were between 26 and 41 years old (52.6%), female (71.4%), and married (66.9%). Married respondents had the highest mild to moderate burden (69.7%), corroborating the findings from the other South Asian studies (Siddiqui & Khalid, 2019).

Anxiety levels were found to be higher in caregivers when the spouse was ill for a shorter period (<10 years) than for relatively longer spells. Perhaps a longer duration of illness results in greater acceptance of the situation and an attitude of being reconciled to the situation. Another study from India reports that caregiver burden increased with the duration of illness (Ampalam et al., 2012). The caregivers of patients with schizophrenia had significantly higher total burden scores as compared to caregivers of those with bipolar disorder. The higher burden was experienced in the lack of external support and disruption of caregivers' routines and relationships with others (Vasudeva et al., 2013).

## 5 Age of Marriage and Its Impact on Mental Health

Age of marriage is an important contingency of the marriage and mental health relationship. Particularly, marriage at an early, non-normative age may not be as salutary as marriage at a more culturally appropriate age. According to the life course perspective, the effect of roles and transitions depends on their timing (Williams & Umberson, 2004). Sometimes, "the timing of an event may be more consequential than its occurrence." This may be especially true for marriage, where there is a widely accepted culturally appropriate time to marry (Settersten & Hagestad, 1996). In particular, it has become increasingly non-normative (both statistically and culturally) to marry at an early age. It is possible that early marriage confers no mental health benefit or even contributes to more mental health problems than other relationship arrangements or not being in a relationship at all. Married couples can benefit from specialisation within their family, economies of scale, and the added insurance an able-bodied partner provides against unexpected events (Waite, 2009).

In South Asian countries, girls are more likely to be married off earlier in life than boys. Child marriage affects girls and boys but disproportionately and more negatively to girls. Child marriage refers to formal marriages and informal unions in which one or both parties are under 18 years of age and live with a partner as if married. Besides being a human rights issue, child marriage has dire reproductive and sexual health consequences for girls, impeding their overall development and well-being. Besides these associated factors, several other factors have also been reported to result from child marriage, such as increased school dropouts, increased marital violence, increased maternal morbidity and mortality, increased risk of unintended pregnancies, decreased utilization of antenatal care and postnatal care services, decreased institutional delivery in health care facilities, and decreased deliveries assisted by skilled birth attendants. In India, Bangladesh, and Nepal, children from low socioeconomic status households are found to be more susceptible to child marriage. Multiple studies from Nepal and Bangladesh reported child marriage as prevalent among Hindus and Muslims (Subramanee et al., 2022).

Marriage may also provide a degree of certainty, finality, and a sense of satisfaction deriving from "accomplishing" one of the tasks involved in transitioning to adulthood, the capstone to adulthood. Waiting until later to marry may do little good in terms of avoiding mental health problems, but much good in terms of improving overall well-being. This latter finding suggests social approval for marriage, which is likely higher for those marrying at ages 22–26 than for those marrying earlier and may be a key mechanism explaining marriage's effect on overall well-being. Strikingly, teenage marriage is selective of those with relatively high psychological distress, suggesting that marriage's mental health benefits in young adulthood are masked by differences in pre-existing psychological distress. Social approval explains some of the age-at-marriage's effects on life satisfaction. It could be further tested to see whether this effect is present in contexts where early marriage is affirmed. Marriage in young adulthood is not detrimental to mental health. Being in any sort of relationship is good for psychological distress, being married or engaged to be married curbs drunkenness, and married young adults, especially those who marry at ages 22–26, are more satisfied with their lives (Uecker, 2008).

## 6 Intimate Partner Violence (IPV)

IPV is defined as "Physical, sexual, or psychological harm by a current or former partner or spouse" (Sugg, 2015b). More than one in three women and one in four men have experienced rape, physical violence, and/or stalking by an intimate partner in their lifetimes. Certain factors, such as young age, female gender, and having a lower income, are associated with higher rates of violence. The highest risk of IPV occurs between the ages of 18 and 24 years. Adolescence (i.e., ages 11–18 years) is also a high-risk time for violence (Breiding et al., 2008a).

The prevalence of violence against women during pregnancy ranges from 0.9% to 20.1%, with most studies being in the 4% to 8% range (Gazmararian, 1996). Psychological and physical consequences experienced by the victims of IPV are described in Table 1

## 7 Marriage & Perceived Social Support

South Asia is home to almost one-third of the world's population, and its diversity of culture and practices makes it a unique region. Due to globalization, countries in this region have undergone massive socio-economic shifts, significantly impacting the family system, including the institution of marriage. Social support is defined as the "availability or existence of people on whom we can rely, people who care about us and love us" (Nawaz et al., 2014). The social support can be of various types like emotional support, instrumental support, informational support, appraisal support and companionship support (Barbour, 2003).

**Table 1** Psychological and physical consequences of the IPV

| Consequences | Evidence & discussing points |
|---|---|
| Increased risk of depression and anxiety | • Women with pre-existing depression are more likely to experience IPV<br>• Not only do depressive symptoms negatively affect QoL, they also hinder people's ability to self-protect (Devries et al., 2013) |
| Post-traumatic stress disorder (PTSD) | • Rate of PTSD diagnosis among female victim of IPV ranges from 31% to 84.4% (Devries et al., 2013)<br>• Depression and PTSD are highly co-morbid conditions |
| Suicidality | • Formerly abused with chronic pain had lifetime prevalence of attempted suicide of 31% (Devries et al., 2013)<br>• A study of urban women found that abused women were nearly 8 times more likely to attempt suicide than non-abused women (Pico-Alfonso et al., 2006) |
| Psychosomatic conditions | • Psycho-physiological mechanisms related to chronic stress related to the IPV lead to gastrointestinal symptoms, like irritable bowel syndrome, gastroesophageal reflux, dyspepsia, etc. (Devries et al., 2013) |
| Risky behaviours | • Individuals who experience IPV are more likely to engage in risky behaviours, such as smoking, that are associated with poorer outcomes for patients with chronic diseases (Breiding et al., 2008b)<br>• Women experiencing current abuse were nearly six times as likely to have a substance abuse diagnosis. Conversely, patients who are diagnosed with alcohol or substance abuse issues are at higher risk of IPV (Bonomi et al., 2009) |
| Contracting sexually transmitted diseases (STDs) | • A significant association between IPV and STD is noted<br>• One of the contributory practices being the control of safe sex choices of the partner<br>• Women experiencing IPV in their current relationship were four times likelihood of having a partner with a known HIV risk factor (Intravenous drug user, recent STD symptoms or diagnosis, recent sex with another man or woman, or known to be HIV-positive) (Wu et al., 2003) |
| Miscellaneous | • Victim of the IPV experience impaired decision-making caused by psychological trauma, PTSD, or substance use (Sugg, 2015a) |
| Physical issues | • Physical injury from IPV can include scratches, bruises, contusions, lacerations, fractured teeth, grievous injuries (e.g., bone fractures, joint dislocations)<br>• Homicide - Women account for 70% of victims killed by an intimate partner<br>– Of special note are the homicide-suicide incidents that occur, in which the perpetrator of the homicide then commits suicide<br>– Most of the homicide victims were female (75%), and in nearly 60% of all homicide-suicide incidents, the victim is a current or former intimate partner of the perpetrator (Sugg, 2015b) |

Social support in marriage includes spouses' efforts to fulfil the immediate needs of their partner provoked by stressful life events and the collective benefits of supportive interactions, such as a sense of security and self-efficacy. There has been a recent progress of interest in the pursuit of social support in marriage, particularly how skills in providing and receiving support may affect the ongoing functioning of the marriage. Recent studies have shown social support to be an important component of marital satisfaction (Patel, 2021). For instance, a study on the impact of spouses' social support behaviour over time in marriage was explored involving 60 newlywed couples. They were asked to participate in problem-solving and social support discussions. For the social support task, couples were asked to have two 10-minute discussions, one in which the husband would discuss a personal problem and the wife would respond (as the helper), and another wherein their roles are reversed. The results indicated that problem-solving and social support discussion tasks appear to enhance couples' social support skills, which in conjunction with their problem-solving skills, has a more positive and lasting impact (Sullivan et al., 1998).

In South Asia, social support has been studied concerning marital satisfaction. For instance, a study in Pakistan explored the relationship between perceived social support and marital satisfaction in love marriage and arranged marriage couples and found that there is a positive relationship between perceived social support and marital satisfaction (Nawaz et al., 2014). Another study from the same country explored the moderating role of social support for marital adjustment, depression, anxiety, and stress in working and non-working women. The results indicated that social support has a positive role in marital adjustment and a negative association concerning the development of anxiety, depression, and stress in working and non-working women. It further moderates marital cohesion and affection, resulting in less stress and depression (Abbas et al., 2019).

## 8 Gender Differences on the Role of Marriage in Mental Health

The gender differences in marriage-related psychological aspects have been assessed in the context of the onset of mental health issues, economic influence, marital timing, and differences in attitudes and beliefs regarding marital experience.

The WHO World Mental Health (WMH) survey initiative conducted a cross-sectional household survey on gender differences in the association of first marriage and being previously married with the subsequent first onset of a range of mental disorders. The survey results were computed using discrete-time survival analysis, the researchers found that marriage was related to reduced risk of the onset of disorders in both genders. In married men, the risk of developing depression and panic disorder was reduced marginally, and in married women, the risk of developing substance use disorder decreased. Both genders who were previously married had a higher risk of developing all the disorders, with an increased risk of developing substance use disorder in women and depression in men (Scott et al., 2010).

A study in South Korea observed how household decision-making affects the mental well-being of Asian immigrant women living with their spouses. The results showed that women in households where their husbands made all the decisions were more likely to experience depression, lower life satisfaction, and lower marital satisfaction compared to women in households where decisions were made together.

Women in households where they made the decisions themselves had somewhat better mental well-being. The study found that one-sided decision-making is a risk for poor mental health, while shared decision-making is protective (Lee et al., 2022).

Gender role expectations also impact the overall experience of marriage. In the South Asian region, the majority of countries have patriarchal societies where gender roles are defined and conformity is required. In a qualitative study, researchers explored gender roles and how they are negotiated in second-generation six South Asian couples through in-depth interviews. Several themes emerged, such as the impact of gender roles, division of labour, breaking down the patriarchy, unconscious bias, financial decisions, becoming parents, discussions about gender roles, and resolving conflicts. The couples had also shared the effect of gender dynamics on their relationship as they strive to create an equal partnership (Patel, 2021).

Marital timing differs by gender, with women marrying earlier in life than men with the average marriage age being higher for men in 114 countries (United Nations, 2011). On average, men marry 3.3 years later than women, with the gap ranging from 1.8 years in North America and Northern Europe to 6.6 years in Western Africa. This gender gap has stayed consistent, even though both men and women are marrying later. This gap affects other areas of life as well. A study in Nepal (2008–2012) examined whether attitudes about marriage age differ by gender. The study found that youth and their parents generally thought women could marry between ages 20 and 25, while men were expected to marry between 23 and 30. The earlier marriage age for women explained a third of the gender gap in marriage timing. Other factors, like neighbours' opinions or potential spouses' views, could also play a role. The study also showed that both genders were less likely to marry if they were much younger than the acceptable marriage age, but this effect was stronger for women (Allendorf et al., 2017).

## 9 Tools to Measure Various Dimensions of Marriage and Relationships

Marriage includes a wide spectrum of behaviours that researchers call family formation and couple unions with legal, economic, social, and spiritual elements. Various instruments have been developed to measure crucial components of marriage and relationships (Table 2). Some of these instruments have been validated in South Asian countries. For instance, Revised Dyadic Adjustment Scale (R-DAS) has been validated in Bangladesh (Shamsun Nahar et al., 2020), in Malaysia (Hamid et al., 2020) & China (Li et al., 2022). Similarly, Kansas Marital Satisfaction Scale (KMSS) has been validated in India (Rani et al., 2019), & Korea (Chung, 2005). Notably, most of the tools mentioned above have been developed with the Western concept of relationship. Hence, the applicability of these tools in South Asia might be doubtful due to differences in culture and systems. This poses the need to develop tools focused specifically on the South Asian population.

**Table 2** Description of tools to measure different aspects of marriage

| S.no | Name of the tool (Author) | Description |
|---|---|---|
| 1 | Dyadic Adjustment Scale (Spanier, 1976) | • The Dyadic Adjustment Scale (DAS) is a self-report questionnaire used to measure the quality of a romantic relationship<br>• It involves satisfaction, consensus, cohesion, and affective expression between partners, with higher scores indicating a more adjusted relationship<br>• It consists of 32 items and is considered one of the most widely used tools to evaluate couple dynamics |
| 2 | Kansas Marital Satisfaction Scale (KMSS) (Schumm et al., 1983) | • The KMMS is a 3-item self-report instrument designed to measure marital quality<br>• Items are rated on a 7-point Likert scale, ranging from 1 (extremely dissatisfied) to 7 (extremely satisfied)<br>• Total score ranges from 3 to 21, with high scores meaning better marital quality |
| 3 | Relationship Commitment Scale (RCS) (Rusbult et al., 1998) | • This is a 7-item scale self-report measure used to assess the relationship between partners<br>• Its domains include: personal commitment (desire to stay in the relationship), structural commitment (investments made in the relationship), and moral commitment (belief in the obligation to stay in the relationship) |
| 4 | Couple rating of relationship elements—(CARE) (Worthington et al., 1997) | • A questionnaire or assessment tool used to evaluate a couple's relationship quality by asking them to rate various aspects of their partnership<br>• Key domains include communication, affection, respect, and emotional support, providing a comprehensive picture of their relationship strengths and areas needing improvement |
| 5 | Religious Commitment Inventory (RCI-10) (Worthington et al., 2003) | • The RCI-10 is a 10-item self-report questionnaire<br>• It is designed to measure the degree to which an individual adheres to their religious values, beliefs, and practices.<br>• It essentially assesses their level of religious commitment by incorporating both internal (intrapersonal) and external (interpersonal) aspects of their religious life, based on Worthington's model of religious commitment |

## 10 Therapeutic Management of Marital Issues

Most of the therapeutic modalities for couples have been developed in the United States and Europe. Relational distress and divorce are linked to a wide range of negative outcomes, including individual psychological disorders, impaired work functioning, and poorer physical health. Given the high prevalence and destructive impact of relational problems and dissolution, mental health professionals have long recognized the need to develop, assess, and implement effective interventions to improve the quality of distressed romantic relationships (Stephenson et al., 2023). Christensen (2010) have given five principles of couple therapy-

I. Shift the couple's conceptualization of problems from individual to interactional

II. Modify emotion-driven, dysfunctional behavioural patterns
III. Elicit avoided and private emotions
IV. Foster productive communication
V. Emphasize strengths and encourage positive behaviour

Below, we have provided some empirically supported approaches to couple therapy (Table 3). Some of these models have found empirical validation in the South Asian population in Canada (Ahmad & Reid, 2016) and Middle East Asia (Soltani et al., 2013), but there is a dearth of research where couple therapy models have been validated in South Asian countries.

## 11 Legal Aspects of Marriage and Mental Health in South Asia

In South Asian countries, legal provisions related to mental illness affecting marriage primarily focus on the capacity for consent and the ability to fulfil marital obligations. The legal framework often provides grounds for annulment or divorce if mental illness is present, though the specifics and thresholds vary by country. For instance, in India, The Special Marriage Act (SMA), 1954 and the Hindu Marriage Act (HMA), 1955 put restrictions on the marriage of PwMI where the presence of an SMI makes marriage voidable, and this makes PwMI vulnerable to be rejected by their partners (Sharma et al., 2015). Similar legal acts in other South Asian countries include the Muslim Family Laws Ordinance of 1961 (Pakistan & Bangladesh), the Marriage Registration Ordinance, 1908 (Sri Lanka), the Civil Code of 2017 (Nepal), etc. (Table 4).

## 12 Long Distance Marital Relationship and Mental Health Issues

Long-distance marital relationships are recently becoming very common mainly due to occupational reasons. In a study conducted in Indonesia, marital satisfaction was assessed in 45 couples with long-distance marriages. The findings indicated that the husbands experienced a medium level of marital satisfaction and wives experienced higher satisfaction levels in long-distance marriages and communication between the partners was associated with marital satisfaction (Putra & Afdal, 2020). A qualitative study in Nepal explored the mental health issues and experiences of 18 wives' whose husbands had left their homes and moved to another city for labour opportunities. The authors identified psychosocial factors like communication (among migrant husbands and their wives), children both as coping and stress-inducing agents, family support and challenges, migration history in the family, and social acceptance of labour migration interact to form a pathway that can either ease or add burden to

**Table 3** Therapy models for couples

| Therapy (Author, year) | Description |
|---|---|
| 1. Traditional Behavioural Couple Therapy (TBCT), Jacobson and Margolin (1979) | • The original scientific basis of TBCT was research suggesting that distressed couples engaged in more negative and fewer positive behaviours with each other compared to satisfied couples and that they also seemed to have more trouble communicating and problem-solving effectively<br>• In line with the dominant behavioural viewpoint of psychologists at the time, the theory underlying TBCT holds that *"current behaviours in the relationship, such as a lack of pleasurable shared activities or deficient skills in communication and problem-solving, cause, and maintain distress for couples."* |
| 2. Cognitive behavioural couple therapy (CBCT), Baucom & Epstein (1990) | • TBCT was expanded to include a focus on thoughts, or 'cognitions,' specifically how partners interpret each other's actions to contribute to distress in relationships<br>• Particular emphasis on 'cognitive distortions': (inaccurate interpretations of events in the world that give rise to unhelpful emotional responses)<br>• Examples of cognitive distortions include unhelpful assumptions ('people don't ever change'), irrational standards ('he should already know why I'm upset'), attentional biases (focusing on negative behaviours while ignoring positive ones), inaccurate attributions ('he forgot about our date because he doesn't care about me'), and overgeneralized expectancies ('she'll never listen to my side of the story') |
| 3. Integrative behavioural couple therapy (IBCT) Christensen & Jacobsen (late 1990s) | • IBCT sought to integrate the components of BCT that are focused on solving problems and 'changing' the behaviours of partners with newer approaches that encourage increased understanding and 'acceptance' of chronic or unsolvable issues in the relationship<br>• The addition of acceptance-based interventions was in line with the burgeoning '3rd wave' of cognitive therapies, which tended to focus on futile and counterproductive attempts to change one's present experience as primary culprits in creating and prolonging suffering |

(continued)

**Table 3** (continued)

| Therapy (Author, year) | Description |
|---|---|
| 4. Emotion Focused Therapy (EFT), Greenberg & Johnson (1988) | • EFT's creators were influenced by experiential, systems, and attachment theories which highlight, respectively, the importance of acknowledging and embracing one's emotions, the costs of inflexible interpersonal behaviour, and the centrality of attachment bonds in romantic relationships<br>• EFT was a response to strict behaviourists and early forms of BCT which were criticized for downplaying the importance of subjective emotional experience |
| 5. Insight-Oriented Couple Therapy, Snyder and Wills (1989) | • Insight-oriented couple therapy (IOCT) represents an integration of psychodynamic theory, which posits that<br>*"Psychological distress is often the result of unconscious conflict between different aspects of the self and cognitive-behavioural tools for improving the quality of relationships."* |
| 6. Systemic Couple Therapy Satir, Minuchin, & Bowen (1970) | • Couple therapy based on systems theory tends to emphasize the patterns of interaction between partners (and often other family members), especially how these patterns serve to maintain balance and stability in the relational 'system.'<br>• Distressing patterns are thought to be maintained by behaviour that is driven primarily by emotions rather than a person's rational decision-making system |
| 7. Gottman-Method Couple Therapy, John and Julie Gottman (1975) | • It includes a range of interventions that mirror multiple aspects of BCT, IBCT, and EFT<br>• 'Rappaport intervention' is similar to the speaker/listener technique used in BCT<br>• Gottman-method couple therapy differs from others<br>1. It focuses more on the description of how distressed couples differ from satisfied couples and less on how relationships change over time<br>2. The treatment includes relatively more aspects of self-help techniques |

wives' mental health (Rai et al., 2023). Spousal migration has been found to increase the risk of depression and has a detrimental effect on the mental well-being of a partner who has been left behind (Tong et al., 2019).

**Table 4** Legal acts related to marriage & divorce in South Asian countries (the laws in bold are specific to marriage in the respective country)

| S.no | Country | Legal Act |
|---|---|---|
| 1 | Afghanistan | • **Civil Code of 1977**<br>• Islamic law<br>• Regional customary law<br>• Traditional ethnic rules<br>• The Mohammedan Law |
| 2 | Bangladesh | • Muslim Marriage and Divorces Act, 1974<br>• Child Marriage Prevention Act, 2014<br>• Child Marriage Restraint Act, 1929<br>• Hindu Marriage Act, 1946<br>• Divorce Act, 1869<br>• Christian Marriage Act, 1872<br>• **Muslim Family Laws Ordinance, 1961**<br>• Dissolution of Muslim Marriages Act, 1939<br>• Special Marriage Act |
| 3 | Bhutan | • Marriage Act of the Kingdom of Bhutan 2017<br>• **Civil and Criminal Procedure Code** |
| 4 | India | • **The Hindu Marriage Act, 1955**<br>• Hindu Succession Act, 1956<br>• Muslim Women's Protection of Rights on Divorce Act, 1986<br>• Parsi Marriage and Divorce Act, 1936<br>• Dowry Prohibition Act, 1961<br>• **The Special Marriage Act, 1954**<br>• The Indian Christian Marriage Act, 1872<br>• Sharia and Mohammedan Law |
| 5 | Maldives | • **Maldives Family Law Act, 2001**<br>• The Mohammedan Law |
| 6 | Nepal | • Marriage Registration Act, 2018<br>• The Social Practices Reform Act, 1976<br>• General Code (Muluki Ain)<br>• **Civil Code, 2017** |
| 7 | Sri Lanka | • Muslim Marriage and Divorce Act<br>• **Marriage Registration Ordinance, 1908 (General Law)**<br>• Kandyan Marriage and Divorce Act<br>• Thesawalamai Law (Tamil inhabitants in Jaffna) |
| 8 | Pakistan | • The Christian Marriage Act, 1872 (Christian)<br>• The Christian Divorce Act, 1869 (Christian)<br>• The Hindu Marriage Act 2017<br>• The Child Marriage Restraint Act 1929<br>• Parsi Marriage and Divorce Act, 1936 (Parsi)<br>• Dissolution of Muslim Marriages Act 1939 (Muslim)<br>• **Muslim Family Laws Ordinance, 1961 (Muslim)**<br>• Family Courts Act, 1964 (Muslim)<br>• Dowry and Bridal Gifts (Restriction) Act 1976 (All citizens of Pakistan)<br>• Guardians and Wards Act (applicable to all citizens of Pakistan but communities may follow their law instead |

## 13 Research Gap and Future Directions

The intersection of marriage and mental health in South Asia is a topic of growing interest, yet it remains underexplored in the academic literature. While there is some research on marital dynamics, mental health issues, and their impact on individuals, other critical issues need to be addressed. These gaps exist due to cultural, social, and methodological challenges that are unique to the region (described below).

### *13.1 Co-Habitation and Mental Health*

Co-habitation has become a global trend, including in South Asia. In countries like India, Pakistan, Bangladesh, and Sri Lanka, co-habitation outside of marriage is still largely stigmatized. For instance, the National Family Health Survey, India (NFHS-5, 2019–2020) reported a significant increase in co-habitation rates among youth in urban areas (Tripathi et al., 2023). Similarly, co-habitation remains uncommon and is strongly discouraged in Pakistan (Halford & Vijver, 2020). Despite its rising occurrence, the relationship between co-habitation and mental health in South Asia remains under-researched.

### *13.2 Same-Sex Marriage & Mental Health*

In South Asia, the intersection of same-sex marriage and mental health has garnered increasing attention, reflecting both societal shifts and the evolving legal landscape. In June 2023, Nepal's Supreme Court recognized same-sex marriages. Studies suggest that legalizing same-sex marriage can lead to improved psychological well-being among sexual minorities (Huang & Liang, 2022). Conversely, in India, the legalization of same-sex marriage is under parliament's discretion. This legal ambiguity continues to impact the mental health of LGBTQ+ individuals in such countries, as the lack of legal recognition may perpetuate societal stigma and discrimination (Devi et al., 2024). Hence, more research on this topic is warranted.

### *13.3 Marital Therapy & Other Forms of Couple Therapy's Impact & Nuances in South Asian Reasons*

Marital and couple therapy in South Asia is evolving to address the unique cultural, social, and familial dynamics prevalent in the region. Traditional values often emphasize family honour and collective well-being, which can influence relationship dynamics and the acceptance of therapeutic interventions. Research indicates that culturally adapted therapeutic models can effectively improve relationship adjustment among South Asian couples (Ahmad & Reid, 2016). Despite the benefits of such interventions, challenges like Stigma, poor help-seeking, and intergenerational trauma (affecting relationship dynamics) persist, which require research exploration.

## 13.4 Impact of Delayed Marriage & Late Childbearing on the Mental Health of Women

Societal expectations in South Asia often place a premium on early marriage and motherhood, leading women considering late marriage to experience social pressure and stigma. This societal disapproval results in feelings of isolation and stress. Moreover, late childbearing is associated with increased health risks related to pregnancy, childbirth, and psychological problems (Sharma & Khurana, 2020). Therefore, the psychosocial determinants of the age of marriage and the mental health consequences thereof need exploration.

## 13.5 Work from Home, Digitalisation, and Impact on Marriage and Mental Health

The rapid adoption of digital technologies and the shift to remote work have significantly impacted South Asia's marriage dynamics and mental health. Here, traditional gender roles often place most household responsibilities on women. The transition to remote work (during/post COVID-19) has intensified this burden, as women are expected to manage both professional and domestic duties, with little change in family support (Kundra et al., 2023). Hence, greater research in this area is required.

## 13.6 Migration & Its Impact on Marriage and Mental Health

Migration significantly influences marital relationships and mental health. Migrating as a family unit can offer emotional support and stability, which are crucial for mental well-being. However, the challenges related to acculturation, coupled with economic pressures, can strain relationships. These stressors may lead to marital conflicts and psychological issues (Zhuang et al., n.d.). In contrast, when only one partner migrates, the separation can lead to feelings of isolation, loneliness, lack of emotional support, labour burden, and anxiety for both individuals; thereby affecting their overall relationship.

## 14 Conclusion

Marriage is typically associated with positive psychological health and well-being; however, this is contextual. Marriage's salutary benefit is determined by the perceived and actual social support and attachment by the partners. Moreover, the mental health benefit of marriage is greater in men as compared to women. Furthermore, it can vary depending on the length-, age, timing of marriage, and emotional or financial support. Marriage's impact on PwMI is complex; therefore, it needs a granular understanding to draw a conclusion. Caregivers of PwMI experience several psychological problems; however, the recovery of the former from mental illness is also determined by the support of the latter. IPV adversely affect the mental well-being of the victim; hence, it requires systematic assessment and interventions, including social interventions. Social support is a key driver of the mental well-being of the partners. Although there are a few tools to measure various dimensions of marriage and marital relationships, culture-specific tools for the SEAR must be developed. The marital and couple therapy requires tailoring as per the culture of the SEAR, including the need to conduct greater research. Legal frameworks around marriage and mental health, though, exist in SEAR; there are variations across the nations, at times lacking clarity, and can put PwMI in disadvantageous positions. Greater research concerning the impact of co-habitation, same-sex marriage, the timing of marriage and childbearing, digitalization and working from home cultures, migration, etc., on marriage and mental health is required.

## References

Abbas, J., Aqeel, M., Abbas, J., Shaher, B., Sundas, J., & Zhang, W. (2019). The moderating role of social support for marital adjustment, depression, anxiety, and stress: Evidence from Pakistani working and nonworking women. *Journal of Affective Disorders, 244*, 231–238. https://doi.org/10.1016/j.jad.2018.07.071

Ahmad, S., & Reid, D. W. (2016). Enhancing the relationship adjustment of South Asian Canadian couples using a systemic-constructivist approach to couple therapy. *Journal of Marital and Family Therapy, 42*(4), 615–629. https://doi.org/10.1111/jmft.12161

Ahmad, S. S., & Koncsol, S. W. (2022). Cultural factors influencing mental health stigma: Perceptions of mental illness (POMI) in Pakistani emerging adults. *Religions, 13*(5), 1–21. https://doi.org/10.3390/rel13050401

Allendorf, K., Thornton, A., Mitchell, C., Young-DeMarco, L., & Ghimire, D. J. (2017). Early women, late men: timing attitudes and gender differences in marriage. *Journal of Marriage and Family, 79*(5), 1478–1496. https://doi.org/10.1111/jomf.12426

Ampalam, P., Gunturu, S., & Padma, V. (2012). A comparative study of caregiver burden in psychiatric illness and chronic medical illness. *Indian Journal of Psychiatry, 54*(3), 239–243. https://doi.org/10.4103/0019-5545.102423

Arafat, S. M. Y., Menon, V., Khan, M. A. S., Htay, M. N. N., Singh, R., Biyyala, D., Krishnamoorthy, Y., & Mynampally, K. (2023). Marital status and suicidal behavior in South Asia: A systematic review and meta-analysis. *Health Science Reports, 6*(12), 1–15. https://doi.org/10.1002/hsr2.1781

Avasthi, A. (2010). Preserve and strengthen family to promote mental health. *Indian Journal of Psychiatry, 52*(2), 113–126. https://doi.org/10.4103/0019-5545.64582

Barbour, A. (2003, August 25). *Social Support and Depression*. Group Research Section. 15th International Congress of the International Association of Group Psychotherapy, Istanbul, Turkey. https://asgpp.org/wp-content/uploads/2020/02/barbour-paper.pdf

Behere, P. B., Rao, T. S. S., & Verma, K. (2011). Effect of marriage on pre-existing psychoses. *Indian Journal of Psychiatry, 53*(4), 287–288. https://doi.org/10.4103/0019-5545.91900

Behere, P. B., Verma, K., Nagdive, A. B., Mansharamani, H., Behere, A. P., Yadav, R., & Fernandes, R. (2020). Is marriage solution for persons with Schizophrenia? *Medical Science, 24*(104), 2663–2674.

Bhandari, A. R., Marahatta, K., Rana, M., Ojha, S. P., & Regmi, M. P. (2017). Caregiving burden among family members of people with mental illness. *Journal of Psychiatrists' Association of Nepal, 4*(1), 36–42. https://doi.org/10.3126/jpan.v4i1.16741

Bonomi, A. E., Anderson, M. L., Reid, R. J., Rivara, F. P., Carrell, D., & Thompson, R. S. (2009). Medical and psychosocial diagnoses in women with a history of intimate partner violence. *Archives of Internal Medicine, 169*(18), 1692–1697. https://doi.org/10.1001/archinternmed.2009.292

Breiding, M. J., Black, M. C., & Ryan, G. W. (2008a). Chronic disease and health risk behaviors associated with intimate partner violence-18 U.S. States/Territories, 2005. *Annals of Epidemiology, 18*(7), 538–544. https://doi.org/10.1016/j.annepidem.2008.02.005

Breiding, M. J., Black, M. C., & Ryan, G. W. (2008b). Chronic disease and health risk behaviors associated with intimate partner violence—18 U.S. States/Territories, 2005. *Annals of Epidemiology, 18*(7), 538–544. https://doi.org/10.1016/j.annepidem.2008.02.005

Brenman, N. F., Luitel, N. P., Mall, S., & Jordans, M. J. D. (2014). Demand and access to mental health services: A qualitative formative study in Nepal. *BMC International Health and Human Rights, 14*(1), 22. https://doi.org/10.1186/1472-698X-14-22

Bursalioglu, F. S., Aydin, N., Yazici, E., & Yazici, A. B. (2013). The correlation between psychiatric disorders and women's lives. *Journal of Clinical and Diagnostic Research, 7*(4), 695–699. https://doi.org/10.7860/JCDR/2013/5635.2884

Christensen, A. (2010). A unified protocol for couple therapy. In K. Hahlweg, M. Grawe-Gerber, & D. H. Baucom (Eds.), *Enhancing couples: The shape of couple therapy to come* (pp. 33–46). Hogrefe Publishing.

Chung, H. (2005). Application and revision of the Kansas marital satisfaction scale for use with Korean couples. *Psychological Reports, 95*, 1015–1022. https://doi.org/10.2466/PR0.95.7.1015-1022

Clarke, P., & Wheaton, B. (2005). Mapping social context on mental health trajectories through adulthood. *Advances in Life Course Research, 9*(04), 269–301. https://doi.org/10.1016/S1040-2608(04)09010-0

Dalui, A., Guha, P., De, A., Chakraborty, S., & Chakraborty, I. (2014). Assessment of stress & related albuminuria in caregivers of severe mentally ill persons. *Indian Journal of Medical Research, 139*(January), 174–177.

Deshmukh, V., Bhagat, A., Shah, N., Sonavane, S., & Desousa, A. (2016). Factors affecting marriage in schizophrenia: A cross-sectional study. *Journal of Mental Health and Human Behavior, 21*(2), 122. https://doi.org/10.4103/0971-8990.193432

Devi, K., Singh, S., & Ts, D. (2024). The intersection of LGBTQ+ mental health and the rise of same-sex marriage: Understanding current trends and implications for LGBTQ+ rights and society Int J Med Res Rev 2024;2(12) 48. *International Journal of Medical Research and Review, 2*, 45–51.

Devries, K. M., Mak, J. Y., Bacchus, L. J., Child, J. C., Falder, G., Petzold, M., Astbury, J., & Watts, C. H. (2013). Intimate partner violence and incident depressive symptoms and suicide attempts: A systematic review of longitudinal studies. *PLoS Medicine, 10*(5). https://doi.org/10.1371/journal.pmed.1001439

Drisya, P., Bindumol, K., Saleem, T. K., & Narayan, D. (2019). Marital problems among partners of patients with bipolar affective disorder. *Indian Journal of Psychological Medicine, 41*(5), 448–454. https://doi.org/10.4103/IJPSYM.IJPSYM_409_18

Eickmeyer, K. J., Manning, W. D., & Brown, S. L. (2019). What's mine is ours? Income pooling in American families. *Journal of Marriage and Family, 81*(4), 968–978. https://doi.org/10.1111/jomf.12565

Elkington, K. S., Hackler, D., Walsh, T. A., Latack, J. A., McKinnon, K., Borges, C., Wright, E. R., & Wainberg, M. L. (2013). Perceived mental illness stigma, intimate relationships, and sexual risk behavior in youth with mental illness. *Journal of Adolescent Research, 28*(3), 378–404. https://doi.org/10.1177/0743558412467686

Gazmararian, J. A. (1996). Prevalence of violence against pregnant women. *JAMA: The Journal of the American Medical Association, 275*(24), 1915. https://doi.org/10.1001/jama.1996.03530480057041

Gurung, D., Poudyal, A., Wang, Y. L., Neupane, M., Bhattarai, K., Wahid, S. S., Aryal, S., Heim, E., Gronholm, P., Thornicroft, G., & Kohrt, B. (2022). Stigma against mental health disorders in Nepal conceptualised with a "what matters most" framework: A scoping review. *Epidemiology and Psychiatric Sciences, 31*,. https://doi.org/10.1017/S2045796021000809

Halford, W. K., & Vijver, F. van de. (2020). Chapter 17—Culture, couple relationship standards, and couple relationship education and therapy. In W. K. Halford & F. van de Vijver (Eds.), *Cross-cultural family research and practice* (pp. 523–563). Academic Press. https://doi.org/10.1016/B978-0-12-815493-9.00017-X

Hamid, N., Muhamad, R., Kueh, C., Zahari, Z., Mohamad, N., Abdullah, N., & Wong, M. S. (2020). Translation of the Revised Dyadic Adjustment Scale (RDAS) into the Malay language and its psychometric qualities among healthy married Malay Women. *Journal of Pharmacy and Bioallied Sciences, 12*(4), 444-448.

Härkönen, J., Brons, M. D., & Dronkers, J. (2021). Family forerunners? Parental separation and partnership formation in 16 countries. *Journal of Marriage and Family, 83*(1), 119–136. https://doi.org/10.1111/jomf.12682

Horwitz, A. V., White, H. R., & Howell-White, S. (1996). Becoming married and mental health: A longitudinal study of a cohort of young adults. *Journal of Marriage and the Family, 58*(4), 895. https://doi.org/10.2307/353978

Hou, C. L., Zang, Y., Rosen, R. C., Cai, M. Y., Li, Y., Jia, F. J., Lin, Y. Q., Ungvari, G. S., Ng, C. H., Chiu, H. F. K., & Xiang, Y. T. (2016). Sexual dysfunction and its impact on quality of life in Chinese patients with schizophrenia treated in primary care. *Comprehensive Psychiatry, 65*, 116–121. https://doi.org/10.1016/j.comppsych.2015.11.002

Huang, Y.-T., & Liang, Z. (2022). Effects of same-sex marriage legalization for sexual minority men in Taiwan: Findings from a prospective study. *International Journal of Public Health, 67*, 1604489. https://doi.org/10.3389/ijph.2022.1604489

Idstad, M., Ask, H., & Tambs, K. (2010). Mental disorder and caregiver burden in spouses: The Nord-Trøndelag health study. *BMC Public Health, 10*. https://doi.org/10.1186/1471-2458-10-516

Uecker, J. E. (2008). Marriage and mental health among young adults. *Journal of Health and Social Behavior, 23*(1), 1–7. https://doi.org/10.1177/0022146511419206.MARRIAGE

Kravdal, Ø., Wörn, J., & Reme, B. A. (2023). Mental health benefits of cohabitation and marriage: A longitudinal analysis of Norwegian register data. *Population Studies, 77*(1), 91–110. https://doi.org/10.1080/00324728.2022.2063933

Kulhara, P., Avasthi, A., Gupta, N., Das, M. K., Nehra, R., Rao, S. A., & Singh, G. (1998). Life events and social support in married schizophrenics. *Indian Journal of Psychiatry, 40*(4), 376–382.

Kumar, P., Sharma, N., Ghai, S., & Grover, S. (2019). Perception about marriage among caregivers of patients with schizophrenia and bipolar disorder. *Indian Journal of Psychological Medicine, 41*(5), 440–447. https://doi.org/10.4103/IJPSYM.IJPSYM_18_19

Kundra, S., Sreen, N., & Dwivedi, R. (2023). Impact of work from home and family support on Indian Women's work productivity during COVID-19. *Vikalpa: The Journal for Decision Makers, 48*(1), 39–53. https://doi.org/10.1177/02560909231162918

Lee, E., Kim, S. I., Jung-Choi, K., & Kong, K. A. (2022). Household decision-making and the mental well-being of marriage-based immigrant women in South Korea. *PLoS ONE, 17*(2), Article e0263642. https://doi.org/10.1371/journal.pone.0263642

Li, M., Chan, C. W. H., Choi, K. C., Zhang, H., Ng, S. N., Huang, L., Zhang, M., & Zhao, W. (2022). The Chinese version of the Revised Dyadic Adjustment Scale for gynaecological cancer patients and their partners: Translation and psychometric evaluation. *Asia-Pacific Journal of Oncology Nursing, 9*(1), 48–54. https://doi.org/10.1016/j.apjon.2021.12.004

Li, X. J., Wu, J. H., Liu, J. B., Li, K. P., Wang, F., Sun, X. H., & Ma, S. H. (2015). The influence of marital status on the social dysfunction of schizophrenia patients in community. *International Journal of Nursing Sciences, 2*(2), 149–152. https://doi.org/10.1016/j.ijnss.2015.04.015

Marcussen, K. (2005). Explaining differences in mental health between married and cohabiting individuals. *Social Psychology Quarterly, 68*(3), 239–257. https://doi.org/10.1177/019027250506800304

Moffitt, P. F., Spence, N. D., & Goldney, R. D. (1986). Mental health in marriage: The roles of need for affiliation, sensitivity to rejection, and other factors. *Journal of Clinical Psychology, 42*(1), 68–76. https://onlinelibrary.wiley.com/doi/10.1002/1097-4679%28198601%2942%3A1%3C68%3A%3AAID-JCLP2270420110%3E3.0.CO%3B2-%23

Nambi, S. (2005). Marriage, mental health and the Indian legislation. *Indian Journal of Psychiatry, 47*(1), 3. https://doi.org/10.4103/0019-5545.46067

Nawaz, S., Javeed, S., Haneef, A., Tasaur, B., & Khalid, I. (2014). Perceived social support and marital satisfaction among love and arranged marriage couples. *International Journal of Academic Research and Reflection, 2*(2), 41–50.

Ohaeri, J. U. (2003). The burden of caregiving in families with a mental illness: A review of 2002. *Current Opinion in Psychiatry, 16*(4), 457–465. https://doi.org/10.1097/01.yco.0000079212.36371.c0

Olsson, A. K., Hjärthag, F., & Helldin, L. (2016). Predicting real-world functional milestones in schizophrenia. *Psychiatry Research, 242*, 1–6. https://doi.org/10.1016/j.psychres.2016.05.015

Patel, D. (2021). *Experience of gender role expectations and negotiation in second generation desi couples*. Antioch University. https://aura.antioch.edu/etds/753

Perelli-Harris, B., Hoherz, S., Lappegård, T., & Evans, A. (2019). Mind the "Happiness" gap: The relationship between cohabitation, marriage, and subjective well-being in the United Kingdom, Australia, Germany, and Norway. *Demography, 56*(4), 1219–1246. https://doi.org/10.1007/s13524-019-00792-4

Pico-Alfonso, M. A., Garcia-Linares, I., Celda-Navarro, N., Blasco-Ros, C., Echeburúa, E., & Martinez, M. (2006). The impact of physical, psychological, and sexual. *Journal of Women's Health, 15*(5), 599–611.

Putra, B. N., & Afdal, A. (2020). Marital satisfaction: An analysis of long distance marriage couples. *International Journal of Research in Counseling and Education, 4*(1), 64. https://doi.org/10.24036/00287za0002

Rai, S., Awale, R., Ghimire, D. J., & Rao, D. (2023). Pathways of association between husbands' migration and mental health of their wives who stay behind. *SSM - Mental Health, 3*, Article 100186. https://doi.org/10.1016/j.ssmmh.2023.100186

Ran, M. S., Chan, C. L. W., Chen, E. Y. H., Xiang, M. Z., Caine, E. D., & Conwell, Y. (2006). Homelessness among patients with schizophrenia in rural China: A 10-year cohort study. *Acta Psychiatrica Scandinavica, 114*(2), 118–123. https://doi.org/10.1111/j.1600-0447.2006.00746.x

Rani, R., Jaiswal, A., Singh, L., & Rashmi, R. (2019). *Standardization and validation of Hindi version of Kansas marital satisfaction scale*.

Ross, C. E. (1995). Reconceptualizing marital status as a continuum of social attachment. *Journal of Marriage and the Family, 57*(1), 129. https://doi.org/10.2307/353822

Salokangas, R. K. R., Honkonen, T., Stengård, E., & Koivisto, A. M. (2001). To be or not to be married—That is the question of quality of life in men with schizophrenia. *Social Psychiatry and Psychiatric Epidemiology, 36*(8), 381–390. https://doi.org/10.1007/s001270170028

Scott, K. M., Wells, J. E., Angermeyer, M., Brugha, T. S., Bromet, E., Demyttenaere, K., De Girolamo, G., Gureje, O., Haro, J. M., Jin, R., Karam, A. N., Kovess, V., Lara, C., Levinson, D., Ormel, J., Posada-Villa, J., Sampson, N., Takeshima, T., Zhang, M., & Kessler, R. C. (2010). Gender and the relationship between marital status and first onset of mood, anxiety and substance use disorders. *Psychological Medicine, 40*(9), 1495–1505. https://doi.org/10.1017/S0033291709991942

Segraves, R. T. (1980). Marriage and mental health. *Journal of Sex and Marital Therapy, 6*(3), 187–198. https://doi.org/10.1080/00926238008406083

Settersten, R. A., & Hagestad, G. O. (1996). What's the latest? II. Cultural age deadlines for educational and work transitions. *Gerontologist, 36*(5), 602–613. https://doi.org/10.1093/geront/36.5.602

Shafiq, S. (2020). Perceptions of Pakistani community towards their mental health problems: A systematic review. *Global Psychiatry, 3*(1), 28–50. https://doi.org/10.2478/gp-2020-0001

Shah, A. A., Sang, A., & Ibupoto, M. H. (2025). Fertility behavior in the context of polygyny in Pakistan with the moderating effect of household wealth status evidences from demographic and health survey 2017–18. *American Journal of Human Biology, 37*(2), 1–10. https://doi.org/10.1002/ajhb.70003

Shamsun Nahar, J., Islam, M., Syed, S.-E., & Islam, Md. M. (2020). Adaptation and validation of the revised dyadic adjustment scale in Bangla (R-DAS Bangla). *Journal of Psychiatry and Psychiatric Disorders, 04*(06). https://doi.org/10.26502/jppd.2572-519X0125

Sharma, M., & Khurana, K. (2020). Psychological concomitants of delayed marriage: A study of millennial. *The International Journal of Indian Psychology, 8*(2), 311–325. https://doi.org/10.25215/0802.038

Sharma, I., Reddy, K., & Kamath, R. (2015). Marriage, mental illness and law. *Indian Journal of Psychiatry, 57*(6), 339. https://doi.org/10.4103/0019-5545.161502

Siddiqui, S., & Khalid, J. (2019). Determining the caregivers' burden in caregivers of patients with mental illness. *Pakistan Journal of Medical Sciences, 35*(5), 1329–1333. https://doi.org/10.12669/pjms.35.5.720

Simon, R. W., & Barrett, A. E. (2010). Nonmarital romantic relationships and mental health in early adulthood: Does the association differ for women and men? *Journal of Health and Social Behavior, 51*(2), 168–182. https://doi.org/10.1177/0022146510372343

Soltani, A., Molazadeh, J., Mahmoodi, M., & Hosseini, S. (2013). A study on the effectiveness of emotional focused couple therapy on intimacy of couples. *Procedia: Social and Behavioral Sciences, 82*, 461–465. https://doi.org/10.1016/j.sbspro.2013.06.293

Srivastava, A. (2013). Marriage as a perceived panacea to mental illness in India: Reality check. *Indian Journal of Psychiatry, 55*(SPEC. SUPPL.), 239–242. https://doi.org/10.4103/0019-5545.105542

Stanley, S., Bhuvaneswari, G. M., & Bhakyalakshmi, S. (2016). Mental health status and perceived burden in caregiving spouses of persons with psychotic illness (A study from India). *Social Work in Mental Health, 14*(5), 530–544. https://doi.org/10.1080/15332985.2015.1064508

Stephenson, K. R., Sullivan, K., & Christensen, A. (2023). Couple therapy. In *Encyclopedia of mental health* (pp. 504–515). Elsevier. https://doi.org/10.1016/B978-0-323-91497-0.00034-5

Subramanee, S. D., Agho, K., Lakshmi, J., Huda, M. N., Joshi, R., & Akombi-Inyang, B. (2022). Child marriage in South Asia: A systematic review. *International Journal of Environmental Research and Public Health, 19*(22). https://doi.org/10.3390/ijerph192215138

Sueyoshi, S., & Ohtsuka, R. (2003). Effects of polygyny and consanguinity on high fertility in the rural Arab population in South Jordan. *Journal of Biosocial Science, 35*(4), 513–526. https://doi.org/10.1017/s0021932003005911

Sugg, N. (2015a). Intimate partner violence. *Medical Clinics of North America, 99*(3), 629–649. https://doi.org/10.1016/j.mcna.2015.01.012

Sugg, N. (2015b). Intimate partner violence: Prevalence, health consequences, and intervention. *Medical Clinics of North America, 99*(3), 629–649. https://doi.org/10.1016/j.mcna.2015.01.012

Sullivan, K. T., Pasch, L. A., Eldridge, K. A., & Bradbury, T. N. (1998). Social support in marriage: Translating research into practical applications for clinicians. *The Family Journal, 6*(4), 263–271. https://doi.org/10.1177/1066480798064002

Thara, R., Kamath, S., & Kumar, S. (2003). Women with schizophrenia and broken marriages—Doubly disadvantaged? Part I: Patient perspective. *International Journal of Social Psychiatry, 49*(3), 225–232. https://doi.org/10.1177/00207640030493008

Thara, R., & Srinivasan, T. N. (2000). How stigmatising is schizophrenia in India? *International Journal of Social Psychiatry, 46*(2), 135–141. https://doi.org/10.1177/002076400004600206

Tong, Y., Chen, F., & Shu, B. (2019). Spousal migration and married adults' psychological distress in rural China: The roles of intimacy, autonomy and responsibility. *Social Science Research, 83*, Article 102312. https://doi.org/10.1016/j.ssresearch.2019.06.003

Tripathi, S., Pathak, V. K., & Lahariya, C. (2023). Key findings from NFHS-5 India report: Observing trends of health indicators between NFHS-4 and NFHS-5. *Journal of Family Medicine and Primary Care, 12*(9), 1759–1763. https://doi.org/10.4103/jfmpc.jfmpc_377_23

Tumin, D., & Zheng, H. (2018). Do the health benefits of marriage depend on the likelihood of marriage? *Journal of Marriage and Family, 80*(3), 622–636. https://doi.org/10.1111/jomf.12471

United Nations. (2011, December). *World Marriage Patterns*. Population Facts. Department of Economic and Social Affairs—Population Division. https://www.un.org/en/development/desa/population/publications/pdf/popfacts/PopFacts_2011-1.pdf

Vasudeva, S., Sekhar, C. K., & Rao, P. G. (2013). Caregivers burden of patients with schizophrenia and bipolar disorder: A sectional study. *Indian Journal of Psychological Medicine, 35*(4), 352–357. https://doi.org/10.4103/0253-7176.122224

Waite, L. J. (2009). Marital history and well-being in later life. *International Handbook of Population Aging, 691–704*. https://doi.org/10.1007/978-1-4020-8356-3_31

Williams, K., & Umberson, D. (2004). Marital status, marital transitions, and health: A gendered life course perspective. *Journal of Health and Social Behavior, 45*(1), 81–98. https://doi.org/10.1177/002214650404500106

Wu, E., El-Bassel, N., Witte, S. S., Gilbert, L., & Chang, M. (2003). Intimate partner violence and HIV risk among urban minority women in primary health care settings. *AIDS and Behavior, 7*(3), 291–301. https://doi.org/10.1023/A:1025447820399

Zhuang, X. Y., Wong, D. F. K., & Ng, T. K. (n.d.). Cultural values of traditionality/modernity: Their differential impacts on marital conflict and marital satisfaction among female and male migrant workers in China. *revista de cercetare si interventie sociala, 45*.

# Chapter 14
# Religion and Mental Health in South Asia

**Ravi Philip Rajkumar**

**Abstract** The relationship between religion and mental health can be studied under at least eight broad categories: (a) the influence of religion on the clinical presentation of mental disorders, (b) the relationship between religion and positive mental health, (c) religion as a risk or protective factor for specific mental disorders, and the ways in which such associations are mediated, (d) religion as a component of explanatory models of mental illness, and of societal attitudes and practices towards them, (e) religion as a factor influencing help-seeking and pathways to care for mental disorders, (f) the effects of religion on the outcome of specific mental disorders, (g) religious coping in the caregivers of persons with mental illness, and (h) religious or spiritual approaches to the treatment of mental disorder. It can be concluded that: (a) there are complex relationships between religion and mental health; (b) religion and spirituality can have positive effects on mental health in both clinical and non-clinical populations; (c) religious coping can have both positive and negative aspects; (d) religion can provide an invaluable source of social support, but can also contribute to stigmatization of the mentally ill; (e) the influence of religion may vary according to the type of mental disorder being considered; and (f) religious and spiritual approaches may be fruitfully integrated with medical or psychological treatments for mental disorder.

**Keywords** Religion · Spirituality · Mental health · Coping · Stigma · Pathways to care · Integrative medicine · Faith healing

## 1 Introduction

Religion and spirituality are as old as humanity. The earliest historical and archaeological records attest to a universal human tendency towards belief in one or more deities, in various forms of ritual worship, and individual or societal practices based

R. P. Rajkumar (✉)
Department of Psychiatry, Jawaharlal Institute of Postgraduate Medical Education and Research (JIPMER), Puducherry, India
e-mail: ravi.psych@gmail.com

 
S. M. Y. Arafat et al. (eds.), *Social Psychiatry in South Asia*, South Asian Perspectives in Mental Health and Psychology , https://doi.org/10.1007/978-981-96-8078-8_14

on these beliefs. South Asia is home to a rich tapestry of diverse religious traditions and customs. Some of these, such as Hinduism and Buddhism, have their origin in South Asian countries, whereas others, such as Islam and Christianity, have spread through inter-cultural contact or colonization. Rates of self-reported religious affiliation and practice are much higher in these countries than in Europe or North America. In a global survey of 106 countries, 100% of respondents from Afghanistan, Bangladesh, India, or Pakistan belonged to a particular religion, 57–96% engaged in daily prayer, and 80–94% considered religion "very important" in their lives (Pew Research Centre, 2018). Religious beliefs, attitudes, customs, and practices influence almost every aspect of individual and social life in this geographical region, including attitudes and practices related to illness and health. Citizens of South Asian countries frequently report turning to God, or seeking help from religious leaders, when exposed to traumatic stressors such as war, civil unrest, natural disasters, or the COVID-19 pandemic (Cardozo et al., 2004; Rajkumar et al., 2008; Riaz et al., 2023; Scholte et al., 2004; Seino et al., 2008). Religion is an important source of strength and support to them when coping with severe illnesses (Banning et al., 2009; Jafree et al., 2024; Khan et al., 2022) or disability (Baniya et al., 2022). They also frequently have recourse to religion or spirituality when dealing with common, stressful life events, such as examinations (Nagabharana et al., 2021; Sharma et al., 2021). Therefore, an intimate relationship between mental health and the different facets of religion in South Asian countries is to be expected (Poudel, 2020).

In 2016, the World Psychiatric Association (WPA) published a position statement on the role of religion and spirituality (often abbreviated R/S) in psychiatry. This statement emphasized the need to take religion into account when considering the prevalence of specific mental disorders, the differentiation between normal and pathological mental states, variations in help-seeking and treatment practices, treatment outcomes, and even the prevention of mental disorders or the promotion of positive mental health. The authors of the statement acknowledged the positive effects of R/S in many of these domains but also highlighted the potential for harm—such as treatment refusal, stigmatization, or negative coping strategies—associated with certain beliefs or customs. In its conclusions, this statement emphasized the need to address religion during history taking, in psychiatric training, in research, and in collaborations between mental health professionals and religious leaders or communities (Moreira-Almeida et al., 2016). Though not specifically developed with any one country or region in mind, the WPA document provides a valuable starting point from which the relationship between religion and mental health in South Asian countries can be examined.

## *1.1 Definitions and Conceptual Issues*

Formal, operationalized definitions of the terms "religion" and "spirituality" remain elusive. The very origins of the word "religion" are obscure. It may be derived from Latin words meaning "to bind" or "to go through in reading, speech or thought", or from an Indo-European root meaning "to have a care for" or "to pay attention to" (Hoyt, 1912). These different roots may capture different facets of religion: its obligatory or "binding" nature, the importance of prayers and religious texts, and the importance accorded by the individual believer to their religious tradition. From a research perspective, "religion" or "religiosity" is generally defined in terms of participation in organized, institutional rituals, while "spirituality" is conceptualized as the individual pursuit of higher purpose or transcendence. It is sometimes stated that spirituality fosters mental well-being, while religion or religiosity can be a source of stress (Dubey et al., 2024). However, the dividing line between religion and spirituality is not always clear, and epidemiological evidence suggests that involvement in religion, rather than "spirituality", is protective against physical and mental illness (Levin, 1996). The apparent differential effects of spirituality and religion on mental health reported in some European and North American samples may not be observed in South Asian cultures, which are characterized by collectivistic values and a more positive attitude towards religious institutions and rituals (Chaudhry, 2008; MacDonald et al., 2015). It is, therefore, important to evaluate the South Asian literature on its own merits, without any preconceived notions derived from research in other countries or continents.

"Religion" or "religiosity" is not a monolithic construct and encompasses several inter-related dimensions. This was illustrated by a factor analysis of responses from over 2000 twin pairs in the United States (Kendler et al., 2003). Data from this sample suggests that religiosity can be decomposed into seven domains, as follows:

- *General religiosity*, which involves the individual's involvement in spiritual issues, their notion of their "place in the universe", and their personal relationship with God.
- *Social religiosity*, which reflects interaction with other religious individuals and attendance at religious services.
- *Involved God,* reflecting a belief that God is actively involved in human life in a benevolent manner (i.e., "theism" instead of "deism").
- *Forgiveness*, involving an individual's "caring, loving and forgiving" attitudes towards the world.
- *God as judge*, a dimension which emphasizes God's role as a ruler, judge, and dispenser of punishment.
- *Unvengefulness/vengefulness*, reflecting whether individuals are likely (or not) to retaliate towards real or perceived insults or injuries directed at themselves.
- *Thankfulness*, encompassing feelings of gratitude towards God and life in general.

Such a "decomposition" allows one to identify aspects of religion that could contribute to positive mental health (for example, forgiveness and thankfulness) or to negative mental health outcomes (such as "God as judge" or vengefulness). This is relevant when considering the distinction between "positive" and "negative" religious coping, as discussed later in this chapter.

Though a factor analysis of this kind is informative and heuristically useful, it is limited by the fact that it was carried out in a "Western" population, drawing predominantly on the Judeo-Christian religious tradition. It is not clear whether similar analyses in South American, Asian, or African populations would yield similar results, or whether the "factor structure" of religiosity in individuals is influenced by the culturally predominant religion. However, preliminary evidence from a study of American, Chinese and Indian patients revealed a five-factor model of spirituality (love, interconnectedness, altruism, contemplative practice, and religious reflection and commitment), suggesting that at least some dimensions of R/S are consistent across religions and cultures (McClintock et al., 2016).

It is beyond the scope of this chapter to make pronouncements on the supernatural aspects of religion, on their relative truth claims, or on the relationship between non-religious belief systems and mental health (Whitley, 2010). The WPA position statement warns psychiatrists against using their position to promote a particular worldview, whether religious or secular, and encourages sensitivity and respect towards diverse religious traditions (Moreira-Almeida et al., 2016). Likewise, it is unwise for the psychiatrist to take an unduly reductionistic stance towards religion and spirituality, or to dismiss religious beliefs and experiences on the basis of evolutionary or neurobiological hypotheses (Verhagen, 2010). While it is possible and fruitful to examine the biological or psychological correlates of religion (Mohandas, 2008; Rim et al., 2019), the latter cannot be reduced to the former. Instead, the emphasis should be on a careful reading and a cautious interpretation of the available evidence, examining both the positive and negative influences of religion on specific mental health outcomes.

The WPA document provides a useful conceptual framework within which research findings on religion and mental health from South Asia can be organized. Broadly speaking, the results of this research can be grouped under eight inter-related headings or questions:

- How does religion influence the presentation of mental illness? This is sometimes referred to as a *pathoplastic* effect, in which religious beliefs or values either the form of psychopathology (as in trance and possession states) or its content (as in religious delusions, hallucinations, or obsessions) (Laroi et al., 2014; Maslowski et al., 1998; Whitwell & Barker, 1980)
- Is there an association between religion and positive mental health? Can religious beliefs and practices enhance psychological resilience in the face of adversity, improve coping with stress, and generally promote flourishing? (Ahrens et al., 2010; Kidwai et al., 2014; Lang et al., 2020)
- Is there an association between religion and the risk of specific mental disorders? Do specific aspects of religiosity act as protective or vulnerability factors for a given condition, such as depression? (Braam & Koenig, 2019; Kendler et al., 2003)
- How does religion influence the way patients, caregivers, and communities understand mental illness? Do religious beliefs contribute to the stigmatization and

isolation of persons with these disorders, or do they facilitate the reintegration of a mentally ill person into their community? (Fabrega, 1991; Grover et al., 2014)

- How does religion influence help-seeking in persons with mental disorders? Do religious beliefs lead these persons to seek non-medical forms of treatment, such as the various forms of faith healing? (Atilola, 2015; van der Watt et al., 2018)
- How does religion influence the course and outcome of specific mental disorders? This includes its effect on measures such as response or remission rates, adherence to treatment, quality of life, and reduction in specific adverse outcomes, such as suicide (Rasic et al., 2009; Stroppa et al., 2018).
- Does religiosity aid coping and adaptation in the caregivers of persons with mental disorder, and more specifically in family caregivers? (Casaleiro et al., 2022; Daliri et al., 2024)
- Are religious and spiritual approaches useful in the management of specific mental disorders? How can these be harmonized with biomedical or psychosocial treatment methods? How can this topic be integrated into the curriculum for the training of mental health professionals? (Bhatti et al., 2024; Hanlon et al., 2014; McGovern et al., 2017)

Relevant evidence from the South Asian literature will be summarized under these broad headings (Fig. 1). Certain additional issues that do not fall into any of the above categories—such as the nature of the religious beliefs held by persons with mental illness and how to distinguish them from psychopathological phenomena—will be considered in a separate section.

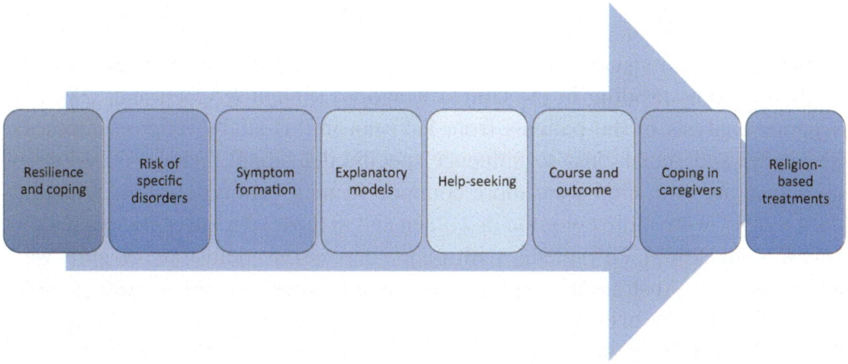


**Fig. 1** Effects of religion on mental health at multiple levels—pathogenesis, phenomenology, outcome, and treatment

## 2 Pathoplastic Effects of Religion and Spirituality in South Asian Patients

Mental illnesses, as defined using standardized criteria—such as the World Health Organization's International Classification of Mental and Behavioural Disorders (ICD-11) or the American Psychiatric Association's Diagnostic and Statistical Manual (DSM-5) have been identified across countries and cultures. However, the form and content of their presentation are significantly influenced by culture, of which religion is an essential component. For example, a traumatic stressor or psychological conflict may result in dissociative identity disorder in a North American patient but in a trance or possession disorder in a South Asian patient. Though the underlying psychobiological mechanism, namely dissociation, is the same in both cases, it takes on different forms depending on whether local culture places an emphasis on individualism and identity, as in the West, or on the importance of spiritual beings, as in the East. In a case series from Sri Lanka, distinct presentations of trance and possession states were identified in Buddhist, Catholic, and Muslim patients, highlighting the complex relations between religion and psychopathology in multi-religious South Asian countries (Hanwella et al., 2012).

Religion can also influence the content of psychopathology. For example, delusions are commonly seen both in affective and non-affective psychoses, but the specific content of these delusions is influenced by local beliefs and values. In a sample of 185 Indian patients with bipolar disorder, nearly 38% reported delusions or hallucinations involving "spiritual" or "supernatural" content (Grover et al., 2016). In a comparative study of British and Pakistani patients with psychotic spectrum disorders, patients from Pakistan were more likely to report delusions with a theme of "black magic", or visual hallucinations of spirits or ghosts (*jinn*) than either white or Indian patients residing in the United Kingdom (Suhail & Cochrane, 2002). In a separate analysis of the patients from Pakistan in this study, religion interacted with gender and social class to influence specific delusional themes: delusions of communicating with God were more common in men, while delusions related to "black magic" were more common in women and in those of a lower socioeconomic status (Suhail, 2003). In patients with major depression, delusions of guilt were more common in Austrian than in Pakistani patients, though ideas of guilt occurred at similar frequencies in both groups (Stompe et al., 2001). In some cases, a mismatch between the patient's delusional beliefs and the actual tenets of their religion can be used to identify "bizarre" delusions, which were formerly considered pathognomonic of schizophrenia. This was illustrated in a study of over 1,900 Indian patients with schizophrenia, in which odd or culturally inappropriate religious beliefs were one of five subtypes or themes of bizarre delusions (De et al., 2013).

Obsessive–compulsive disorder (OCD) frequently presents with obsessive fears or doubts related to contamination, blasphemy, or other "forbidden" thoughts with a religious theme. The specific content of these obsessions can vary according to the patient's belief system. For example, following attendance at a traditional Hindu funeral, an Indian patient developed obsessive fears related to contamination with ashes from the funeral pyre, which subsequently generalized to firewood in general. These symptoms failed to respond to pharmacotherapy but reduced significantly after exposure and response therapy (ERP) involving graded exposure to ashes and, eventually, self-exposure to burial grounds (Nath et al., 2016). In a sample of 50 Indian patients with OCD, self-reported religiosity was associated with higher levels of guilt (Rakesh et al., 2021).

Finally, religious beliefs can also result in atypical or unusual presentations of otherwise well-characterized mental disorders. In a series of three children from Sri Lanka, who presented with claims of "having been reincarnated" and "recalling past lives", the underlying diagnosis in all cases was autism spectrum disorder (ASD). The authors of this case series hypothesized that disturbances in theory of mind and sense of self, combined with increased imaginative or "fantasy" thinking, interacted with cultural beliefs about rebirth or reincarnation, leading to this presentation (Chandradasa & Champika, 2018). Similarly, an Indian patient with schizophrenia was reported to maintaining his left hand in a closed-fist position for several months, leading to contractures and skin ulceration. On clarification, this was found to result from a delusion in which this posture was a ritual (*sadhana*) that he could release only when God appeared to him. Both the delusion and the associated behaviour gradually improved following antipsychotic treatment (Mukherjee et al., 2015). In some cases, these religious-themed symptoms can lead to significant disability or morbidity. This was vividly illustrated by a case report from India, in which a patient with an acute psychotic episode engaged in auto-enucleation of both eyes out of a delusional belief that he had to offer his eyes to God. This belief was noted to be similar to a Hindu legend in which a hunter offered his eyes to Lord Shiva as a sign of his fervent devotion (Harish et al., 2012).

Overall, though the South Asian literature on this topic is sparse, there is some evidence that religious beliefs and practices can influence either the form or the content of psychopathology in several conditions, including conversion and dissociative disorders, psychotic disorders, and OCD. Such presentations may be particularly common in patients with schizophrenia or bipolar disorder and may sometimes be associated with a significant risk of harm to oneself. Mental health professionals from South Asia should be aware of this, particularly when distinguishing between religious and delusional beliefs, or between "normal" ritualistic behaviour and "bizarre" or "disorganized" psychotic behaviour.

## 3 Religion and Positive Mental Health in South Asia

There is substantial evidence that certain facets of religion or spirituality are associated with positive mental health in South Asian populations. This can be seen both in community samples, where religiosity and religious coping are associated with lower psychological distress, and in persons undergoing adversity, such as severe illnesses or natural disasters. Before reviewing South Asian research in this field, it is important to understand that religious coping strategies can be either adaptive or maladaptive. Research by Kenneth Pargament and his colleagues has helped to operationalize this distinction and has led to the adoption of the terms "positive" and "negative" religious coping in the wider literature (Pargament et al., 2000). Though the finer details of these two forms of religious coping vary across religions, cross-national research has shown that positive religious coping is more common than negative coping regardless of religious affiliation (Abu-Raiya & Pargament, 2015). Broadly speaking, positive religious coping covers attitudes and themes such as forgiveness, spiritual connection, and collaboration with others based on religious values, and interpreting situations in a positive or "benevolent" light. Negative coping includes such approaches as a lack of spiritual contentment or satisfaction, views of God as vengeful or punitive, discord with others over religious beliefs, and beliefs related to demonic causes of adversity or trauma (Pargament et al., 1998). These two forms of coping generally have opposite effects on mental health outcomes, but both can coexist in the same person—for example, a patient with depression may believe that his symptoms are demonic in origin, but can also believe in God's forgiveness as contributing to his healing, or seek support from others in his religious community. When they are both used, they may interfere with each other in complex ways (Ghorbani et al., 2021).

## *3.1 Religion and Positive Mental Health in the General Population*

There is evidence from several South Asian countries that religious or spiritual beliefs and practices are associated with improved general mental health, as measured either by improved psychological well-being or by a lesser risk of sub-syndromal symptoms of anxiety or depression. In a sample of engineering students from India, self-reported spirituality was negatively correlated with self-reported stress (Yadav et al., 2017). Similarly, self-reported spiritual and religious practice was positively correlated subjective happiness, life satisfaction, and a sense of meaning or purpose in life in South Indian postgraduate students, though these correlations were weak in magnitude (Deb et al., 2020). Similar results were obtained in university students from Pakistan (Saleem & Saleem, 2017). In a study involving young adults from both India and Israel, scores on a measure of spiritual intelligence were positively correlated with life satisfaction (Walter et al., 2024). In medical faculty from an Indian teaching hospital, the statement "My religious or spiritual beliefs strongly influence my work" was associated with higher ratings of personal accomplishment, but not with job stress or satisfaction (Lal et al., 2020). Positive religious coping has been associated with greater mental well-being in engineers from Pakistan (Fatima et al., 2024).

Religiosity may also have a positive effect on mental health in the elderly, who are at a high risk of depression due to medical comorbidities and socioeconomic difficulties. In a survey of over 31,000 respondents aged 60 years and above from

India, those who perceived religion as "very important" had fewer subthreshold depressive symptoms. There was an apparent "dose–response" relationship in this sample, as even those who perceived religion as "somewhat important" had fewer symptoms than those who considered it unimportant, but the magnitude of this effect was smaller (Saravanakumar et al., 2022). In a sample of South Indian elderly adults, religiosity was negatively correlated with two measures of psychological distress and was considered a valuable resource in coping with stressors (Chokkanathan, 2009). A study of older adults from Nepal found that prayer was associated with lower levels of depressive symptoms in men but not in women (Gautam et al., 2007).

There is no clear-cut evidence that any particular religion has a greater protective effect than another. In a study of Bangladeshi students entering college, self-reported religious practice was associated with fewer depressive symptoms, but there was no difference in these symptoms between Hindu and Muslim respondents (Siddik et al., 2023). In adolescent girls from India, there was a weak association between Hindu religious affiliation and greater self-reported academic stress, implying a protective association with other religious affiliations: however, other variables, such as parental education, choice of subject for secondary examinations and individual personality traits, were more strongly predictive of stress in this sample (Rentala et al., 2019). In a study of older adults from India, self-reported religious affiliation (Hindu, Muslim, Sikh or "other") was not associated with variations in psychological distress, though factors such as income, education, living with one's spouse, physical health and experiences of elder abuse predicted variations in this variable (Srivastava et al., 2021). In a similar study involving older adults from Nepal, Christian religious affiliation was associated with a lower quality of life (QoL) than Hinduism or Buddhism, while Buddhist affiliation was associated with a higher QoL than Hinduism. The authors acknowledged that there was no clear or obvious explanation for this result (Yadav et al., 2020).

Paradoxical associations have also been reported in this field. Thus, in a sample of rural older adults from Bangladesh, "religiosity" was negatively associated with overall quality of life (QoL). This study used a single instrument to measure the strength of religious belief (Uddin et al., 2017). A similar result was obtained in elderly adults from Bhutan, in whom scores on a locally developed measure of spirituality, addressing practices such as prayer and meditation, was negatively associated with QoL (Dorji et al., 2017). One explanation for this finding is that elderly adults with a poor QoL due to other factors, such as illness or disability, may seek solace in religious or spiritual practices. Neither of these studies specifically examined relationships with the psychological domain of QoL.

### 3.2 Religion and Positive Mental Health in South Asian Persons Facing Stress, Trauma, or Adversity

Exposure to chronic or traumatic stress is a risk factor for several mental disorders. The causal pathway from such an event (e.g., childhood physical abuse) to a particular syndrome (e.g., depression or post-traumatic stress disorder) is not linear and can be mediated through or moderated by several factors, including religiosity or religious coping. For example, in young adults from Afghanistan, Islamic positive religious coping was associated with lower levels of anxiety and depressive symptoms after experiencing childhood sexual abuse. This association was significant only in those participants who had a high baseline level of Muslim "experiential religiousness", characterized by a "close and loving" attitude towards God and acceptance of His will. There was also evidence of interference between positive and negative religious coping: in respondents who reported both forms, the latter reduced the protective effects of the former (Ghorbani et al., 2021). Similar beneficial effects of positive religious coping have examined using qualitative research methods, and have been reported in Bangladeshi healthcare workers testing positive during the COVID-19 pandemic (Arefin et al., 2022), in fishing communities from South India affected by the 2004 Asian tsunami (Rajkumar et al., 2008) and in parents bereaved during the civil unrest in Kashmir (Khursheed & Shahnawaz, 2020). In some cases, individuals reported a stronger connection to God and greater resilience in the aftermath of these events, suggesting that religious coping could contribute to post-traumatic growth.

Null or inverse results have also been obtained in this domain by some researchers. For instance, in a sample of 588 healthcare students living through the COVID-19 pandemic, the use of religion as a coping strategy was not significantly associated with levels of sub-syndromal anxiety or depression; however, this study did not formally test for a statistical association between these variables (Mishra et al., 2023). In a study of earthquake survivors from Nepal, religious coping was more commonly reported by those with post-traumatic stress disorder (PTSD), whereas active coping was used by those without PTSD. However, as this was a cross-sectional study, the direction of the association was unclear (Adhikari Baral & Bhagawati, 2019). Similar results have been reported in tsunami survivors from Sri Lanka (Hollifield et al., 2008). It is possible that those with PTSD symptoms resorted to religious coping to deal with distressing symptoms and that it serves as a "protective shield" against such symptoms (Zukerman & Korn, 2014).

Religious coping also plays a central role in patients suffering from chronic, life-threatening, or terminal illnesses, such as cancer. In these cases, the relationship between religiosity and mental health in South Asian patients is bidirectional, and may depend on variables such as the stage of the illness. Depression or anxiety was linked to reduced spiritual well-being in Indian patients with advanced cancer receiving hospice care (Kandasamy et al., 2011), while Hindu religiosity was positively associated with emotional well-being in Indian women with breast cancer undergoing surgery (Pandey et al., 2005). A similar positive relationship between spirituality and quality of life was observed in a mixed population of Stage I and

II cancers (oral, breast or lung) from a northeastern state of India (Bhattacharjee & Ghosh, 2024). The bidirectional nature of this relationship was also noted in a mixed population of cancer patients from Pakistan, 61% of whom had advanced cancer (Stage III or IV). In these patients, Muslim religiosity was associated with reduced fears related to death, but depression was negatively associated with Muslim religiosity. Subsequent analysis of this data showed that optimism and depression mediated the link between religiosity and death anxiety in these patients (Abbas et al., 2022). In women from Bangladesh with metastatic breast cancer, the use of religion as a coping strategy was associated with higher levels of active coping and acceptance of the illness but the strength of these correlations was modest (Islam et al., 2023). Similar protective effects may be seen in other terminal illnesses. In a qualitative study of patients with advanced hepatitis C from Pakistan, respondents stated that religion helped them to come to terms with their prognosis, and expressed a desire for greater participation in religious practices (Ahmad et al., 2024). In contrast to these findings, a study of metastatic cancer patients from Bangladesh found no association between spiritual well-being and either anxiety or depression (Rahman et al., 2024).

There is little research from South Asia on the relationship between religion or spirituality and resilience in the face of disability, such as that caused by a stroke or spinal cord injury. A study of Hindu male patients from India, hospitalized for various general medical or surgical conditions, found a positive association between spirituality and both overall and psychological QoL (Nandika & Nagalakshmi, 2021). In patients from Pakistan with disability due to limb loss, religiosity was positively correlated with self-efficacy and negatively associated with depressive symptoms (Batool & Nawaz, 2016). Spirituality was also associated with reduced psychological distress in Pakistani patients with extensive burns (Jibeen et al., 2018). The perceived benefit of R/S activities was associated with lower levels of depression in Sri Lankan patients with traumatic spinal cord injuries (Xue et al., 2016). However, in persons with a spinal cord injury following an earthquake in Nepal, there was no significant correlation between self-reported spirituality and psychological resilience (Bhattarai et al., 2018).

Overall, the evidence of these studies, though mixed, suggests that religiosity or spirituality can be an important "general resistance resource" for mental health in South Asians (Chokkanathan, 2009; Levin, 2003) (Table 1). Religious and spiritual practice appear to "buffer" the effects of life stressors, promote mental well-being, and aid adaptation to adverse life situations, even if these are traumatic. However, the magnitude of these effects is weak to moderate in most studies, and the presence of divergent results in the literature suggests that they are not universal.

**Table 1** Effects of religion on positive mental health

| Processes | Beneficial outcomes |
|---|---|
| Overall level of religiosity or spirituality<br>Importance of religion in one's life<br>Positive religious coping<br>Prayer | Lower psychological distress<br>Better subjective mental well-being<br>Greater life satisfaction<br>Lower levels of depression and anxiety<br>Better coping with trauma or stress<br>Post-traumatic growth |

# 4 Religion as a Risk or Protective Factor for Mental Illness in the South Asian Population

## *4.1 Religion as a Protective Factor*

Epidemiological research from countries across the globe suggests that religious involvement is protective against both physical and mental illness (Levin, 1996; VanderWeele & Ouyang, 2025). In South Asian populations, these effects have been demonstrated most specifically for common mental disorders (CMD), namely depression and anxiety. In a survey of over 4000 adolescent or adult respondents from Bhutan, self-identifying as "very spiritual" and giving importance to the role of *karma* in daily life were both associated with lower levels of CMD symptomatology (Sithey et al., 2018). In adults residing in a rural area of South India, several measures of R/S—spiritual intelligence, engagement in religious practices, and intrinsic religiosity—were associated with lower rates of depression (Rajan et al., 2024). A case–control study from India found that self-reported religiosity and spirituality were higher in healthy controls than in patients with depression (Dua et al., 2021). Muslim religiosity was associated with lower rates of CMD symptoms in Pakistani students during the COVID-19 pandemic (Saleem et al., 2021). In contrast, a study of high school students from India found that religious coping was approximately two times more common in those with depression or anxiety, though whether this was a cause or a consequence of these disorders could not be assessed (Sharma et al., 2021).

In the elderly, there is some evidence that religious practices are protective against late-life depression, just as it is against subthreshold depressive symptoms. In a sample of elderly adults from Bangladesh without any self-reported medical illness, engagement in these practices was associated with a two-fold reduction in the risk of depression (Disu et al., 2019).

There is also some evidence that affiliation with specific religious groups—more specifically, with the "majority" religion—is associated with a lower risk of CMD. This has been demonstrated (a) in Indian adolescents from an urban slum, where depression was more common in Muslim than in Hindu youth (Chauhan & Dhar, 2020), in Indian women following childbirth, where the same result was observed (Mishra et al., 2020; Singh et al., 2021), (b) in adults from Eastern Nepal, where depression was less common in Hindus and Buddhists than in adherents of folk (Kirat) religion (Sherchand et al., 2018), (c) in adolescents in Pakistan, where depression was more common in religious minorities (Hindus and Christians) than in Muslims (Iqbal et al., 2012), and (d) in school-age children in Sri Lanka, where behavioural problems were more common in Hindu than in Buddhist children (Prior et al., 2005). As all these studies were cross-sectional, no definitive conclusion can be drawn from them, though it is possible that social factors related to minority status—sometimes termed "minority stress" —may have contributed to this outcome (Buckner et al., 2022; Iqbal et al., 2012).

Religious beliefs and practices may have protective effects against suicide or self-harm. Certain religions, such as Christianity or Islam, may have strong proscriptions against suicide; in contrast, Hinduism and Buddhism disapprove of suicide but may either tolerate it or adopt an ambivalent attitude towards it in some cases (Utyasheva et al., 2022; Vijayakumar & John, 2018). In a sample of 172 community respondents from India, suicidal behaviours were reported less frequently by Muslims than by Hindus. This may reflect the above differences in religious attitudes towards suicide (Thimmaiah et al., 2016). A similar differential effect of Hinduism and Islam has been observed in community and population-level surveys (Kar et al., 2024; Kuttichira, 2018). However, religion is only one of many factors influencing suicide risk. In Muslim-majority countries such as Pakistan, negative life events, poor social support, and fixed risk factors such as gender may "override" religious prohibitions (Eskin et al., 2021; Khan et al., 2008). In a case–control, psychological autopsy study of suicides from Pakistan, completed suicides were found to have lower levels of participation in religious and spiritual activities than controls (Ali & Saleem, 2024). In Afghan students living through civil unrest, trust in a higher power—a measure of religious belief—was associated with lower levels of suicidal ideation in those with PTSD (Mehrabi et al., 2023). These findings suggests that religious belief and practice, rather than simple affiliation, may protect against suicidality. Though suicide is proscribed in Christianity, Indian Christians have been observed to have higher suicide rates than Hindus (Arya et al., 2019).

A small number of studies have reported associations between religious affiliation and addictive disorders. Tobacco use has been reported to be lower in Sikhs in northern India (Darshan et al., 1981) and in Hindus in a slum in North-Eastern India (Sarkar et al., 2019), Alcohol use was more common in Buddhist than in Hindu or folk religion adherents in Nepal (Rathod et al., 2018), and less common in Muslims in an urban slum in India (Kim et al., 2013). A single study from India examined the association between religion and Internet addiction in adolescents during the COVID-19 pandemic and found lower scores on the Internet Addiction Test in Hindus than in non-Hindus (Ramakrishna et al., 2023). However, whether these findings can be specifically attributed to a protective effect of religion are unknown.

In summary, there is some evidence that religious and spiritual practices may protect against common mental disorders, both in the general population and in the elderly (Table 2). Preliminary evidence suggests that certain religious beliefs and practices may protect against suicide attempts, but the strength and consistency of this evidence is modest. Evidence for differential protective effects of specific

**Table 2** Protective effects of religion against mental disorders

| Disorder(s) | Strength of evidence |
|---|---|
| Common mental disorders | ++ |
| Depression | ++ |
| Late-life depression | + |
| Self-harm | + |
| Substance use disorders | ± |

Legend: ++ protective effects in multiple studies; + protective effects in a single study, or more positive than negative studies; ± equivocal or inconsistent results

religions is unclear, and may result from the confounding effect of socioeconomic factors.

## *4.2 Religion as a Risk Factor*

Though certain facets of religion and spirituality appear to be protective against disorders such as depression, associations in the other direction have also been reported from several Asian countries. This may occur in one of four ways (Fig. 2).

First, certain types of negative religious coping, as discussed in the preceding section, may have a harmful effect on mental health. In a study of adults affected by an earthquake in north-western Pakistan, those who believed that they were being punished for their sins, or for lack of adequate spirituality, had higher levels of

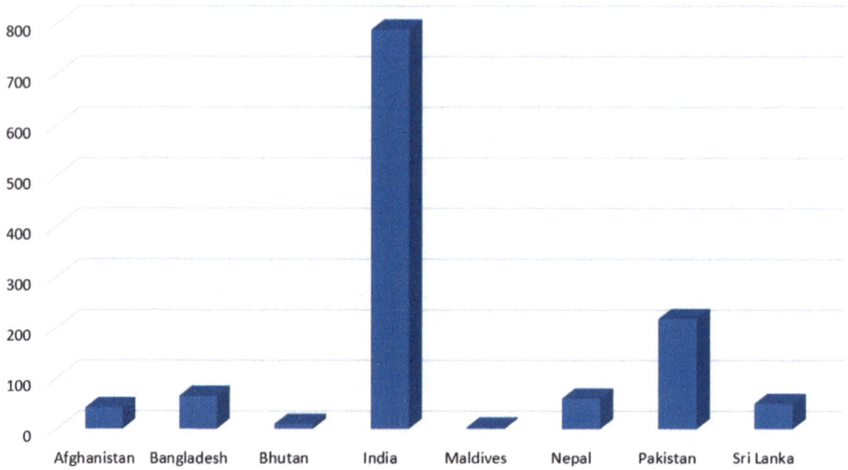


**Fig. 2** Number of published articles on religion and spirituality in relation to mental health from all eight South Asian countries, as retrieved from the PubMed database

PTSD. There was no protective effect of positive religious coping against PTSD. This may be explained by the fact that there was a weak positive correlation between positive and negative religious coping in these respondents (Feder et al., 2013). A similar association between negative ("passive") religious coping and PTSD was observed in female survivors of the 2004 Asian tsunami in Sri Lanka (Wickrama et al., 2017). Negative religious coping was also associated with an increased rate of suicide attempts in Indian patients with depression (Dua et al., 2021).

Second, religious values or obligations can come into conflict with individuals' wishes, leading to the activation of psychological defence mechanisms that lead to specific symptom presentations. For example, in a case series of young women from Pakistan, it was found that a conflict between religious proscriptions and sexual or romantic desires facilitated the emergence of conversion disorder (Bokharey et al., 2023).

Third, certain attitudes or traditional practices associated with specific religions may have negative effects on the mental health of certain groups. For example, traditional beliefs regarding the inferiority of certain castes, leading to their exclusion or marginalization in society, have been associated with elevated levels of depression and anxiety in members of "lower" or Scheduled Castes (Goghari & Kusi, 2023). Strict forms of seclusion related to menstruation have been associated with increased levels of stress and negative emotions in adolescent girls and women from Nepal (Baumann et al., 2021; Sharma et al., 2022). Beliefs about traditional gender roles and women's status, leading to increased rates of intimate partner violence (IPV) or abuse, have been associated with increased rates of depression and anxiety in women from Pakistan (Niaz, 2004). In Sri Lanka, IPV was more common in women from Christian, Hindu, or Muslim than Buddhist religious backgrounds (Bandara et al., 2022). Beliefs and practices about the inferiority of a particular gender or community lie at the interface between religion and culture, have deep roots in communities, and are often difficult to address in clinical or public health practice (Baumann et al., 2021).

More rarely, specific religious or spiritual practices can trigger an episode of mental illness, particularly in vulnerable individuals. In a case series from India, two male patients who attempted to practice *Kundalini yoga*, an ancient Hindu mystical practice, without appropriate training or supervision developed psychotic episodes. In both cases, consultation between the psychiatric team and a yoga expert made it clear that the patient was suffering from a mental illness and not from a spiritual experience. Both patients responded well to pharmacotherapy (Suchandra et al., 2021). Even more rarely, religious beliefs can result in the social contagion of specific psychiatric symptoms or disorders, particularly those resulting from somatization or dissociation. Such religion-themed "mass hysteria" has been reported in a rural Indian extended family, affecting ten of the 31 members. Interestingly, two of these patients also had bipolar disorder, which was recognized by the rest of the family as a mental illness and was not ascribed to any spiritual or supernatural cause (Mattoo et al., 2002).

Overall, there is inconsistent evidence for a harmful effect of R/S on mental health in South Asian populations. When such an effect is observed, it may be due either to the use of negative religious coping, to religious beliefs or customs that lead to the marginalization of a particular group, or because of a conflict between traditional religious values and those of modernity. The latter issue may be increasingly significant in the coming decade due to the ongoing phenomenon of "Westernization" in South Asian countries (Renner et al., 2014).

## 5 Religion and Explanatory Models of Mental Illness in South Asian Communities

Prior to the development of psychological and biomedical models of mental illness, religious or spiritual explanations of "madness" were common in both the East and the West. According to these models, neurological and mental illnesses could be seen as the result of fate, demonic possession, black magic, curses, or even divine punishment (Brizzi et al., 2016). These models are endorsed by local faith healers and community members, leading to a cycle of repeated help-seeking outside the healthcare system (Shohel et al., 2022). Such explanatory models of mental illness are even endorsed in films or television serials (Pinto, 2016). These models can contribute significantly to the stigmatization, exclusion, and even ill-treatment of persons with mental illness, though not invariably (Ran et al., 2021). Even in the present day, an association between religiosity and negative attitudes towards mental illness and psychiatry has been documented in medical students (Al-Natour et al., 2021). However, religion is not the only source of explanatory models of mental illness in South Asian cultures. In a comparative study of Nigerian, Bangladeshi and white British people residing in the United Kingdom, respondents from Bangladesh were less likely to endorse magical explanations of depression than the Nigerian group, and were more likely to attribute this disorder to interpersonal or family problems (Lavender et al., 2006). Religious beliefs may influence the labelling of behaviour as normal or pathological, and these beliefs may interact with variables such as gender and social status in making this determination (Wilce, 1998).

Religious or supernatural explanatory models may be particularly prominent in those conditions popularly labelled as "madness"—severe mental illnesses such as schizophrenia and bipolar disorder. For example, in patients with a first episode of schizophrenia from South India, 73% believed that their illness was due to "spiritual or mystical causes", including black magic, demonic possession, *karma*, or punishment for past sins (Saravanan et al., 2007). A nearly identical result was obtained from a North Indian sample of patients with schizophrenia, in which 66% of patients endorsed one or more "supernatural" causes for their illness, and 62% reported that these beliefs were common in their community. Rural residence and a lower educational level were positively correlated with religious explanatory models (Kate et al., 2012).

Apart from severe mental illnesses, religious or magical explanatory models may be endorsed in the case of CMD or psychosomatic disorders. In a sample of 200 individuals from a rural community in South India who were presented with a case vignette of depression, 23.5% believed that the condition described was due to black magic, and 21% attributed it to evil spirits, in contrast to 39% who thought it was due to "stress" or "tension" (Hegde & Karkal, 2022). In community-dwelling rural men from another South Indian state, about of those suffering from erectile dysfunction, 8% reported that their condition was due to divine punishment for former sins (Vivekanandan et al., 2019). In a mixed sample of patients seeking help at a tertiary hospital in North India, the majority of whom had stress-related, somatoform or mood disorders, 6% endorsed supernatural explanations for their illness (Mishra et al., 2011). In caregivers of children with attention-deficit/hyperactivity disorder (ADHD), 18% endorsed a religious explanatory model, stating that their child's illness was "fate" or "God's will" (Wilcox et al., 2007).

There is little research on the extent to which religious explanatory models contribute to stigmatization or other adverse outcomes, such as physical abuse, in persons with mental illness. In a survey of city dwellers from India, neither religious affiliation nor strength of religious belief were associated with levels of perceived stigma against the mentally ill (Böge et al., 2018), and in another study involving inhabitants of two Indian cities, religious devotion was associated with lower perceived stigma (Zieger et al., 2016). In contrast, the endorsement of supernatural explanatory models, such as black magic or divine punishment, was associated with negative attitudes towards the mentally ill in university students from Pakistan (Waqas et al., 2014).

In summary, religion does have a significant influence on explanatory models for certain mental illnesses in South Asia, and most particularly for schizophrenia. These models are endorsed by members of the community, caregivers, and even patients themselves, and may be external (e.g., black magic, evil spirits) or internal (e.g., punishment for past sins or *karma*). However, there is inconsistent evidence on the extent to which these models contribute to the stigma against the mentally ill. Religious explanatory models likely interact with other factors, such as education, culture, and the gender of the patient, to determine outcomes such as stigmatization or exclusion in South Asian countries (Maharjan & Panthee, 2019; Waqas et al., 2014; Zieger et al., 2016).

In some cases, distinguishing between unusual forms of religious experience and psychopathology can pose a genuine challenge to clinicians. A historically important example of this sort, reported from India in the nineteenth century, is the case of a patient named Tajuddin who was hospitalized with a diagnosis of cannabis-induced "insanity" or "melancholia", characterized by disorganized speech and behaviour. During his stay in a mental asylum, he was reputed to have special or miraculous powers and was subsequently considered to be a "saint" or *fakir*, whose legacy within Islam continues to this day in the Indian sub-continent. The hospital where he was once admitted houses a shrine in his honour. Cases of this sort illustrate the dangers of "pathologizing" the more extreme forms of spiritual experience or ascetic behaviour, as well as the fine line between those labelled saints and "madmen" (Huddar et al., 2021).

## 6 Religion and Help-Seeking for Mental Disorders in South Asia

Help-seeking for mental disorders is significantly influenced by religious beliefs and practices in South Asian patients. A high level of stigma against mental illness, which can be associated with some religious explanatory models, can impede help-seeking. Alternatively, religious beliefs can lead individuals or their families to seek help from faith healers or through magico-religious rituals, leading to delays in care or even in a refusal to seek medical treatment (Lauber & Rössler, 2007; Rathinavel et al., 2010). However, such associations are not universal: in a study of respondents from 16 Muslim-majority countries, self-reported religiosity was associated with positive attitudes towards seeking professional help for a mental disorder (Fekih-Romdhane et al., 2023).

In a qualitative study of patients with mental illness and their caregivers from Bangladesh, help-seeking from a faith healer (*Kabiraj* or *Fakir*) was common, especially in those with lower levels of education and from rural backgrounds. It was common for these patients to consult many such healers and to seek psychiatric help only after several unsuccessful attempts at treatment (Shohel et al., 2022). Sometimes, religious or spiritual treatment may be preferentially sought even if explanatory models are not explicitly religious. Thus, in a survey of post-partum women in Afghanistan, mothers with post-partum depression attributed their illness to interpersonal or health-related factors, but were more likely to obtain a traditional protective amulet (*tawiz*) from a religious leader than to seek psychiatric care (Newbrander et al., 2014).

A useful way of examining the influence of religion on help-seeking in mental disorders is by studying the pathways to care of these patients. From whom do they initially and subsequently seek help, and how many such contacts occur before they enter the mental healthcare system? In a sample of patients eventually seeking help at a general hospital psychiatry unit in North India, faith healers were the first contact in 8% of patients, as opposed to 45% for psychiatrists and 44% for other physicians. Of those who sought help from faith healers, 75% endorsed supernatural explanatory models; of those who sought help from psychiatrists, nearly 90% believed that their condition should be treated by a mental health professional (Mishra et al., 2011). In two similar surveys of psychiatric outpatients in Bangladesh, "native or religious healers" were the first form of help sought by 22–23% of patients, and faith healing was associated with a delay of around 4 to 8 months in obtaining psychiatric care. In the second of these studies, 25% of patients and caregivers endorsed religious explanatory models of their illness. Caregivers played a key role in determining whether religious or medical treatment was sought: overall, the pathway to care was determined by caregivers in 72% of cases (Giasuddin et al., 2012; Nuri et al., 2018). In a multi-centre study from Nepal, faith healers accounted for over 28% of first contacts for mental illness, but the median time to psychiatric care (around 1 month) was significantly shorter than in Bangladesh (Gupta et al., 2021). In a community survey of 16 provinces in Afghanistan, 21% of those seeking help for a mental illness consulted a local religious leader (*Imam*) or faith healer (Kovess-Masfety et al., 2022). In cross-national research involving cities in India, Bangladesh, and Nepal, faith healers were the first source of help sought for mental illness in 14–22% of patients (Hashimoto et al., 2015).

Another way of assessing the impact of religion on the utilization of mental health care is to examine the perceived barriers to its use. In a survey of respondents from Pakistan, nearly two-thirds (66%) of a sample of 3500 community dwellers reported "religious fatalism" as a barrier to seeking psychiatric care: this was the third most common perceived barrier, next to "lack of faith in psychiatric treatment" (76%) and "prior personal experience" (72%) (Husain, 2020). In a qualitative study of mothers from Pakistan experiencing post-partum depression, religious beliefs were identified as a barrier to seeking and continuing treatment (Sakina et al., 2021). In rural Indian patients with schizophrenia who had never sought treatment, religious explanatory models were cited as the reason for not seeking help by 56% of caregivers (Reddy et al., 2014). In patients with substance use disorders from Afghanistan and Bangladesh, religious prohibitions of substance use did act as a barrier to seeking substance use treatment or harm reduction services, but these were less important than factors such as treatment cost, lack of adequate services, or criminalization of substance use (Al-Ghafri et al., 2023).

The level of religious belief can influence attitudes not only towards the causes of mental illness but also towards psychiatric medication or treatment in general, and this can serve as a further barrier to professional help-seeking, even if faith healing is not formally sought. In a survey of the general population from five large Indian cities, self-reported "strong religious beliefs" were associated with more negative attitudes towards psychiatrists and psychiatric treatment. In this sample, negative attitudes were more common among Hindu and Muslim respondents than among Christians, but the latter finding should be interpreted with caution due to the small number of Christian participants (Zieger et al., 2017). Among patients with schizophrenia in a rural Indian community, 14% of treatment refusal or avoidance was due to "magico-religious beliefs" about the illness and its treatment (Kumar et al., 2016). In another study of Indian patients with schizophrenia, 47% believed that prayer could relieve their symptoms, nearly 10% believed that magico-religious rituals could cure their illness, and 25% had had such a ritual performed by their family members during their most recent episode (Kate et al., 2012).

Overall, religious treatment is the first form of care sought by over 20% of South Asian patients with mental illness. There is some evidence of an association between religious explanatory models and recourse to faith healing, but this is not invariable. Certain religious beliefs can act as a barrier to care, both in general and for specific conditions such as schizophrenia or substance use disorders. These associations may be influenced by factors such as education, individual religiosity, mental health literacy, and the ease of access to mental health services (Amarasuriya et al., 2015; Usman Shah et al., 2018).

## 7 Religion and the Course and Outcome of Mental Illness in South Asian Patients

Given the evidence for a protective effect of R/S against some forms of mental illness in South Asia, it is natural to postulate a similar beneficial effect of religious belief or practice on their course and outcome. There is some evidence of this from studies outside Asia: in Brazilian patients being treated for bipolar disorder, religiosity was associated with better QoL over a period of two years (Stroppa et al., 2018). Similarly, positive religious coping, involving belief in a God who is concerned with the individual's well-being, was associated with better response to pharmacotherapy in patients from the United States hospitalized for major depression (Murphy & Fitchett, 2009). On the other hand, effects in the opposite direction can also occur: in the first of these studies, negative religious coping was associated with more depressive symptoms.

Research from India suggests that R/S has beneficial effects on several course and outcome variables in schizophrenia. In North Indian patients with chronic schizophrenia, spirituality was significantly associated with better QoL in the domains of psychological well-being, social relationships, and independent functioning (Shah et al., 2011). Measures of religiosity and positive religious coping were also associated with better adherence to medications in Indian patients with this disorder (Triveni et al., 2021). In a qualitative study of caregivers of patients being treated for schizophrenia, religious behaviours such as prayer, visiting religious shrines and participation in rituals were reported to have a positive effect on recovery (Gandhi & Jones, 2020).

Evidence for such an effect in other disorders is sparse. In patients from North India seeking treatment for depression, religiosity was negatively associated with suicidal ideation: however, this study purposefully selected subjects with "high" and "low" religiosity for comparison, introducing a significant risk of bias (Gupta et al., 2011). In patients with remitted bipolar disorder attending an outpatient clinic in a tertiary hospital in India, 15% of patients reported that religiosity and religious explanatory models had prevented them from attempting suicide even when they experienced suicidal ideation (Grover et al., 2016). In Indian patients with opioid or alcohol dependence seeking help at an addiction treatment centre, Hindu religious affiliation was associated with a lower risk of relapse (Sau et al., 2013).

At this point in time, the evidence for a beneficial effect of religiosity in this domain is strongest for schizophrenia. More research is required in this area, both to replicate existing findings and to identify the component(s) of R/S that are most beneficial to persons with mental illness.

## 8 Religiosity in the Caregivers of Persons with Mental Illness in South Asia

In South Asia, most persons with mental illness are cared for by their family members or spouses. In patients' severe mental illnesses, the responsibility for seeking and administering treatment, and handling the patient's behavioural problems, often falls on one or two family members, who are usually parents, spouses, or children. Family caregivers in South Asian countries experience a substantial burden affecting most domains of their lives, including physical and mental health, social relationships, employment, and economic security (Cham et al., 2022). In 20–40% of caregivers, this burden is perceived to be severe. In the face of these difficulties, many caregivers have recourse to religious or spiritual beliefs and practices (Gupta et al., 2022; Walke et al., 2018). Such strategies have been found to enhance caregivers' coping abilities and acceptance of severe mental illnesses. On the other hand, many caregivers in this situation report spiritual needs or concerns that are not adequately addressed by mental health professionals (Casaleiro et al., 2022; Issac et al., 2022). Such a felt need is mirrored by a relative paucity of literature examining the links between R/S, coping and resilience in this caregiver population, both in developed countries (Baronet, 1999) and in South Asia.

Indian caregivers of patients with schizophrenia use both positive and negative religious coping methods, and negative religious coping has been associated with greater psychological distress. Interestingly, higher scores for negative and overall symptoms of schizophrenia in patients were associated with lower positive coping and higher negative coping in Indian caregivers (Rao et al., 2020). In a qualitative study of Indian caregivers of patients with schizophrenia, caregivers reported explanatory models that reflected negative religious coping, such as "evil spirits" or "the patient's *karma*"; however, they also reported that religion and spirituality were important in helping them cope and adapt to their relative's illness (Soni et al., 2024).

Two studies from India have examined religious coping in caregivers of persons with mental illness without a focus on any specific diagnosis. In the first, it was found that religious coping was the most frequently used method adopted by caregivers, followed by planning and active coping, but associations between coping methods and caregiver well-being were not examined (Walke et al., 2018). The second was a qualitative study of young adult caregivers whose parents had chronic psychiatric or medical illnesses. In this mixed sample, caregivers reported that religious belief and rituals served as a source of support, provided a sense of meaning in life, and fostered resilience (Hebbani & Srinivasan, 2016).

The importance of R/S to caregivers of children with neurodevelopmental disorders has been examined in parents from India and Pakistan. In a quantitative study of Indian parents of children with autism spectrum disorders, the majority reported that belief in a "supreme being" and attendance at religious services were important coping mechanisms. Most of these parents received high scores on a measure of resilience, but the correlation between religious coping and resilience was not assessed (Das et al., 2017). In a qualitative study of Pakistani parents of children with intellectual disability, R/S was reported to be an important source of comfort and resilience (Lakhani et al., 2024).

## 9 Religious Approaches to the Treatment of Mental Disorder in South Asian Patients

There is sufficient evidence to suggest that religion and spirituality should be addressed during the training of mental health professionals and that psychiatrists should incorporate elements of religion and spirituality into their patient assessments and management plans (Verhagen, 2010). Such a need may be particularly acute in South Asian countries, where religious values and practices play a prominent role in individual and community life (Chaudhry, 2008). In the South Asian context, two specific questions arise regarding the management of mental illness in relation to R/S:

- Is it possible for mental health professionals and faith healers/traditional healers to collaborate constructively in the management of individual patients?
- Are psychosocial treatment approaches grounded in local religious beliefs, ideas and practices feasible and effective? Do they offer advantages over "standard" forms of psychotherapy in terms of efficacy and acceptability to patients and caregivers?

Though the answer to both these questions is probably affirmative, such approaches require a careful consideration of each country or region's religious beliefs, values, customs and rituals. It should also be acknowledged that in a multi-religious or multi-cultural society (for example, India), an intervention based on one religious tradition may not be accepted by adherents of another. Even in countries with a single dominant religion (for example, Nepal or Pakistan), there may be local or regional variations in religious customs and rituals, which should be considered when designing religiously informed psychosocial interventions. In brief, when attempting to integrate religion and spirituality into psychotherapy, one size does not fit all.

### *9.1 Collaboration Between Mental Health Professionals and Traditional Healers in South Asia*

Research on the efficacy of faith healing for mental disorders in South Asian countries is limited. In a systematic review of thirty-two relevant studies examining this outcome, only three were from this region—two from India and one from Pakistan (Nortje et al., 2016). In a subsequent systematic review of qualitative research on the perceived effectiveness of faith healing for mental illness, only two of sixteen studies—both from India—were from this region (van der Watt et al., 2018). The available evidence suggests that faith healing is efficacious in reducing psychological distress and symptoms of CMD—depression and anxiety—but not in severe mental illnesses. Research from Nepal suggests that magico-religious methods of healing have positive effects on psychosocial processes such as constructing a sense of meaning, facilitating catharsis, modifying maladaptive cognitions, and making use of local beliefs regarding interpersonal relationships and illness (Pham et al., 2021a). Such findings lend credence to the idea that traditional healers could handle persons with CMD if this is their preference, while referring patients with severe mental disorders, such as schizophrenia, to community or hospital-based psychiatry services. Alternatively, faith healers could collaborate with mental health professionals both in treating CMD and in deciding which patients have more severe illnesses requiring psychiatric care.

Is there evidence from real-world settings that such approaches are feasible and effective? A theoretical analysis by Sax (2014) suggests that combined treatment may not be feasible due to ideological and systemic barriers. In contrast with this, a survey of Indian physicians found that nearly 70% were "satisfied" with faith healing for mental disorders, and 73% reported that integrating faith healing with "allopathic" medicine could reduce the stigma associated with them. Conversely, ritual healers in India have shown an increasing willingness to engage with psychological concepts: in the words of a faith healer from Kerala, "…I read our traditional books and compare them with psychology and develop my theory" (Lang, 2014) (Ramakrishnan et al., 2014). In a survey of traditional healers, community dwellers and doctors from Nepal, these stakeholders concurred on the importance of mental health literacy for traditional healers, the facilitation of referrals in both directions, and the need for open dialogue between traditional healers and mental health professionals (Pham et al., 2021b). In interviews with patients with schizophrenia, traditional healers and primary healthcare staff from Pakistan, the need to combine spiritual and medical approaches in the rehabilitation of this disorder were emphasized (Khattak et al., 2022). All these findings suggest that such collaboration is feasible both in principle and in practice.

Evidence on the implementation of such combined treatments is limited but promising. In a community-based camp for the treatment of substance use disorders, religious activities focusing on faith in God, optimism towards recovery and religious music were combined with pharmacological and group therapies and were perceived positively by patients (Chavan & Priti, 1999). In the Indian state of Gujarat, a government-sponsored pilot project has examined the efficacy and acceptability of combined psychiatric treatment and faith healing for mental disorders. Patients receiving combined treatment reported a synergy between religious practices and pharmacotherapy, easier access to treatment and good subjective outcomes. However, certain barriers to this approach were identified: (a) long-term adherence to treatment, (b) difficulty in convincing certain faith healers about the benefits of medical treatment, (c) high employee turnover, and (d) lack of infrastructure in terms of space and medication availability (Saha et al., 2021). Overall, regardless of the difficulties identified both in theory and in practice, such approaches may offer substantial benefits to patients, caregivers, and communities. More importantly, they may be a valuable mental health asset in settings where resources for psychiatric treatment are limited (Mathias et al., 2024).

## 9.2 Religious and Spiritually Informed Approaches to Psychosocial Treatment for Mental Illness in South Asia

Psychotherapeutic approaches developed in Europe or North America may not always be accepted by South Asian patients, and even therapists may encounter difficulties in applying them directly (Jacob & Krishna, 2003). A fruitful way of integrating R/S into mental health care is to incorporate concepts from traditional religious texts or belief systems, or specific religious practices, into psychological treatments such as cognitive-behavioural therapy. Experts from South Asia have suggested several ways in which this could be done, based on the coherence between specific religious and psychotherapeutic concepts. These are summarized in Table 3. Overall, the adoption of such concepts could lead to a "localization" or "Asianization" of psychiatry and clinical psychology, making them more sensitive to local beliefs and grounding them in traditional sources of wisdom (Avasthi et al., 2013).

Though rigorous, randomized controlled trials in this field have yet to be conducted on a large scale, there is already evidence that such religiously informed psychological interventions are beneficial in South Asian populations—both in healthy individuals and in those with common mental disorders. Examples of such interventions are given in Table 4.

Though results of this sort need replication, they suggest that the addition of religious or spiritual elements to psychotherapy may be beneficial both in healthy individuals exposed to psychosocial risk factors and in patients with depression or anxiety. One limitation of this research is that it is not known whether these effects are maintained over a longer follow-up period. Other such interventions are being developed and tested. These include a counselling module for Indian patients with CMD based on the *Ramayana* (Kurhade et al., 2024) and a culturally adapted form of problem-solving in Pakistani adolescents with self-harm, designed to be used in collaboration with religious leaders (Husain et al., 2022). Even where formal clinical trials are not possible, a skilled therapist may be able to include religious or spiritual practices within a psychotherapy framework. An example is the report by de Zoysa (2011) of using Buddhist mindfulness techniques in combination with CBT for the treatment of depression.

**Table 3** Conceptual overlaps between religious and psychotherapeutic concepts in South Asia

| Concept or approach | Description |
|---|---|
| Therapist-patient relationship | It can be based on the story of Lord Krishna and Arjuna in the *Bhagavad Gita* (Reddy, 2012) or on the traditional Indian relationship between the spiritual teacher (*guru*) and disciple (*chela*) (Neki, 1973). Such a relationship is collaborative, supportive, and educational |
| Self-awareness and emotional awareness | Buddhist and Hindu concepts of the self, involving non-dualistic views of mind and body, can be used to facilitate self-awareness, self-regulation, and lifestyle modification (*Jnana yoga*) (Keshavan & Bhargav, 2024; Rajagopal, 2024). Awareness of positive and negative emotions and their relationship to one's beliefs and conduct is emphasized in the *Bhagavad Gita* (Dhillon, 2023) and in the Sikh *Guru Granth Sahib* (Kalra et al., 2012) |
| Mindfulness and meditation | Buddhist teachings emphasize "non-judgmental awareness" of current thoughts and situations, as does the Hindu concept of *Dhyana* or meditation. These can aid in relaxation, anxiety reduction, and regulation of other negative affects, such as anger (Chandradasa & Kuruppuarachchi, 2019; Dhillon, 2023; Varambally & Gangadhar, 2012) |
| Narrative approaches to therapy | Narratives shape individuals' self-perception, cognition, and behaviour, and culturally derived narratives may provide a sense of meaning, identity, and purpose in life. Anecdotes from religious texts, such as the *Ramayana*, may be used to this end in specific therapeutic contexts (Jacob & Krishna, 2003) |
| Behavioural techniques | Approaches such as "mindfulness of breathing" (in Buddhism) and specific *yoga* techniques (in Hinduism) positively modulate parasympathetic activity and stress responses, and may be useful in a wide range of mental disorders characterized by autonomic and hypothalamic–pituitary–adrenal (HPA) axis dysregulation (Chandradasa & Kuruppuarachchi, 2019; Varambally & Gangadhar, 2012) |
| Psychoeducation | Some experts have seen connections between the educational role of the mental health professional and the liberating value of knowledge in Hindu (*Advaita*) philosophy (Rajagopal, 2024) |
| Mind–body medicine | The close link between mind and body, between emotions and mental and physical health, has been emphasized in Buddhist, Hindu, Islamic and Sikh traditions (e.g., "heart talk" in Islam). This acts as a corrective to Western models of mind based on Cartesian dualism, and facilitates the adoption of mind–body interventions (Hussain, 2013; Kalra et al., 2012; Varambally & Gangadhar, 2012) |
| Positive psychology | Concepts of "doing good well" (*Karma yoga*) overlap with Western positive psychology models based on flourishing and virtue. These can be used to develop resilience and positive personality traits or behaviour patterns beyond a simple "treatment" paradigm (Keshavan et al., 2024) |

**Table 4** Research on religion-based psychological interventions in South Asia

| Intervention | Target population | Description | Outcome |
|---|---|---|---|
| Islamic patterned art therapy (Hajra & Saleem, 2021) | University students ($n$ = 60) | Art therapy using an Islamic colouring book and calligraphy, 30–45 min/day for 2 weeks | Significant improvements (≈30–60%) in measures of depression, anxiety, stress, and psychological well-being. No effect of baseline self-reported religiosity (high vs. low) on intervention efficacy |
| *Surah-al-Rahman* for depression (Rafique et al., 2019) | Women hospitalized for severe major depression ($n$ = 12; 6 in treatment and control groups) | Listening to recitation of Quranic verses for 22 min, twice a day for 4 weeks (treatment); instrumental music (control). Both groups received pharmacological treatment | Significant improvement over 4 weeks in both groups, but recitation > music in terms of percentage of symptom reduction |
| "The Hero Lab" (Sundar et al., 2016) | Hindu youth in a slum ($n$ = 50, age 8–14) | Culturally appropriate activities aimed at developing "positive psychology" domains such as resilience, empathy, and gratitude, delivered by a community Hindu leader for 6 months | Significant increases (≈50–70%) in measures of life satisfaction, empathy, and sense of meaning in life |
| *Yagna* pathy (Balkrishna et al., 2024) | Persons with symptoms of common mental disorders ($n$ = 426) | Inhalation of specific fumes using a traditional fire pit (*Hawan*) along with the chanting of two traditional mantras, 45 min/day for 30 days | Significant reduction (>60%) in scores on measures of stress, anxiety, and depression |

## 10 Other Issues of Clinical or Public Health Relevance

There are certain other topics or questions regarding religion and mental health which are of specific relevance to the South Asian context, but which do not fit neatly into the categories listed above. The list given below is not meant to be exhaustive but is derived from the existing South Asian and global literature, and illustrates the depth and complexity of the relationship between religion and mental health.

- What are the biological and psychological correlates of religious and spiritual practice in relation to mental health? Can research in this field facilitate a rapprochement between religion and science, which is more conceivable in South Asian than in Western cultures? (Rosmarin et al., 2022).
- What is the relationship between R/S and temperamental or personality traits in South Asian countries? (Arora & Varma, 1982; Butt et al., 2023). Can religious beliefs or practices shape personality development, and thereby influence the risk of subsequent mental illness?
- Can religion- or spirituality-based therapies be developed for conditions other than depression and anxiety, particularly in conditions such as OCD (Besiroglu et al., 2014) and dissociative disorder (Gaw et al., 1998) where religion influences symptom presentation?
- What are the benefits of religion and spirituality in the long-term rehabilitation of persons with chronic mental disorders? Can positive results obtained in specific institutions be generalized to other South Asian communities? (Chaudhry & Mirza, 1983)
- How can mental health workers collaborate with religious leaders in reducing mental health stigma in South Asian communities, particularly where it is associated with religious, supernatural, or superstitious beliefs (Fekih-Romdhane et al., 2023)?
- How can national mental health programmes in South Asian countries draw upon religious traditions and institutions as a mental health "asset" and incorporate it into community- and hospital-based mental health initiatives? (Mathias et al., 2024)
- How can the structural and systemic barriers that hinder collaboration between mental health professionals and traditional/faith healers be surmounted in the South Asian context? (Sax, 2014)
- What role will be played by religious beliefs, traditions, and institutions in supporting mental health in the face of increasing secularization, "Westernization" and medicalization in South Asian countries? (Avasthi et al., 2013; Halliburton, 2005)
- How can R/S be used to promote positive mental health in South Asians, both at the population level (e.g., in schools and colleges) and in at-risk populations with significant religious or spiritual needs (e.g., the elderly or socioeconomically deprived)? (Housen et al., 2019; Ramakrishnan et al., 2018).

## 11 Limitations of the Available Evidence

The literature reviewed in this chapter suggests that there are several significant links, both positive and negative—though mainly the former—between R/S and mental health in South Asia. However, from an evidence-based perspective, most of the reviewed studies have important conceptual and methodological limitations, which limit the extent to which firm conclusions can be drawn from them.

Perhaps the most important limitation is methodological in nature and has to do with the fact that most of the existing research is cross-sectional. While cross-sectional studies are useful at identifying or confirming associations, they cannot tell us much about either causality or its direction. Thus, if a study finds an association between religious practices and lower levels of depression, we cannot be sure if this association is causal, due to a confounding or interacting factor, or simply a "chance" association due to statistical issues (e.g., sample sizes, failure to correct for multiple comparisons). Moreover, even if a causal relationship exists, what is its direction? Do people who pray or attend temple rituals regularly suffer from less depression, or are people likely to pray or visit temples more if they are less depressed (in view of depressive symptoms such as fatigue and lack of interest in daily activities)?

The second most important limitation, which is both conceptual and methodological, has to do with defining and operationalizing religion and spirituality for research purposes. Though a variety of instruments have been used by researchers in the field, ranging from simple yes/no questionnaires to complex psychometric instruments, there is little correspondence between them. For example, a four-item, yes–no questionnaire, as used in the Pew Research Survey of 108 nations, will yield quite different information from a scale meant to measure religious coping or spiritual intelligence. Because of this, it is difficult to compare the results of research in this area or to conduct formal meta-analyses. Moreover, such heterogeneity makes it difficult to assess which facets of religion or spirituality have benefits on specific mental health domains.

Another important limitation has to do with potential confounding factors. Are the associations between R/S and mental health in South Asian countries still significant after correcting for demographic variables (such as age, sex, or income) or other cultural variables (such as social capital or social support)? Most research in this area is observational in nature, and many reports do not include multivariate or other analyses that would permit the measurement of a specific association with religious belief or practice.

Apart from these challenges, there are also practical difficulties in conducting research in this area. Religion and spirituality are sensitive topics that are difficult to explore in the span of a brief research interview, and mental health researchers may not receive adequate training in these areas. Moreover, there can be marked cross-national variations in mental health infrastructure, funding, and manpower that influence research output. This can be appreciated by examining Fig. 2, which illustrates the approximate number of publications on R/S in relation to mental health from each South Asian country. It can be seen from this figure that the majority of relevant publications are from India, with the next substantial contribution from Pakistan, modest numbers from Afghanistan, Bangladesh, Nepal, and Sri Lanka, and few or no reports from Bhutan and the Maldives. This unequal distribution probably reflects variations in mental health funding, infrastructure, and trained personnel, and is an important limitation when attempting to generalize from country-level to regional findings. A key challenge for South Asian mental health experts and policymakers is to ensure that other countries in the region have the chance to "catch up" and generate locally relevant data on the links between R/S and mental health. This could be done through cross-national research or other forms of regional collaboration that facilitate knowledge transfer and resource sharing in this field.

## 12 Conclusions

Religion and spirituality are an integral part of the lives of South Asians, and influence their mental health irrespective of age, gender, socioeconomic status, or specific religious affiliation. Despite certain limitations of the existing literature, there is ample evidence to suggest that religious beliefs and practices can promote positive mental health, facilitate coping with adversity, protect against common mental diseases, and provide support and solace to the caregivers of persons with severe mental disorders. These benefits must be weighed against the potential harm caused by negative religious coping or by supernatural explanatory models of mental illness that increase stigmatization and hinder access to mental health care. In the South Asian context, religion and spirituality are an important resource that can potentially improve community mental health and reduce the treatment gap for common mental disorders. Leveraging this "asset" in a way that benefits all stakeholders, and that respects both the spiritual and scientific paradigms, is a vital future task for mental health practitioners, researchers, and policymakers in this region.

## References


Abbas, Q., Kanwal, U., Saeed, W., Khan, M. U., Shahzadi, M., & Faran, M. (2022). Relationship of Muslim religiosity and death anxiety with the mediating effect of optimism and depression among cancer patients in Pakistan. *Journal of Religion and Health, 61*(2), 1418–1436. https://doi.org/10.1007/s10943-021-01415-2

Abu-Raiya, H., & Pargament, K. I. (2015). Religious coping among diverse religions: Commonalities and divergences. *Psychology of Religion and Spirituality, 7*(1), 24–33. https://doi.org/10.1037/a0037652

Adhikari Baral, I., & Bhagawati, K. C. (2019). Post traumatic stress disorder and coping strategies among adult survivors of earthquake, Nepal. *BMC Psychiatry, 19*(1), 118. https://doi.org/10.1186/s12888-019-2090-y

Ahmad, A., Asim, M., Malik, N., Safdar, M. R., Sher, F., & Sohail, M. M. (2024). Between life and death: How do Muslim terminal patients in Pakistan cope with hepatitis C utilizing their beliefs and social support? *Journal of Religion and Health, 63*(5), 3455–3473. https://doi.org/10.1007/s10943-023-01828-1

Ahrens, C. E., Abeling, S., Ahmad, S., & Hinman, J. (2010). Spirituality and well-being: The relationship between religious coping and recovery from sexual assault. *Journal of Interpersonal Violence, 25*(7), 1242–1263. https://doi.org/10.1177/0886260509340533

Al-Ghafri, Q., Radcliffe, P., & Gilchrist, G. (2023). Barriers and facilitators to accessing inpatient and community substance use treatment and harm reduction services for people who use drugs in the Muslim communities: A systematic narrative review of studies on the experiences of people who receive services and service providers. *Drug and Alcohol Dependence, 244*, Article 109790. https://doi.org/10.1016/j.drugalcdep.2023.109790

Al-Natour, A., Abuhammad, S., & Al-Modallal, H. (2021). Religiosity and stigma toward patients with mental illness among undergraduate university students. *Heliyon, 7*(3), Article e06565. https://doi.org/10.1016/j.heliyon.2021.e06565

Ali, S. A., & Saleem, T. (2024). Psychological autopsies: religious and spiritual factors for suicide in cases and controls. *Frontiers in Psychiatry, 15*, 1419669. https://doi.org/10.3389/fpsyt.2024.1419669

Amarasuriya, S. D., Jorm, A. F., & Reavley, N. J. (2015). Depression literacy of undergraduates in a non-western developing context: The case of Sri Lanka. *BMC Research Notes, 8*, 593. https://doi.org/10.1186/s13104-015-1589-7

Arefin, S., Rashid, T., Bhattacharjee, M., Habib, M. D., Islam, M. A., & Rahaman, M. A. (2022). "The whole sky has broken down on me. I might die alone": A qualitative study on the lived experiences of COVID-19 positive frontline workers in Bangladesh. *Frontiers in Sociology, 7*, 1054921. https://doi.org/10.3389/fsoc.2022.1054921

Arora, M. M., & Varma, V. K. (1982). Relationship of psychoticism with certain socio-economic variables. *Indian Journal of Psychiatry, 24*(2), 164–168.

Arya, V., Page, A., Dandona, R., Vijayakumar, L., Mayer, P., & Armstrong, G. (2019). The geographic heterogeneity of suicide rates in India by religion, caste, tribe, and other backward classes. *Crisis, 40*(5), 370–374. https://doi.org/10.1027/0227-5910/a000574

Atilola, O. (2015). Level of community mental health literacy in sub-Saharan Africa: Current studies are limited in number, scope, spread, and cognizance of cultural nuances. *Nordic Journal of Psychiatry, 69*(2), 93–101. https://doi.org/10.3109/08039488.2014.947319

Avasthi, A., Kate, N., & Grover, S. (2013). Indianization of psychiatry utilizing Indian mental concepts. *Indian Journal of Psychiatry, 55*(Suppl 2), S136–S144. https://doi.org/10.4103/0019-5545.105508

Balkrishna, A., Gupta, A., Ghosh, S., & Arya, V. (2024). An application of *Yagna Pathy*: A spiritual, cost-effective, indigenous low-intensity psychological intervention to manage common mental disorders: A cross-sectional pilot study in India. *Journal of Evidence-Based Integrative Medicine, 29*, 2515690X241284280. https://doi.org/10.1177/2515690X241284280

Bandara, P., Knipe, D., Munasinghe, S., Rajapakse, T., & Page, A. (2022). Socioeconomic and geographic correlates of intimate partner violence in Sri Lanka: Analysis of the 2016 demographic and health survey. *Journal of Interpersonal Violence, 37*(21–22), NP20569–NP20601. https://doi.org/10.1177/08862605211055146

Baniya, M., Kitrungrote, L., & Damkliang, J. (2022). Prevalence, severity, and self-management of depressive mood among community-dwelling people with spinal cord injury in Nepal. *Belitung Nursing Journal, 8*(2), 101–107. https://doi.org/10.33546/bnj.1991

Banning, M., Hafeez, H., Faisal, S., Hassan, M., & Zafar, A. (2009). The impact of culture and sociological and psychological issues on Muslim patients with breast cancer in Pakistan. *Cancer Nursing, 32*(4), 317–324. https://doi.org/10.1097/NCC.0b013e31819b240f

Baronet, A. M. (1999). Factors associated with caregiver burden in mental illness: A critical review of the research literature. *Clinical Psychology Review, 19*(7), 819–841. https://doi.org/10.1016/s0272-7358(98)00076-2

Batool, S. S., & Nawaz, S. (2016). Factors affecting disability-related depression in patients with lost limbs: A mediational model. *Journal of Religion and Health, 55*(4), 1381–1393. https://doi.org/10.1007/s10943-015-0098-2

Baumann, S. E., Merante, M. M., Wiltrout, C. T., Cutlip, T., Finkel, M., Maharjan, B., Lhaki, P., & Burke, J. G. (2021). Is criminalization the answer? Perspectives of community members and police on menstrual seclusion policy in Far-West Nepal. *Health Policy and Planning, 36*(7), 1003–1012. https://doi.org/10.1093/heapol/czab032

Besiroglu, L., Karaca, S., & Keskin, I. (2014). Scrupulosity and obsessive compulsive disorder: The cognitive perspective in Islamic sources. *Journal of Religion and Health, 53*(1), 3–12. https://doi.org/10.1007/s10943-012-9588-7

Bhattacharjee, A., & Ghosh, T. (2024). Predictors of quality of life of cancer patients: A psycho-oncological study conducted at Tripura, North-East India. *Indian Journal of Cancer, 61*(1), 105–113. https://doi.org/10.4103/ijc.ijc_389_21

Bhattarai, M., Maneewat, K., & Sae-Sia, W. (2018). Psychosocial factors affecting resilience in Nepalese individuals with earthquake-related spinal cord injury: A cross-sectional study. *BMC Psychiatry, 18*(1), 60. https://doi.org/10.1186/s12888-018-1640-z

Bhatti, M. M., Siddiqi, N., Jennings, H., Afaq, S., Arsh, A., & Khan, B. A. (2024). Effectiveness, barriers, and facilitators of interventions delivered by traditional healers for the treatment of common mental disorders: A systematic review. *Transcultural Psychiatry, 61*(6), 885–904. https://doi.org/10.1177/13634615241273001

Böge, K., Zieger, A., Mungee, A., Tandon, A., Fuchs, L. M., Schomerus, G., Tam Ta, T. M., Dettling, M., Bajbouj, M., Angermeyer, M., & Hahn, E. (2018). Perceived stigmatization and discrimination of people with mental illness: A survey-based study of the general population in five metropolitan cities in India. *Indian Journal of Psychiatry, 60*(1), 24–31. https://doi.org/10.4103/psychiatry.IndianJPsychiatry_406_17

Bokharey, I. Z., Fahim, U., Tahir, K., & Shireen, Z. (2023). Addressing the elephant in the room: Understanding functional neurological symptom disorder through the lens of culture and religion. *Frontiers in Neurology, 14*, 1174364. https://doi.org/10.3389/fneur.2023.1174364

Braam, A. W., & Koenig, H. G. (2019). Religion, spirituality and depression in prospective studies: A systematic review. *Journal of Affective Disorders, 257*, 428–438. https://doi.org/10.1016/j.jad.2019.06.063

Brizzi, K., Deki, S., Tshering, L., Clark, S. J., Nirola, D. K., Patenaude, B. N., McKenzie, E. D., McLane, H. C., Cash, S. S., Dorji, C., & Mateen, F. J. (2016). Knowledge, attitudes and practices regarding epilepsy in the Kingdom of Bhutan. *International Health, 8*(4), 286–291. https://doi.org/10.1093/inthealth/ihw017

Buckner, J. D., Morris, P. E., Shepherd, J. M., & Zvolensky, M. J. (2022). Ethnic-racial identity and hazardous drinking among black drinkers: A test of the minority stress model. *Addictive Behaviors, 127*, Article 107218. https://doi.org/10.1016/j.addbeh.2021.107218

Butt, D. S., Majeed, A., Khawar, R., Asad, S., & Hussain, S. (2023). Personality, religiosity and satisfaction with life in young Muslim and Christian women in Pakistan. *Journal of Religion and Health, 62*(5), 3382–3398. https://doi.org/10.1007/s10943-023-01779-7

Cardozo, B. L., Bilukha, O. O., Crawford, C. A., Shaikh, I., Wolfe, M. I., Gerber, M. L., & Anderson, M. (2004). Mental health, social functioning, and disability in postwar Afghanistan. *JAMA, 292*(5), 575–584. https://doi.org/10.1001/jama.292.5.575

Casaleiro, T., Caldeira, S., Cardoso, D., & Apóstolo, J. (2022). Spiritual aspects of the family caregivers' experiences when caring for a community-dwelling adult with severe mental illness: A systematic review of qualitative evidence. *Journal of Psychiatric and Mental Health Nursing, 29*(2), 240–273. https://doi.org/10.1111/jpm.12816

Cham, C. Q., Ibrahim, N., Siau, C. S., Kalaman, C. R., Ho, M. C., Yahya, A. N., Visvalingam, U., Roslan, S., Abd Rahman, F. N., & Lee, K. W. (2022). Caregiver burden among caregivers of patients with mental illness: A systematic review and meta-analysis. *Healthcare (Basel, Switzerland), 10*(12), 2423. https://doi.org/10.3390/healthcare10122423

Chandradasa, M., & Champika, L. (2018). Reincarnation type presentations of children with high-functioning autism in Sri Lanka. *Explore, 14*(3), 230–233. https://doi.org/10.1016/j.explore.2017.09.011

Chandradasa, M., & Kuruppuarachchi, K. A. L. A. (2019). Confluence of western psychotherapy and religious teachings in mental healthcare of an Asian Buddhist community: Sri Lanka. *Journal of Religion and Health, 58*(5), 1471–1476. https://doi.org/10.1007/s10943-018-0674-3

Chaudhry, H. R.2008 Psychiatric care in Asia: Spirituality and religious connotations. *International Review of Psychiatry (Abingdon, England), 20*(5), 477–483. https://doi.org/10.1080/09540260802397602

Chaudhry, M. R., & Mirza, L. (1983). Fountain house, lahore—A unique experiment in cross-cultural collaboration. *Indian Journal of Psychiatry, 25*(4), 322–327.

Chauhan, S. K., & Dhar, M. (2020). Prevalence and predictors of mental health disorder among the adolescent living in the slums of Lucknow, India: A cross-sectional study. *Community Mental Health Journal, 56*(3), 383–392. https://doi.org/10.1007/s10597-019-00452-2

Chavan, B. S., & Priti, A. (1999). Treatment of alcohol and drug abuse in camp setting. *Indian Journal of Psychiatry, 41*(2), 140–144.

Chokkanathan S. (2009). Resources, stressors and psychological distress among older adults in Chennai, India. *Social Science & Medicine (1982), 68*(2), 243–250. https://doi.org/10.1016/j.socscimed.2008.10.008

Daliri, D. B., Aninanya, G. A., Laari, T. T., Abagye, N., & Afaya, A. (2024). Coping strategies used by informal family caregivers of individuals living with mental illness in the Upper East Region of Ghana: A qualitative study. *British Medical Journal Open, 14*(7), Article e084791. https://doi.org/10.1136/bmjopen-2024-084791

Darshan, S., Neki, J. S., & Mohan, D. (1981). Drug abuse in a farm community: A brief appraisal of a research work. *Drug and Alcohol Dependence, 7*(4), 347–366. https://doi.org/10.1016/0376-8716(81)90050-8

Das, S., Das, B., Nath, K., Dutta, A., Bora, P., & Hazarika, M. (2017). Impact of stress, coping, social support, and resilience of families having children with autism: A North East India-based study. *Asian Journal of Psychiatry, 28*, 133–139. https://doi.org/10.1016/j.ajp.2017.03.040

De, S., Bhatia, T., Thomas, P., Chakraborty, S., Prasad, S., Nagpal, R., Nimgaonkar, V. L., & Deshpande, S. N. (2013). Bizarre delusions: A qualitative study on Indian schizophrenia patients. *Indian Journal of Psychological Medicine, 35*(3), 268–272. https://doi.org/10.4103/0253-7176.119484

de Zoysa, P. (2011). The use of Buddhist mindfulness meditation in psychotherapy: A case report from Sri Lanka. *Transcultural Psychiatry, 48*(5), 675–683. https://doi.org/10.1177/1363461511418394

Deb, S., Thomas, S., Bose, A., & Aswathi, T. (2020). Happiness, meaning, and satisfaction in life as perceived by Indian University students and their association with spirituality. *Journal of Religion and Health, 59*(5), 2469–2485. https://doi.org/10.1007/s10943-019-00806-w

Dhillon, M. (2023). Weaving together the ancient and the contemporary: intersections of the Bhagavad Gita with modern psychology. *Pastoral Psychology*, 1–13. Advance online publication. https://doi.org/10.1007/s11089-023-01070-2

Disu, T. R., Anne, N. J., Griffiths, M. D., & Mamun, M. A. (2019). Risk factors of geriatric depression among elderly Bangladeshi people: A pilot interview study. *Asian Journal of Psychiatry, 44*, 163–169. https://doi.org/10.1016/j.ajp.2019.07.050

Dorji, N., Dunne, M. P., Seib, C., & Deb, S. (2017). Quality of life among senior citizens in Bhutan. *Asia-Pacific Journal of Public Health, 29*(1), 35–46. https://doi.org/10.1177/1010539516685609

Dua, D., Padhy, S., & Grover, S. (2021). Comparison of religiosity and spirituality in patients of depression with and without suicidal attempts. *Indian Journal of Psychiatry, 63*(3), 258–269. https://doi.org/10.4103/psychiatry.IndianJPsychiatry_246_20

Dubey, M. J., Ghosh, R., Das, G., Roy, D., Das, S., Chakraborty, A. P., Chatterjee, S., Dubey, S., & Benito-León, J. (2024). Beyond belief and practice: An exploratory literature review and discussion of the differential impact of spirituality and religiosity on mental health disorders. *Journal of Religion and Health*. https://doi.org/10.1007/s10943-024-02090-9

Eskin, M., Baydar, N., Harlak, H., Hamdan, M., Mechri, A., Isayeva, U., Abdel-Khalek, A. M., Rezaeian, M., Asad, N., El-Nayal, M., Buhairan, F. A., Noor, I. M., Khader, Y., Khan, A., Sayyari, A. A., Khader, A., Behzadi, B., Öztürk, C. Ş, Agha, H., … Khan, M. M. (2021). Cultural and interpersonal risk factors for suicide ideation and suicide attempts among Muslim college students from 11 nations. *Journal of Affective Disorders, 294*, 366–374. https://doi.org/10.1016/j.jad.2021.07.050

Fabrega, H., Jr. (1991). Psychiatric stigma in non-Western societies. *Comprehensive Psychiatry, 32*(6), 534–551. https://doi.org/10.1016/0010-440x(91)90033-9

Fatima, S., Arshad, S., Farooq, Z., & Sharif, S. (2024). "Religious coping fosters mental health": Does psychological capital enable Pakistani engineers to translate religious coping into mental wellbeing? *Journal of Religion and Health*. https://doi.org/10.1007/s10943-024-02075-8

Feder, A., Ahmad, S., Lee, E. J., Morgan, J. E., Singh, R., Smith, B. W., Southwick, S. M., & Charney, D. S. (2013). Coping and PTSD symptoms in Pakistani earthquake survivors: Purpose in life, religious coping and social support. *Journal of Affective Disorders, 147*(1–3), 156–163. https://doi.org/10.1016/j.jad.2012.10.027

Fekih-Romdhane, F., Daher-Nashif, S., Stambouli, M., Alhuwailah, A., Helmy, M., Shuwiekh, H. A. M., Mohamed Lemine, C. M. F., Radwan, E., Saquib, J., Saquib, N., Fawaz, M., Zarrouq, B., Naser, A. Y., Obeid, S., Saleh, M., Haider, S., Miloud, L., Badrasawi, M., Hamdan-Mansour, A., … Hallit, S. (2023). Mental illness stigma as a moderator in the relationship between religiosity and help-seeking attitudes among Muslims from 16 Arab countries. *BMC Public Health, 23*(1), 1671. https://doi.org/10.1186/s12889-023-16622-7

Gandhi, S., & Jones, D. (2020). Family caregivers' perspective on factors affecting recovery from schizophrenia. *East Asian Archives of Psychiatry: Official Journal of the Hong Kong College of Psychiatrists = Dong Ya jing shen ke xue zhi : Xianggang jing shen ke yi xue yuan qi kan, 30*(4), 113–119. https://doi.org/10.12809/eaap1941

Gautam, R., Saito, T., & Kai, I. (2007). Leisure and religious activity participation and mental health: Gender analysis of older adults in Nepal. *BMC Public Health, 7*, 299. https://doi.org/10.1186/1471-2458-7-299

Gaw, A. C., Ding, Q., Levine, R. E., & Gaw, H. (1998). The clinical characteristics of possession disorder among 20 Chinese patients in the Hebei province of China. *Psychiatric Services (Washington, D.C.), 49*(3), 360–365. https://doi.org/10.1176/ps.49.3.360

Ghorbani, N., Chen, Z. J., Ghafari, F., Watson, P. J., & Liu, G. (2021). Recollections of childhood sexual abuse: Complexities of religious coping and Muslim religious and psychological adjustment in Afghanistan. *Journal of Religion and Health, 60*(6), 4209–4226. https://doi.org/10.1007/s10943-021-01349-9

Giasuddin, N. A., Chowdhury, N. F., Hashimoto, N., Fujisawa, D., & Waheed, S. (2012). Pathways to psychiatric care in Bangladesh. *Social Psychiatry and Psychiatric Epidemiology, 47*(1), 129–136. https://doi.org/10.1007/s00127-010-0315-y

Goghari, V. M., & Kusi, M. (2023). An introduction to the basic elements of the caste system of India. *Frontiers in Psychology, 14*, 1210577. https://doi.org/10.3389/fpsyg.2023.1210577

Grover, S., Davuluri, T., & Chakrabarti, S. (2014). Religion, spirituality, and schizophrenia: A review. *Indian Journal of Psychological Medicine, 36*(2), 119–124. https://doi.org/10.4103/0253-7176.130962

Grover, S., Hazari, N., Aneja, J., Chakrabarti, S., & Avasthi, A. (2016). Influence of religion and supernatural beliefs on clinical manifestation and treatment practices in patients with bipolar disorder. *Nordic Journal of Psychiatry, 70*(6), 442–449. https://doi.org/10.3109/08039488.2016.1151930

Gupta, S., Avasthi, A., & Kumar, S. (2011). Relationship between religiosity and psychopathology in patients with depression. *Indian Journal of Psychiatry, 53*(4), 330–335. https://doi.org/10.4103/0019-5545.91907

Gupta, A. K., Joshi, S., Kafle, B., Thapa, R., Chapagai, M., Nepal, S., Niraula, A., Paudyal, S., Sapkota, P., Poudel, R., Gurung, B. S., Pokhrel, P., Jha, R., Pandit, S., Thapaliya, S., Shrestha, S., Volpe, U., & Sartorius, N. (2021). Pathways to mental health care in Nepal: A 14-center nationwide study. *International Journal of Mental Health Systems, 15*(1), 85. https://doi.org/10.1186/s13033-021-00509-4

Gupta, P., Bharti, P., Bathla, M., Singh, A. H., & Bhusri, L. (2022). A cross-sectional study to assess the caregiver burden and the quality of life of caregivers of the patients suffering with psychiatric illness. *Industrial Psychiatry Journal, 31*(1), 151–157. https://doi.org/10.4103/ipj.ipj_228_20

Hajra, B., & Saleem, T. (2021). The use of Islamic patterned art therapy: healing of psychological problems among university students. *Journal of Religion and Health, 60*(6), 4361–4386. https://doi.org/10.1007/s10943-021-01240-7

Halliburton, M. (2005). "Just some spirits": The erosion of spirit possession and the rise of "tension" in South India. *Medical Anthropology, 24*(2), 111–144. https://doi.org/10.1080/01459740590933849

Hanlon, C., Luitel, N. P., Kathree, T., Murhar, V., Shrivasta, S., Medhin, G., Ssebunnya, J., Fekadu, A., Shidhaye, R., Petersen, I., Jordans, M., Kigozi, F., Thornicroft, G., Patel, V., Tomlinson, M., Lund, C., Breuer, E., De Silva, M., & Prince, M. (2014). Challenges and opportunities for implementing integrated mental health care: A district level situation analysis from five low- and middle-income countries. *PLoS ONE, 9*(2), Article e88437. https://doi.org/10.1371/journal.pone.0088437

Hanwella, R., de Silva, V., Yoosuf, A., Karunaratne, S., & de Silva, P. (2012). Religious beliefs, possession states, and spirits: Three case studies from Sri Lanka. *Case Reports in Psychiatry, 2012*, Article 232740. https://doi.org/10.1155/2012/232740

Harish, T., Chawan, N., Rajkumar, R. P., & Chaturvedi, S. K. (2012). Bilateral self-enucleation in acute transient psychotic disorder: The influence of sociocultural factors on psychopathology. *Comprehensive Psychiatry, 53*(5), 576–578. https://doi.org/10.1016/j.comppsych.2011.07.001

Hashimoto, N., Fujisawa, D., Giasuddin, N. A., Kenchaiah, B. K., Narmandakh, A., Dugerragchaa, K., Tamrakar, S. M., Adhikari, S. R., & Sartorius, N. (2015). Pathways to mental health care in Bangladesh, India, Japan, Mongolia, and Nepal. *Asia-Pacific Journal of Public Health, 27*(2), NP1847–NP1857. https://doi.org/10.1177/1010539510379395

Hebbani, S., & Srinivasan, K. (2016). "I take up more responsibilities for my family's wellbeing"—A qualitative approach to the cultural aspects of resilience seen among young adults in Bengaluru, India. *Asian Journal of Psychiatry, 22*, 28–33. https://doi.org/10.1016/j.ajp.2016.04.003

Hegde, S., & Karkal, R. (2022). Explanatory models of depression in a rural community of coastal Karnataka, India: A cross-sectional survey. *Indian Journal of Psychological Medicine, 44*(4), 371–377. https://doi.org/10.1177/02537176211051001

Hollifield, M., Hewage, C., Gunawardena, C. N., Kodituwakku, P., Bopagoda, K., & Weerarathnege, K. (2008). Symptoms and coping in Sri Lanka 20–21 months after the 2004 tsunami. *The British Journal of Psychiatry: the Journal of Mental Science, 192*(1), 39–44. https://doi.org/10.1192/bjp.bp.107.038422

Housen, T., Ara, S., Shah, A., Shah, S., Lenglet, A., & Pintaldi, G. (2019). Dua Ti Dawa Ti: Understanding psychological distress in the ten districts of the Kashmir Valley and community mental health service needs. *Conflict and Health, 13*, 59. https://doi.org/10.1186/s13031-019-0243-8

Hoyt, S. F. (1912). The etymology of religion. *Journal of the American Oriental Society, 32*(2), 126–129. https://doi.org/10.2307/3087765

Huddar, A., Raja, T., Jain, S., & Singh, S. P. (2021). From schizophrenia to sainthood—Tajuddin Fakir. *Asian Journal of Psychiatry, 55*, Article 102465. https://doi.org/10.1016/j.ajp.2020.102465

Husain, N., Tofique, S., Chaudhry, I. B., Kiran, T., Taylor, P., Williams, C., Memon, R., Aggarwal, S., Alvi, M. H., Ananiadou, S., Ansari, M. A., Aseem, S., Beck, A., Alam, S., Colucci, E., Davidson, K., Edwards, S., Emsley, R., Green, J., … Chaudhry, N. (2022). Youth culturally adapted manual assisted problem solving training (YCMAP) in Pakistani adolescent with a history of self-harm: Protocol for multicentre clinical and cost-effectiveness randomised controlled trial. *British Medical Journal Open, 12*(5), Article e056301. https://doi.org/10.1136/bmjopen-2021-056301

Husain, W. (2020). Barriers in seeking psychological help: Public perception in Pakistan. *Community Mental Health Journal, 56*(1), 75–78. https://doi.org/10.1007/s10597-019-00464-y

Hussain, F. (2013). 'Heart-talk:' considering the role of the heart in therapy as evidenced in the Quran and medical research. *Journal of Religion and Health, 52*(4), 1203–1210. https://doi.org/10.1007/s10943-011-9560-y

Iqbal, S., Ahmad, R., & Ayub, N. (2012). Level of depression among adolescents of religious minorities and their dominant counterparts in Pakistan. *Journal of Child and Adolescent Mental Health, 24*(2), 163–171. https://doi.org/10.2989/17280583.2012.735506

Islam, N., Bhuiyan, A. K. M. M. R., Alam, A., Chowdhury, M. K., Biswas, J., Banik, P. C., Molla, M. M. A., Kowshik, M. M., Sarker, M., & Ahmed, N. (2023). Coping strategy among the women with metastatic breast cancer attending a palliative care unit of a tertiary care hospital of Bangladesh. *PLoS ONE, 18*(1), Article e0278620. https://doi.org/10.1371/journal.pone.0278620

Issac, A., Nayak, S. G., Yesodharan, R., & Sequira, L. (2022). Needs, challenges, and coping strategies among primary caregivers of schizophrenia patient: A systematic review & meta-synthesis. *Archives of Psychiatric Nursing, 41*, 317–332. https://doi.org/10.1016/j.apnu.2022.09.001

Jacob, K. S., & Krishna, G. S. (2003). The Ramayana and psychotherapy. *Indian Journal of Psychiatry, 45*(4), 200–204.

Jafree, S. R., Naveed, A., Ahsan, H., Burhan, S. K., Khan, M. A., Khawar, A., & Fischer, F. (2024). Mental health and quality of life in patients with chronic liver disease: A single-center structural equation model. *BMC Gastroenterology, 24*(1), 193. https://doi.org/10.1186/s12876-024-03268-x

Jibeen, T., Mahfooz, M., & Fatima, S. (2018). Spiritual transcendence and psychological adjustment: The moderating role of personality in burn patients. *Journal of Religion and Health, 57*(5), 1618–1633. https://doi.org/10.1007/s10943-017-0484-z

Kalra, G., Bhui, K. S., & Bhugra, D. (2012). Sikhism, spirituality and psychiatry. *Asian Journal of Psychiatry, 5*(4), 339–343. https://doi.org/10.1016/j.ajp.2012.08.011

Kandasamy, A., Chaturvedi, S. K., & Desai, G. (2011). Spirituality, distress, depression, anxiety, and quality of life in patients with advanced cancer. *Indian Journal of Cancer, 48*(1), 55–59. https://doi.org/10.4103/0019-509X.75828

Kar, S. K., Naskar, C., Marthoenis, M., Tomer, S., Menon, V., & Arafat, S. M. Y. (2024). Suicide and Socio-demography: An ecological study from India. *Indian Journal of Psychological Medicine*, 02537176241262696. Advance online publication. https://doi.org/10.1177/02537176241262696

Kate, N., Grover, S., Kulhara, P., & Nehra, R. (2012). Supernatural beliefs, aetiological models and help seeking behaviour in patients with schizophrenia. *Industrial Psychiatry Journal, 21*(1), 49–54. https://doi.org/10.4103/0972-6748.110951

Kendler, K. S., Liu, X. Q., Gardner, C. O., McCullough, M. E., Larson, D., & Prescott, C. A. (2003). Dimensions of religiosity and their relationship to lifetime psychiatric and substance use disorders. *The American Journal of Psychiatry, 160*(3), 496–503. https://doi.org/10.1176/appi.ajp.160.3.496

Keshavan, M. S., & Bhargav, H. (2024). Know thyself (Jnana Yoga): Psychotherapeutic insights from the east. *Asian Journal of Psychiatry, 92*, Article 103907. https://doi.org/10.1016/j.ajp.2023.103907

Keshavan, M. S., Hegde, S., & Bhargav, H. (2024). Doing good well (Karma Yoga, the path of selfless action): Psychotherapeutic lessons from the East. *Asian Journal of Psychiatry, 101*, Article 104201. https://doi.org/10.1016/j.ajp.2024.104201

Khan, K. I., Sabir, Q. U. A., Shafqat, A., & Aslam, M. (2022). Exploring the psychological and religious perspectives of cancer patients and their future financial planning: A Q-methodological approach. *BMC Palliative Care, 21*(1), 186. https://doi.org/10.1186/s12904-022-01079-z

Khan, M. M., Naqvi, H., Thaver, D., & Prince, M. (2008). Epidemiology of suicide in Pakistan: Determining rates in six cities. *Archives of Suicide Research: Official Journal of the International Academy for Suicide Research, 12*(2), 155–160. https://doi.org/10.1080/13811110701857517

Khattak, M. I., Dikomitis, L., Khan, M. F., Haq, M. U., Saeed, U., Awan, N. R., Haq, Z. U., Shepherd, T., Mallen, C. D., & Farooq, S. (2022). Patients' and healthcare professionals' perspectives on a community-based intervention for schizophrenia in Pakistan: A focus group study. *PLoS ONE, 17*(8), Article e0273286. https://doi.org/10.1371/journal.pone.0273286

Khursheed, M., & Shahnawaz, M. G. (2020). Trauma and post-traumatic growth: Spirituality and self-compassion as mediators among parents who lost their young children in a protracted conflict. *Journal of Religion and Health, 59*(5), 2623–2637. https://doi.org/10.1007/s10943-020-00980-2

Kidwai, R., Mancha, B. E., Brown, Q. L., & Eaton, W. W. (2014). The effect of spirituality and religious attendance on the relationship between psychological distress and negative life events. *Social Psychiatry and Psychiatric Epidemiology, 49*(3), 487–497. https://doi.org/10.1007/s00127-013-0723-x

Kim, S., Rifkin, S., John, S. M., & Jacob, K. S. (2013). Nature, prevalence and risk factors of alcohol use in an urban slum of Southern India. *The National Medical Journal of India, 26*(4), 203–209.

Kovess-Masfety, V., Karam, E., Keyes, K., Sabawoon, A., & Sarwari, B. A. (2022). Access to care for mental health problems in Afghanistan: A national challenge. *International Journal of Health Policy and Management, 11*(8), 1442–1450. https://doi.org/10.34172/ijhpm.2021.46

Kumar, C. N., Thirthalli, J., Suresha, K. K., Venkatesh, B. K., Kishorekumar, K. V., Arunachala, U., & Gangadhar, B. N. (2016). Reasons for schizophrenia patients remaining out of treatment: Results from a prospective study in a rural South Indian community. *Indian Journal of Psychological Medicine, 38*(2), 101–104. https://doi.org/10.4103/0253-7176.178767

Kurhade, C. S., Jagannathan, A., Varambally, S., Shivana, S., Sudhir, P., & Gangadhar, B. N. (2024). Development of a Ramayana-based counseling module for persons with common mental health disorders. *Indian Journal of Psychological Medicine*, 02537176241245073. Advance online publication. https://doi.org/10.1177/02537176241245073

Kuttichira, P. (2018). The phenomenon of family suicides: An explorative study into consecutive 32 incidents in Kerala. *Indian Journal of Psychological Medicine, 40*(2), 108–112. https://doi.org/10.4103/IJPSYM.IJPSYM_109_17

Lakhani, A., Ali, T. S., Kramer-Roy, D., & Ashraf, D. (2024). Informal social support for families with children with an intellectual disability in Karachi, Pakistan: A qualitative exploratory study design. *Heliyon, 10*(20), Article e39221. https://doi.org/10.1016/j.heliyon.2024.e39221

Lal, A., Tharyan, A., & Tharyan, P. (2020). The prevalence, determinants and the role of empathy and religious or spiritual beliefs on job stress, job satisfaction, coping, burnout, and mental health in medical and surgical faculty of a teaching hospital: A cross-sectional survey. *La Revue De Medecine Interne, 41*(4), 232–240. https://doi.org/10.1016/j.revmed.2019.12.005

Lang, C. (2014). Trick or treat? Muslim Thangals, psychologisation and pragmatic realism in northern Kerala, India. *Transcultural Psychiatry, 51*(6), 904–923. https://doi.org/10.1177/1363461514525221

Lang, M., Krátký, J., & Xygalatas, D. (2020). The role of ritual behaviour in anxiety reduction: An investigation of Marathi religious practices in Mauritius. *Philosophical Transactions of the Royal Society of London. Series B, Biological Sciences, 375*(1805), 20190431. https://doi.org/10.1098/rstb.2019.0431

Laroi, F., Luhrmann, T. M., Bell, V., Christian, W. A., Jr., Deshpande, S., Fernyhough, C., Jenkins, J., & Woods, A. (2014). Culture and hallucinations: Overview and future directions. *Schizophrenia Bulletin, 40*(S4), S213–S220. https://doi.org/10.1093/schbul/sbu012

Lauber, C., & Rössler, W. (2007). Stigma towards people with mental illness in developing countries in Asia. *International Review of Psychiatry (Abingdon, England), 19*(2), 157–178. https://doi.org/10.1080/09540260701278903

Lavender, H., Khondoker, A. H., & Jones, R. (2006). Understandings of depression: An interview study of Yoruba, Bangladeshi and White British people. *Family Practice, 23*(6), 651–658. https://doi.org/10.1093/fampra/cml043

Levin J. S. (1996). How religion influences morbidity and health: Reflections on natural history, salutogenesis and host resistance. *Social Science & Medicine (1982), 43*(5), 849–864. https://doi.org/10.1016/0277-9536(96)00150-5

Levin, J. (2003). Spiritual determinants of health and healing: An epidemiologic perspective on salutogenic mechanisms. *Alternative Therapies in Health and Medicine, 9*(6), 48–57.

MacDonald, D. A., Friedman, H. L., Brewczynski, J., Holland, D., Salagame, K. K., Mohan, K. K., Gubrij, Z. O., & Cheong, H. W. (2015). Spirituality as a scientific construct: Testing its universality across cultures and languages. *PLoS ONE, 10*(3), Article e0117701. https://doi.org/10.1371/journal.pone.0117701

Maharjan, S., & Panthee, B. (2019). Prevalence of self-stigma and its association with self-esteem among psychiatric patients in a Nepalese teaching hospital: A cross-sectional study. *BMC Psychiatry, 19*(1), 347. https://doi.org/10.1186/s12888-019-2344-8

Maslowski, J., Jansen van Rensburg, D., & Mthoko, N. (1998). A polydiagnostic approach to the differences in the symptoms of schizophrenia in different cultural and ethnic populations. *Acta Psychiatrica Scandinavica, 98*(1), 41–46. https://doi.org/10.1111/j.1600-0447.1998.tb10040.x

Mathias, K., Bunkley, N., Pillai, P., Ae-Ngibise, K. A., Kpobi, L., Taylor, D., Joag, K., Rawat, M., Hammoudeh, W., Mitwalli, S., Kagee, A., van Rensburg, A., Bemme, D., Burgess, R. A., Jain, S., Kienzler, H., & Read, U. M. (2024). Inverting the deficit model in global mental health: An examination of strengths and assets of community mental health care in Ghana, India, Occupied Palestinian territories, and South Africa. *PLOS Global Public Health, 4*(3), Article e0002575. https://doi.org/10.1371/journal.pgph.0002575

Mattoo, S. K., Gupta, N., Lobana, A., & Bedi, B. (2002). Mass family hysteria: A report from India. *Psychiatry and Clinical Neurosciences, 56*(6), 643–646. https://doi.org/10.1046/j.1440-1819.2002.01069.x

McClintock, C. H., Lau, E., & Miller, L. (2016). Phenotypic dimensions of spirituality: Implications for mental health in China, India, and the United States. *Frontiers in Psychology, 7*, 1600. https://doi.org/10.3389/fpsyg.2016.01600

McGovern, T. F., McMahon, T., Nelson, J., Bundoc-Baronia, R., Giles, C., & Schmidt, V. (2017). A descriptive study of a spirituality curriculum for general psychiatry residents. *Academic Psychiatry: the Journal of the American Association of Directors of Psychiatric Residency Training and the Association for Academic Psychiatry, 41*(4), 471–476. https://doi.org/10.1007/s40596-017-0687-3

Mehrabi, A., Naghavi, A., Afsharzada, M. E., Afsharzada, M. S., Brailovskaia, J., & Teismann, T. (2023). Trust in higher guidance and suicidality in Afghan students under the Taliban regime. *International Journal of Clinical and Health Psychology: IJCHP, 23*(4), Article 100398. https://doi.org/10.1016/j.ijchp.2023.100398

Mishra, N., Nagpal, S. S., Chadda, R. K., & Sood, M. (2011). Help-seeking behavior of patients with mental health problems visiting a tertiary care center in north India. *Indian Journal of Psychiatry, 53*(3), 234–238. https://doi.org/10.4103/0019-5545.86814

Mishra, K., Mohapatra, I., & Rout, R. N. (2020). An epidemiological study on depression among women during postpartum period in an urban slum of Bhubaneswar. *Journal of Family Medicine and Primary Care, 9*(9), 4736–4740. https://doi.org/10.4103/jfmpc.jfmpc_793_20

Mishra, J., Samanta, P., Panigrahi, A., Dash, K., Behera, M. R., & Das, R. (2023). Mental health status, coping strategies during Covid-19 pandemic among undergraduate students of healthcare profession. *International Journal of Mental Health and Addiction, 21*(1), 562–574. https://doi.org/10.1007/s11469-021-00611-1

Mohandas, E. (2008). Neurobiology of spirituality. *Mens Sana Monographs, 6*(1), 63–80. https://doi.org/10.4103/0973-1229.33001

Moreira-Almeida, A., Sharma, A., van Rensburg, B. J., Verhagen, P. J., & Cook, C. C. (2016). WPA position statement on spirituality and religion in psychiatry. *World Psychiatry: Official Journal of the World Psychiatric Association (WPA), 15*(1), 87–88. https://doi.org/10.1002/wps.20304

Mukherjee, N., Umesh, S., & Mondal, G. (2015). Dermatological manifestations resulting from 'sadhana': An acting out of delusion in a patient of schizophrenia. *Asian Journal of Psychiatry, 14*, 82–83. https://doi.org/10.1016/j.ajp.2015.02.005

Murphy, P. E., & Fitchett, G. (2009). Belief in a concerned god predicts response to treatment for adults with clinical depression. *Journal of Clinical Psychology, 65*(9), 1000–1008. https://doi.org/10.1002/jclp.20598

Nagabharana, T. K., Joseph, S., Rizwana, A., Krishna, M., Barker, M., Fall, C., Kumaran, K., & Krishnaveni, G. V. (2021). What stresses adolescents? A qualitative study on perceptions of stress, stressors and coping mechanisms among urban adolescents in India. *Wellcome Open Research, 6*, 106. https://doi.org/10.12688/wellcomeopenres.16818.1

Nandika, S. R., & Nagalakshmi, K. (2022). Spirituality as intrinsic motivational factor and health related quality of life among hospitalized male patients practicing Hinduism in India. *Industrial Psychiatry Journal, 31*(1), 120–125. https://doi.org/10.4103/ipj.ipj_222_20

Nath, K., Victor, R., & Naskar, S. (2016). An atypical and resistant case of obsessive compulsive disorder responding satisfactorily with an unusual way of exposure and response prevention therapy. *Journal of Clinical and Diagnostic Research: JCDR, 10*(3), VD03–VD04. https://doi.org/10.7860/JCDR/2016/18633.7481

Neki, J. S. (1973). Guru-chela relationship: The possibility of a therapeutic paradigm. *The American Journal of Orthopsychiatry, 43*(5), 755–766. https://doi.org/10.1111/j.1939-0025.1973.tb00847.x

Newbrander, W., Natiq, K., Shahim, S., Hamid, N., & Skena, N. B. (2014). Barriers to appropriate care for mothers and infants during the perinatal period in rural Afghanistan: A qualitative assessment. *Global Public Health, 9 Suppl 1*(Suppl 1), S93–S109. https://doi.org/10.1080/17441692.2013.827735

Niaz, U. (2004). Women's mental health in Pakistan. *World Psychiatry: Official Journal of the World Psychiatric Association (WPA), 3*(1), 60–62.

Nortje, G., Oladeji, B., Gureje, O., & Seedat, S. (2016). Effectiveness of traditional healers in treating mental disorders: A systematic review. *The Lancet Psychiatry, 3*(2), 154–170. https://doi.org/10.1016/S2215-0366(15)00515-5

Nuri, N. N., Sarker, M., Ahmed, H. U., Hossain, M. D., Beiersmann, C., & Jahn, A. (2018). Pathways to care of patients with mental health problems in Bangladesh. *International Journal of Mental Health Systems, 12*, 39. https://doi.org/10.1186/s13033-018-0218-y

Pandey, M., Thomas, B. C., SreeRekha, P., Ramdas, K., Ratheesan, K., Parameswaran, S., Mathew, B. S., & Rajan, B. (2005). Quality of life determinants in women with breast cancer undergoing treatment with curative intent. *World Journal of Surgical Oncology, 3*, 63. https://doi.org/10.1186/1477-7819-3-63

Pargament, K. I., Koenig, H. G., & Perez, L. M. (2000). The many methods of religious coping: Development and initial validation of the RCOPE. *Journal of Clinical Psychology, 56*(4), 519–543. https://doi.org/10.1002/(SICI)1097-4679(200004)56:4%3C519::AID-JCLP6%3E3.0.CO;2-1

Pargament, K. I., Smith, B. W., Koenig, H. G., & Perez, L. (1998). Patterns of positive and negative religious coping with major life stressors. *Journal for the Scientific Study of Religion, 37*(4), 710–724. https://doi.org/10.2307/1388152

Pew Research Center. (2018). *The age gap in religion around the world*. Pew Research Center, June 13, 2018. Available online at https://www.pewresearch.org/religion/2018/06/13/the-age-gap-in-religion-around-the-world/

Pham, T. V., Kaiser, B. N., Koirala, R., Maharjan, S. M., Upadhaya, N., Franz, L., & Kohrt, B. A. (2021a). Traditional healers and mental health in Nepal: A scoping review. *Culture, Medicine and Psychiatry, 45*(1), 97–140. https://doi.org/10.1007/s11013-020-09676-4

Pham, T. V., Koirala, R., & Kohrt, B. A. (2021b). Traditional and biomedical care pathways for mental well-being in rural Nepal. *International Journal of Mental Health Systems, 15*(1), 4. https://doi.org/10.1186/s13033-020-00433-z

Pinto, S. (2016). "The tools of your chants and spells": Stories of madwomen and Indian practical healing. *Medical Anthropology, 35*(3), 263–277. https://doi.org/10.1080/01459740.2015.1081902

Poudel, A. (2020). Role of spirituality in mental health in Nepal. *JNMA: Journal of the Nepal Medical Association, 58*(226), 439–441. https://doi.org/10.31729/jnma.5110

Prior, M., Virasinghe, S., & Smart, D. (2005). Behavioural problems in Sri Lankan schoolchildren: Associations with socio-economic status, age, gender, academic progress, ethnicity and religion. *Social Psychiatry and Psychiatric Epidemiology, 40*(8), 654–662. https://doi.org/10.1007/s00127-005-0942-x

Rafique, R., Anjum, A., & Raheem, S. S. (2019). Efficacy of Surah Al-Rehman in managing depression in Muslim women. *Journal of Religion and Health, 58*(2), 516–526. https://doi.org/10.1007/s10943-017-0492-z

Rahman, R., Mariam, L., Su, R., Malhotra, C., & Ozdemir, S. (2024). Quality of life and its predictors among patients with metastatic cancer in Bangladesh: The approach survey. *BMC Palliative Care, 23*(1), 2. https://doi.org/10.1186/s12904-023-01301-6

Rajagopal, S. (2024). The spiritual philosophy of *Advaita*: Basic concepts and relevance to psychiatry. *Indian Journal of Psychiatry, 66*(2), 202–207. https://doi.org/10.4103/indianjpsychiatry.indianjpsychiatry_368_23

Rajan, V., Saya, G. K., Menon, V., & Raghavan, B. (2024). Prevalence of depressive symptoms and its association with religiosity and spiritual intelligence among adults in rural Puducherry, India: A community-based study. *Journal of Religion and Health*, https://doi.org/10.1007/s10943-024-02063-y. Advance online publication. https://doi.org/10.1007/s10943-024-02063-y

Rajkumar, A. P., Premkumar, T. S., & Tharyan, P. (2008). Coping with the Asian tsunami: Perspectives from Tamil Nadu, India on the determinants of resilience in the face of adversity. *Social Science & Medicine (1982), 67*(5), 844–853. https://doi.org/10.1016/j.socscimed.2008.05.014

Rakesh, K., Arvind, S., Dutt, B. P., Mamta, B., Bhavneesh, S., Kavita, M., Navneet, K., Shrutika, G., Priyanka, B., Arun, K., Harkamal, K., & Jagdeep, K. (2021). The role of religiosity and guilt in symptomatology and outcome of obsessive compulsive disorder. *Psychopharmacology Bulletin, 51*(3), 38–49.

Ramakrishna, S. K., Vranda, M. N., Sharma, M. K., Majhi, G., Gunasekaren, D., & Cicil, R. V. (2023). A retrospective study of life skills promotes healthy Internet use among adolescents. *Journal of Family Medicine and Primary Care, 12*(10), 2307–2312. https://doi.org/10.4103/jfmpc.jfmpc_279_23

Ramakrishnan, P., Rane, A., Dias, A., Bhat, J., Shukla, A., Lakshmi, S., Ansari, B. K., Ramaswamy, R. S., Reddy, R. A., Tribulato, A., Agarwal, A. K., SatyaPrasad, N., Mushtaq, A., Rao, P. H., Murthy, P., & Koenig, H. G. (2014). Indian health care professionals' attitude towards spiritual healing and its role in alleviating stigma of psychiatric services. *Journal of Religion and Health, 53*(6), 1800–1814. https://doi.org/10.1007/s10943-014-9822-6

Ramakrishnan, P., Baccari, A., Ramachandran, U., Ahmed, S. F., & Koenig, H. G. (2018). Teachers' and parents' perspectives on a curricular subject of "religion and spirituality" for Indian schools: A pilot study toward school mental health program. *Journal of Religion and Health, 57*(4), 1330–1349. https://doi.org/10.1007/s10943-017-0474-1

Ran, M. S., Hall, B. J., Su, T. T., Prawira, B., Breth-Petersen, M., Li, X. H., & Zhang, T. M. (2021). Stigma of mental illness and cultural factors in Pacific Rim region: A systematic review. *BMC Psychiatry, 21*(1), 8. https://doi.org/10.1186/s12888-020-02991-5

Rao, P., Grover, S., & Chakrabarti, S. (2020). Coping with caregiving stress among caregivers of patients with schizophrenia. *Asian Journal of Psychiatry, 54*, Article 102219. https://doi.org/10.1016/j.ajp.2020.102219

Rasic, D. T., Belik, S. L., Elias, B., Katz, L. Y., Enns, M., Sareen, J., & Swampy Cree Suicide Prevention Team. (2009). Spirituality, religion and suicidal behavior in a nationally representative sample. *Journal of Affective Disorders, 114*(1–3), 32–40. https://doi.org/10.1016/j.jad.2008.08.007

Rathinavel, I., Prashanth, N. R., Kasthuri, P., Kumar, C. N., & Chandrashekar, H. (2010). Why do mentally ill patients seek religious places for treatment? *Indian Journal of Psychiatry, 52*(3), 280–281. https://doi.org/10.4103/0019-5545.71002

Rathod, S. D., Luitel, N. P., & Jordans, M. J. D. (2018). Prevalence and correlates of alcohol use in a central Nepal district: Secondary analysis of a population-based cross-sectional study. *Global Mental Health (Cambridge, England), 5*, Article e37. https://doi.org/10.1017/gmh.2018.28

Reddy, M. S. (2012). Psychotherapy—Insights from Bhagavad Gita. *Indian Journal of Psychological Medicine, 34*(1), 100–104.

Reddy, S. K., Thirthalli, J., Channaveerachari, N. K., Reddy, K. N., Ramareddy, R. N., Rawat, V. S., Narayana, M., Ramkrishna, J., & Gangadhar, B. N. (2014). Factors influencing access to

psychiatric treatment in persons with schizophrenia: A qualitative study in a rural community. *Indian Journal of Psychiatry, 56*(1), 54–60. https://doi.org/10.4103/0019-5545.124714
Renner, W., Ramalingam, P., & Pirta, R. S. (2014). Moral universals, ancient culture and Indian youth: Part II—Facing the challenge of Westernization. *Journal of the Indian Academy of Applied Psychology, 40*(1), 9–19.
Rentala, S., Nayak, R. B., Patil, S. D., Hegde, G. S., & Aladakatti, R. (2019). Academic stress among Indian adolescent girls. *Journal of Education and Health Promotion, 8*, 158. https://doi.org/10.4103/jehp.jehp_116_19
Riaz, B. K., Islam, M. Z., Ahmed, H. U., Akhtar, K., Haque, A., Amin, K. M. B., Mahmood, F., Refat, M. N. H., & Islam, F. (2023). Post-traumatic stress disorders and coping strategies of health professionals during COVID-19 pandemic in Bangladesh: Findings of a countrywide cross-sectional study. *The Lancet Regional Health. Southeast Asia, 11*, Article 100131. https://doi.org/10.1016/j.lansea.2022.100131
Rim, J. I., Ojeda, J. C., Svob, C., Kayser, J., Drews, E., Kim, Y., Tenke, C. E., Skipper, J., & Weissman, M. M. (2019). Current understanding of religion, spirituality, and their neurobiological correlates. *Harvard Review of Psychiatry, 27*(5), 303–316. https://doi.org/10.1097/HRP.0000000000000232
Rosmarin, D. H., Kaufman, C. C., Ford, S. F., Keshava, P., Drury, M., Minns, S., Marmarosh, C., Chowdhury, A., & Sacchet, M. D. (2022). The neuroscience of spirituality, religion, and mental health: A systematic review and synthesis. *Journal of Psychiatric Research, 156*, 100–113. https://doi.org/10.1016/j.jpsychires.2022.10.003
Saha, S., Chauhan, A., Hamlai, M., Saiyad, V., Makwana, S., Shah, K., & Pandya, A. (2021). Unique collaboration of modern medicine and traditional faith-healing for the treatment of mental illness: Best practice from Gujarat. *Journal of Family Medicine and Primary Care, 10*(1), 521–526. https://doi.org/10.4103/jfmpc.jfmpc_979_19
Sakina, R., Chaudhry, A. G., & Khan, S. E. (2021). An exploration of illness narratives of mothers with maternal depression in semi-urban areas. *The Psychiatric Quarterly, 92*(1), 147–159. https://doi.org/10.1007/s11126-020-09781-y
Saleem, S., & Saleem, T. (2017). Role of religiosity in psychological well-being among medical and non-medical students. *Journal of Religion and Health, 56*(4), 1180–1190. https://doi.org/10.1007/s10943-016-0341-5
Saleem, M., Bakar, A., Durrani, A. K., & Manzoor, Z. (2021). Impact of perceived severity of COVID-19 (SARS-COV-2) on mental health of university students of Pakistan: The mediating role of Muslim religiosity. *Frontiers in Psychiatry, 12*, Article 560059. https://doi.org/10.3389/fpsyt.2021.560059
Saravanakumar, P., Muhammad, T., & Srivastava, S. (2022). Cross-sectional associations of personal efforts and beliefs and depressive symptoms among older adults in India. *Scientific Reports, 12*(1), 13194. https://doi.org/10.1038/s41598-022-17578-1
Saravanan, B., Jacob, K. S., Johnson, S., Prince, M., Bhugra, D., & David, A. S. (2007). Belief models in first episode schizophrenia in South India. *Social Psychiatry and Psychiatric Epidemiology, 42*(6), 446–451. https://doi.org/10.1007/s00127-007-0186-z
Sarkar, A., Roy, D., & Nongpiur, A. (2019). A population-based study on tobacco consumption in urban slums: Its prevalence, pattern, and determinants. *Journal of Family Medicine and Primary Care, 8*(3), 892–898. https://doi.org/10.4103/jfmpc.jfmpc_42_19
Sau, M., Mukherjee, A., Manna, N., & Sanyal, S. (2013). Sociodemographic and substance use correlates of repeated relapse among patients presenting for relapse treatment at an addiction treatment center in Kolkata, India. *African Health Sciences, 13*(3), 791–799. https://doi.org/10.4314/ahs.v13i3.39
Sax, W. (2014). Ritual healing and mental health in India. *Transcultural Psychiatry, 51*(6), 829–849. https://doi.org/10.1177/1363461514524472
Scholte, W. F., Olff, M., Ventevogel, P., de Vries, G. J., Jansveld, E., Cardozo, B. L., & Crawford, C. A. (2004). Mental health symptoms following war and repression in eastern Afghanistan. *JAMA, 292*(5), 585–593. https://doi.org/10.1001/jama.292.5.585

Seino, K., Takano, T., Mashal, T., Hemat, S., & Nakamura, K. (2008). Prevalence of and factors influencing posttraumatic stress disorder among mothers of children under five in Kabul, Afghanistan, after decades of armed conflicts. *Health and Quality of Life Outcomes, 6*, 29. https://doi.org/10.1186/1477-7525-6-29

Shah, R., Kulhara, P., Grover, S., Kumar, S., Malhotra, R., & Tyagi, S. (2011). Contribution of spirituality to quality of life in patients with residual schizophrenia. *Psychiatry Research, 190*(2–3), 200–205. https://doi.org/10.1016/j.psychres.2011.07.034

Sharma, A., McCall-Hosenfeld, J. S., & Cuffee, Y. (2022). Systematic review of menstrual health and hygiene in Nepal employing a social ecological model. *Reproductive Health, 19*(1), 154. https://doi.org/10.1186/s12978-022-01456-0

Sharma, K. K., Meena, P. S., Jhilowa, C. S., Jhanwar, S., Rohilla, J., Tak, P., & Jain, M. (2021). A study comparing depression, anxiety, and coping styles between high school students attending and not attending coaching class for medical entrance examination. *Journal of Education and Health Promotion, 10*, 283. https://doi.org/10.4103/jehp.jehp_1281_20

Sherchand, O., Sapkota, N., Chaudhari, R. K., Khan, S. A., Baranwal, J. K., Pokhrel, T., Das, B. K. L., & Lamsal, M. (2018). Association between vitamin D deficiency and depression in Nepalese population. *Psychiatry Research, 267*, 266–271. https://doi.org/10.1016/j.psychres.2018.06.018

Shohel, T. A., Nasrin, N., Farjana, F., Shovo, T. E., Asha, A. R., Heme, M. A., Islam, A., Paul, P., & Hossain, M. T. (2022). 'He was a brilliant student but became mad like his grandfather': An exploratory investigation on the social perception and stigma against individuals living with mental health problems in Bangladesh. *BMC Psychiatry, 22*(1), 702. https://doi.org/10.1186/s12888-022-04359-3

Siddik, M. A. B., Hasan, M. N., Mahmud, A., Munmun, M. S., Milad, M. H., Ali, A., Ahmed, Z., & Uddin, M. J. (2023). Prevalence of depression and its associated factors among undergraduate admission candidates in Bangladesh: A nation-wide cross-sectional study. *PLoS ONE, 18*(11), Article e0295143. https://doi.org/10.1371/journal.pone.0295143

Singh, G., Ranjan, A., Agarwal, N., & Kumar, P. (2021). Assessment of magnitude and predictors of postpartum depression among mothers attending immunization clinics in Bihar, India. *Journal of Family Medicine and Primary Care, 10*(1), 312–320. https://doi.org/10.4103/jfmpc.jfmpc_1676_20

Sithey, G., Li, M., Wen, L. M., Kelly, P. J., & Clarke, K. (2018). Socioeconomic, religious, spiritual and health factors associated with symptoms of common mental disorders: A cross-sectional secondary analysis of data from Bhutan's Gross National Happiness Study, 2015. *British Medical Journal Open, 8*(2), Article e018202. https://doi.org/10.1136/bmjopen-2017-018202

Soni, A., Kumar, R., & Das, A. (2024). Experiences of the family caregivers of persons with schizophrenia in north Indian region: A qualitative inquiry. *Archives of Psychiatric Nursing, 51*, 17–24. https://doi.org/10.1016/j.apnu.2024.05.005

Srivastava, S., Purkayastha, N., Chaurasia, H., & Muhammad, T. (2021). Socioeconomic inequality in psychological distress among older adults in India: A decomposition analysis. *BMC Psychiatry, 21*(1), 179. https://doi.org/10.1186/s12888-021-03192-4

Stompe, T., Ortwein-Swoboda, G., Chaudhry, H. R., Friedmann, A., Wenzel, T., & Schanda, H. (2001). Guilt and depression: A cross-cultural comparative study. *Psychopathology, 34*(6), 289–298. https://doi.org/10.1159/000049327

Stroppa, A., Colugnati, F. A., Koenig, H. G., & Moreira-Almeida, A. (2018). Religiosity, depression, and quality of life in bipolar disorder: A two-year prospective study. *Revista brasileira de psiquiatria (Sao Paulo, Brazil: 1999), 40*(3), 238–243. https://doi.org/10.1590/1516-4446-2017-2365

Suchandra, H. H., Bojappen, N., Rajmohan, P., Phurailatpam, S., Murali, L. P., Salam Ok, A., Pahuja, E., Bhargav, H., Mehta, U. M., Manjunatha, N., & Thirthalli, J. (2021). Kundalini-like experience as psychopathology: A case series and brief review. *Complementary Therapies in Clinical Practice, 42*, Article 101285. https://doi.org/10.1016/j.ctcp.2020.101285

Suhail, K. (2003). Phenomenology of delusions in Pakistani patients: Effect of gender and social class. *Psychopathology, 36*(4), 195–199. https://doi.org/10.1159/000072789

Suhail, K., & Cochrane, R. (2002). Effect of culture and environment on the phenomenology of delusions and hallucinations. *International Journal of Social Psychiatry, 48*(2), 126–138. https://doi.org/10.1177/002076402128783181
Sundar, S., Qureshi, A., & Galiatsatos, P. (2016). A positive psychology intervention in a Hindu community: The pilot study of the hero lab curriculum. *Journal of Religion and Health, 55*(6), 2189–2198. https://doi.org/10.1007/s10943-016-0289-5
Thimmaiah, R., Poreddi, V., Ramu, R., Selvi, S., & Math, S. B. (2016). Influence of religion on attitude towards suicide: An Indian perspective. *Journal of Religion and Health, 55*(6), 2039–2052. https://doi.org/10.1007/s10943-016-0213-z
Triveni, D., Grover, S., & Chakrabarti, S. (2021). Does religiosity in persons with schizophrenia influence medication adherence. *Indian Journal of Psychiatry, 63*(3), 228–232. https://doi.org/10.4103/psychiatry.IndianJPsychiatry_413_20
Uddin, M. A., Soivong, P., Lasuka, D., & Juntasopeepun, P. (2017). Factors related to quality of life among older adults in Bangladesh: A cross sectional survey. *Nursing & Health Sciences, 19*(4), 518–524. https://doi.org/10.1111/nhs.12385
Usman Shah, H. B., Atif, I., Nabeel, M., Qureshi, H., Sadiq, S. M., Ahmed, W., Raheem, A., & Bukhari, H. (2018). Perceptions about treatment of psychiatric disorders by faith healers/psychiatrists among general public of urban and rural areas of Rawalpindi District. *Journal of Ayub Medical College, Abbottabad: JAMC, 30*(2), 223–228.
Utyasheva, L., Robertson, G., & Sharma, J. R. (2022). Perception of the criminality of attempted suicide in Nepal and its impact on suicide reporting. *International Journal of Law and Psychiatry, 83*, Article 101796. https://doi.org/10.1016/j.ijlp.2022.101796
van der Watt, A. S. J., van de Water, T., Nortje, G., Oladeji, B. D., Seedat, S., Gureje, O., & Partnership for Mental Health Development in Sub-Saharan Africa (PaM-D) Research Team. (2018). The perceived effectiveness of traditional and faith healing in the treatment of mental illness: A systematic review of qualitative studies. *Social Psychiatry and Psychiatric Epidemiology, 53*(6), 555–566. https://doi.org/10.1007/s00127-018-1519-9
VanderWeele, T. J., & Ouyang, S. T. (2025). Religion and mental health: Is the relationship causal? *Journal of Religion and Health*. https://doi.org/10.1007/s10943-025-02266-x
Varambally, S., & Gangadhar, B. N. (2012). Yoga: A spiritual practice with therapeutic value in psychiatry. *Asian Journal of Psychiatry, 5*(2), 186–189. https://doi.org/10.1016/j.ajp.2012.05.003
Verhagen, P. J. (2010). The case for more effective relationships between psychiatry, religion and spirituality. *Current Opinion in Psychiatry, 23*(6), 550–555. https://doi.org/10.1097/YCO.0b013e32833d8b04
Vijayakumar, L., & John, S. (2018). Is Hinduism ambivalent about suicide? *The International Journal of Social Psychiatry, 64*(5), 443–449. https://doi.org/10.1177/0020764018777523
Vivekanandan, K. S., Thangadurai, P., Prasad, J., & Jacob, K. S. (2019). Sexual dysfunction among men in rural Tamil Nadu: Nature, prevalence, clinical features, and explanatory models. *Indian Journal of Psychological Medicine, 41*(1), 81–86. https://doi.org/10.4103/IJPSYM.IJPSYM_153_18
Walke, S. C., Chandrasekaran, V., & Mayya, S. S. (2018). Caregiver burden among caregivers of mentally ill individuals and their coping mechanisms. *Journal of Neurosciences in Rural Practice, 9*(2), 180–185. https://doi.org/10.4103/jnrp.jnrp_312_17
Walter, O., Kasler, J., & Routray, S. (2024). Emotional intelligence, spiritual intelligence, depression and anxiety, and satisfaction with life among emerging adults in Israel and India: The impact of gender and individualism/collectivism. *BMC Psychology, 12*(1), 332. https://doi.org/10.1186/s40359-024-01806-6
Waqas, A., Zubair, M., Ghulam, H., Wajih Ullah, M., & Zubair Tariq, M. (2014). Public stigma associated with mental illnesses in Pakistani university students: A cross sectional survey. *PeerJ, 2*, Article e698. https://doi.org/10.7717/peerj.698
Whitley, R. (2010). Atheism and mental health. *Harvard Review of Psychiatry, 18*(3), 190–194. https://doi.org/10.3109/10673221003747674

Whitwell, F. D., & Barker, M. G. (1980). 'Possession' in psychiatric patients in Britain. *The British Journal of Medical Psychology, 53*(4), 287–295. https://doi.org/10.1111/j.2044-8341.1980.tb02554.x

Wickrama, T., Wickrama, K. A. S., Banford, A., & Lambert, J. (2017). PTSD symptoms among tsunami exposed mothers in Sri Lanka: The role of disaster exposure, culturally specific coping strategies, and recovery efforts. *Anxiety, Stress, and Coping, 30*(4), 415–427. https://doi.org/10.1080/10615806.2016.1271121

Wilce, J. M., & Jr,. (1998). The pragmatics of "madness": Performance analysis of a Bangladeshi woman's "aberrant" lament. *Culture, Medicine and Psychiatry, 22*(1), 1–54. https://doi.org/10.1023/a:1005323231400

Wilcox, C. E., Washburn, R., & Patel, V. (2007). Seeking help for attention deficit hyperactivity disorder in developing countries: A study of parental explanatory models in Goa, India. *Social Science & Medicine (1982), 64*(8), 1600–1610. https://doi.org/10.1016/j.socscimed.2006.11.032

Xue, S., Arya, S., Embuldeniya, A., Narammalage, H., da Silva, T., Williams, S., & Ravindran, A. (2016). Perceived functional impairment and spirituality/religiosity as predictors of depression in a Sri Lankan spinal cord injury patient population. *Spinal Cord, 54*(12), 1158–1163. https://doi.org/10.1038/sc.2016.56

Yadav, R., Khanna, A., & Singh, D. (2017). Exploration of relationship between stress and spirituality characteristics of male and female engineering students: A comprehensive study. *Journal of Religion and Health, 56*(2), 388–399. https://doi.org/10.1007/s10943-015-0174-7

Yadav, U. N., Thapa, T. B., Mistry, S. K., Ghimire, S., Yadav, K. K., Boateng, G. O., & O'Callaghan, C. (2020). Biosocial and disease conditions are associated with good quality of life among older adults in rural eastern Nepal: Findings from a cross-sectional study. *PLoS ONE, 15*(11), Article e0242942. https://doi.org/10.1371/journal.pone.0242942

Zieger, A., Mungee, A., Schomerus, G., Ta, T. M., Dettling, M., Angermeyer, M. C., & Hahn, E. (2016). Perceived stigma of mental illness: A comparison between two metropolitan cities in India. *Indian Journal of Psychiatry, 58*(4), 432–437. https://doi.org/10.4103/0019-5545.196706

Zieger, A., Mungee, A., Schomerus, G., Ta, T. M. T., Weyers, A., Böge, K., Dettling, M., Bajbouj, M., von Lersner, U., Angermeyer, M. C., Tandon, A., & Hahn, E. (2017). Attitude toward psychiatrists and psychiatric medication: A survey from five metropolitan cities in India. *Indian Journal of Psychiatry, 59*(3), 341–346. https://doi.org/10.4103/psychiatry.IndianJPsychiatry_190_17

Zukerman, G., & Korn, L. (2014). Post-traumatic stress and world assumptions: The effects of religious coping. *Journal of Religion and Health, 53*(6), 1676–1690. https://doi.org/10.1007/s10943-013-9755-5

# Chapter 15
# Regional Conflict and Mental Health in South Asia

**Sheikh Shoib, Tushar Kanti Bhadra, and Fahimeh Saeed**

**Abstract** This chapter focuses on the profound impact of regional conflicts on mental health within South Asia, a region marred by decades of strife in countries like Afghanistan, Bangladesh, India, and Sri Lanka. These conflicts have led to a high prevalence of mental health disorders such as post-traumatic stress disorder (PTSD), depression, and substance abuse, significantly affecting the well-being of the population. This chapter highlights the psychological and social consequences, including refugee crises, community breakdown, and intergenerational trauma, with specific risks to women, children, and ethnic/religious minorities. Cultural and systemic barriers to mental healthcare, such as stigma, inequitable resource allocation, and workforce shortages, are also discussed. While local and international initiatives have attempted to address these issues through community-based programs and partnerships, significant gaps remain. The chapter advocates for strengthening mental health structures through training, increased funding, and collaborative research. It also emphasizes the importance of peacebuilding to foster cooperation, respect, and moral courage, ultimately improving mental health outcomes in the region.

**Keywords** Regional conflict · South Asia · Mental health · PTSD · Refugee crises

S. Shoib (✉)
Department of Health Services, Srinagar, Kashmir, India
e-mail: Sheikhshoib22@gmail.com

T. K. Bhadra
Dhaka Medical College and Hospital, Dhaka, Bangladesh

F. Saeed
Psychosis Research Center, University of Social Welfare and Rehabilitation Sciences, Tehran, Iran
e-mail: Fa.saeed@uswr.ac.ir

 
S. M. Y. Arafat et al. (eds.), *Social Psychiatry in South Asia*, South Asian Perspectives in Mental Health and Psychology , https://doi.org/10.1007/978-981-96-8078-8_15

## 1 Introduction

South Asia has been marred by several regional conflicts for decades. Sri Lanka saw large anti-Tamil riots in the late 1950s (followed by more in the late 1970s and 1980s) and brutal insurgencies thereafter aimed at overthrowing the regimes. The ethnic conflict between the Sinhalese and Tamils in May 2009 killed over 100,000 people (Riaz et al., 2019). Afghanistan, which is located on the periphery of South Asia, is a prime example of longstanding external incursion and internal conflict. Kashmir has been a source of strife since 1947, with multiple crises and wars between India and Pakistan. Bangladesh also witnessed a violent war. It gained its independence after 9-month war with Pakistan (Paul, 2010). Bangladesh also witnessed Rohingya refugee crisis.

Regional conflicts have long term disastrous effects on mental health and well-being of nations. According to WHO, mean comorbidity adjusted age standardized point prevalence was recorded as 13% for mild forms of depression, anxiety and post-traumatic stress disorder (PTSD) and 4% for moderate forms in conflict ridden population (Charlson et al., 2019). For South Asian nations which had undergone brutal armed dispute, mental health problem is a burning issue for them. This chapter aims to give some perspectives regarding impact of regional conflicts on mental health in South Asia and propose additional interventions.

## 2 Historical Context of Conflicts

South Asia comprises 8 countries: Sri Lanka, India, Afghanistan, Pakistan, Bangladesh, Nepal, Maldives, and Bhutan. Sri Lanka experienced a three decade long conflict. Violent part of this dispute started in early 1980s when the Sinhalese political elite tried to marginalize the Tamil minority and deny them equal citizenship rights, and the Tamil minority started to seek more power sharing. Ultimately, the Liberation Tigers of Tamil Eelam (LTTE) were formed in 1983, which started an insurgency in the northeast. The Sinhalese then started military repression. In April 2009, the LTTE was defeated. The primary causes of this conflict were Sri Lanka's failure to meet the Tamil minority's political and economic demands (Paul, 2010).

Kashmir is a disputed region between India, Pakistan, and China. The Kashmir conflict dates to 1947. India and Pakistan fought their first war over Kashmir in 1947–1948. A ceasefire was reached on January 1, 1949, India controlling 65% of the land and Pakistan controlling the rest. War broke out again in 1965, but the truce was negotiated that September. The status quo was mostly preserved until 1989, when insurgency broke out there (A Brief History of the Kashmir Conflict, 2001). Since 1989, unrest in Indian-controlled Kashmir has claimed tens of thousands of lives. In 1999, Kargil conflict broke out. The Indian government revoked Kashmir's seven-decade-old special autonomy article 370 on August 4, 2019. Prior to the announcements, tens of thousands of additional Indian troops were stationed in the area and a lockdown was imposed (Kashmir Conflict Since Partition, 2021).

Last 50 years of Afghanistan include the Soviet invasion in 1979, a ten-year savage struggle with US- and Pakistani-supported mujahidin, return of Taliban in 1996, U.S. led war which saw Taliban's ouster and longstanding war since 2002 between allies and Taliban that ended on 2021 (Paul, 2010).

In 1947, Pakistan was formed as a single sovereign state after splitting of India. But soon disparities and divisions begin to appear between western and eastern part of Pakistan. The non-Bengali ruling class of West Pakistan posed a threat to Bengali language and culture. In 1970, the Awami League got an overwhelming victory in the first free election of Pakistan, which was undermined by the West Pakistan leadership. Instead, they launched a military campaign throughout East Pakistan, which started the liberation war, and Bangladesh gained independence on December 16, 1971. This nine-months-long war has seen massacres, rapes, tortures, forced displacements (Totten & Parsons, 2013). The Rohingya's predicament has existed for two centuries. Due to anti-Rohingya military campaign, the Rohingya have been continuously fleeing to safer neighbouring countries, where they now live as stateless refugees (Milton et al., 2017). In Bangladesh, Protests against job quotas began in July 2024 and swiftly spread, with demands for an end to the ruling government. According to reports, the July violence and retaliatory violence claimed the lives of about 1000 individuals, including more than 100 children (Human Rights Watch, 2024).

## *2.1 Case Studies*

### 2.1.1 Case Study 1

Security worries are among the prominent issues in the minds of those living in Kashmir. Thousands have become widows and orphans, and thousands have lost their lives. Many people got disappeared and massive property destruction was done. Mental health in Kashmir was ignored for a long time (Shoib & Arafat, 2020). Due to ongoing conflict, there has been rise in psychiatric illnesses. Torture, beatings, rape, and threats to one's life act as stressors in this conflict. Among young people, suicide rate and substance abuse in Kashmir is rising. There is a shortage of mental health staff. The tertiary level is severely strained by the primary and secondary level service shortages (Shoib, Chandradasa, et al., 2021; Shoib, Islam, et al., 2021).

### 2.1.2 Case Study 2

The three decade long civil war in Sri Lanka is the most brutal internal conflict which has occurred in the country. This civil war took heavy toll on mental health (Dissanayake et al., 2023).After war, Sri Lanka experienced tough job of rebuilding nation. As health structures were damaged, providing health care service to all was not easy. Apart from that, lack of budget worsens the problem in mental health care delivery system.

# 3 Psychological and Social Impact of Conflict

## 3.1 *Social Dimensions of Conflict in South Asia*

### 3.1.1 Serious Social Crises Are Underway in the Disputed Areas

Refugee crises in Bangladesh and Pakistan: Due to long standing violence, population residing in conflict prone areas had to leave their homeland and become refugees. The worldwide refugee population is now 43.7 million by mid-2024.Without gaining peace, return of refugees to homeland becomes a difficult job (Paul, 2010). The Rohingya refugee crisis in Bangladesh has become one of the longest-lasting in the world. They have endured terrible living conditions marked by a lack of access to basic healthcare, movement restriction, violence. Cox's Bazar district is worst affected in this crisis (Milton et al., 2017). Due to the ongoing conflict in neighbouring Afghanistan during the past forty years, a large number of people have migrated from Afghanistan to Pakistan which also created a similar refugee crisis for Pakistan (Malik et al., 2019).

Breakdown of community structure: People have succeeded in creating a network of mutually beneficial relationships and duties, a dynamic equilibrium, harmony within the family and community, ritualistic practices, and life patterns. More than the external conditions, those ties and relationships give them a sense of strength and worth. This feeling of contentment is disrupted by the conflict, which is perceived as an external imposition (Somasundaram, 2010).

Intergenerational trauma: Horrific experiences of war create a chilling effect in conflict-affected populations that can be long-lasting. Trauma experienced by one generation can be transmitted to their children and thus has a bad impact on their mental health (Tarabay & Golm, 2024).

### 3.1.2 Specific Population at Risk

Women and Children: Substantial evidence persists that armed conflict has a devastating effect on women and children. It increases indirect mortality in women and children. Also, famine can occur due to these conflicts, which causes malnutrition in children. In times of war, sexual assault against women and children is more common (Bendavid et al., 2021).

Ethnic and Religious Minorities: Regional conflicts also create havoc for ethnic and religious minorities. Often, they had to leave their home and become refugees in such conflicts. Not only that they also experience genocide.

### 3.2 *Mental Health Consequences*

The mental health of people in conflict areas is at risk (Shoib, Javed et al., 2022). The most prevalent disorders are PTSD, Depression, substance use disorder, and suicidal behaviours consciously.

PTSD is a chronic impairing disorder that occurs after exposure to stressful situations. It can cause disruption in family and individual functioning (Miao et al., 2018). In 2019, 316 million adult war veterans worldwide experienced PTSD (Hoppen et al., 2021).

The most prevalent mental health consequence associated with war is depression. Many populations in armed conflicts suffer from torture, rape, abduction, displacement. All these things make them vulnerable to depression (Anbesaw et al., 2024).

Substance abuse is rampant in war torn areas. In a state of instability and weak rule of law, there is a lack of proper border control, which results in new routes of trafficking and increased access to drugs (Hanna, 2017).Violent experiences of war also increases risk of suicide in these areas.

## 4 Cultural and Systemic Barriers to Mental Health Care

South Asia faces numerous obstacles in the field of mental health, such as widespread stigma, ignorance, a paucity of resources, a significant treatment gap, and inadequate financing (Jahan et al., 2024). Ensuring and maintaining food and water security is a priority for every government during conflict. In such circumstances, policies related to promoting mental health lose their relevance (Shoib, Rathnayake, et al., 2022). High social stigma associated with mental illness has a negative impact on help-seeking behaviour. This stigma arises from myths of mental illness. As a result, people affected by mental illness face social isolation and discrimination.

South Asia suffers from health inequities. It lacks in the field of mental health due to inadequate financial support and poor infrastructure. Shortage of mental health experts is big limiting factor for developing mental health services (Trivedi et al., 2007).

In the post-war period, mental health care faced considerable limits. Post-conflict interventions were considered politically troublesome and a threat to national security. Strict restrictions on NGO operations and increased security measures hampered necessary initiatives (Salih et al., 2025).

### *4.1 Policy Changes*

Though mental health problem in South Asia is a big issue, there is a large gap remains in local and international efforts to address them. Most mental health care delivery systems remain concentrated in urban areas. Apart from that, fund shortage, lack of trained mental health experts, absence of a proper healthcare delivery system, etc. are making this problem worse (Islam & Biswas, 2015).

## 5 Strategies for Mitigation and Intervention

It is essential to investigate a wide range of solutions and interventions in order to solve the complex issues in mental health care in places that are prone to conflict (Jahan et al., 2024). In India, general hospital psychiatry departments began in the 1960s, followed by the formulation of the national mental health program in 1982. A host of other initiatives, such as the establishment of community or satellite clinics, domiciliary care programs, and training of schoolteachers, volunteers, and village leaders in early detection of mental problems, also helped energize the community programs. Non-governmental organizations (NGOs) also contributed to community mental health care. They are actively involved in mental health-related work, including rehabilitation, outreach, life skills training, providing psychological support, and building resilience around societal concerns (Thara & Padmavati, 2013).

Government and International health organizations played a significant role in improving health of the conflict affected South Asian region. For example, Sri Lankan government provided huge financial support in redeveloping health structure after war. International medical organizations, including Médecins Sans Frontières, have partnered with the government to provide mental health services, in conflict-affected areas of Pakistan (David et al., 2017).

## 6 Future Directions and Recommendations

### *6.1 Strengthening Mental Health Structures*

Training and Capacity building should be given priority as they are highly essential. Existing primary care physicians in the community are often not ready or inclined to treat the mentally ill. While training enhances their skills, they should be sufficiently motivated to take on the duty of caring for people with mental health disorders. More funding must be set aside for community-based mental health care. Telepsychiatry holds significant potential for addressing the mental health needs of underserved regions, particularly considering the inequitable distribution of mental health professionals, the challenges of reaching remote areas, and the critical need for timely intervention (Shoib, Armiya'u, et al., 2022). Special programs are needed for marginalized and vulnerable communities such as women and children, and people with disability, especially in rural areas (Thara & Padmavati, 2013).

South Asia still lags in mental health research. There is lack of research regarding the impact of regional conflicts on the mental health of the affected population and the effectiveness of targeted interventions which needs to be addressed. Psychiatric rehabilitation, major depression treatment, culturally acceptable psychotherapy, mental health service delivery, epidemiological studies, burden of care, mental disorder course and outcome, classification systems, and psychoeducation are some possible research collaboration areas in this region. Also, local and international organizations need to contribute more to the research field (Trivedi et al., 2007).

Peacebuilding promotes healthy cooperation among actors at both the local and international levels and focuses on relationships in complex contexts (Lemon & Pinet, 2018).It can be used in building honest relationships that teach people to respect the inherent worth of others and in forming a character based on humility, moral courage, and a calming presence and thus improves the mental health situation (Srof et al., 2023).

## 7 Conclusion

This chapter has tried to give an outline of the impact of longstanding conflict on mental health in South Asian people. Efforts are ongoing from both local and international communities to address this problem. But more need to be done, like ensuring long-lasting peace, building cooperation among South Asian countries in mental health research, allocating more budget in building trained mental health workers, and establishing an accessible healthcare delivery system. The international community should come forward in this regard to maintain peace in this region.

## References

A Brief History of the Kashmir Conflict. (2001). *The Telegraph*. https://www.telegraph.co.uk/news/1399992/A-brief-history-of-the-Kashmir-conflict.html

Anbesaw, T., Kassa, M. A., Yimam, W., Kassaw, A. B., Belete, M., Abera, A., Abebe, G., Yimer, N., Melkam, M., & Ayano, G. (2024). Factors associated with depression among war-affected population in Northeast, Ethiopia. *BMC Psychiatry, 24*(1), 376. https://doi.org/10.1186/s12888-024-05812-1

Bendavid, E., Boerma, T., Akseer, N., Langer, A., Malembaka, E. B., Okiro, E. A., Wise, P. H., Heft-Neal, S., Black, R. E., & Bhutta, Z. A. (2021). The effects of armed conflict on the health of women and children. *The Lancet, 397*(10273), 522–532. https://doi.org/10.1016/S0140-6736(21)00131-8

Charlson, F., van Ommeren, M., Flaxman, A., Cornett, J., Whiteford, H., & Saxena, S. (2019). New WHO prevalence estimates of mental disorders in conflict settings: A systematic review and meta-analysis. *The Lancet, 394*(10194), 240–248. https://doi.org/10.1016/S0140-6736(19)30934-1

David, S., Gazi, R., Mirzazada, M. S., Siriwardhana, C., Soofi, S., & Roy, N. (2017). Conflict in South Asia and its impact on health. *BMJ*. https://doi.org/10.1136/bmj.j1537

Dissanayake, L., Jabir, S., Shepherd, T., Helliwell, T., Selvaratnam, L., Jayaweera, K., Abeysinghe, N., Mallen, C., & Sumathipala, A. (2023). The aftermath of war; mental health, substance use and their correlates with social support and resilience among adolescents in a post-conflict region of Sri Lanka. *Child and Adolescent Psychiatry and Mental Health, 17*(1), 101. https://doi.org/10.1186/s13034-023-00648-1

Hanna, F. B. (2017). Alcohol and substance use in humanitarian and postconflict situations. *Information for Authors, 23*(3). http://www.emro.who.int/emhj-volume-23-2017/volume-23-issue-3/alcohol-and-substance-use-in-humanitarian-and-post-conflict-situations.html

Hoppen, T. H., Priebe, S., Vetter, I., & Morina, N. (2021). Global burden of post-traumatic stress disorder and major depression in countries affected by war between 1989 and 2019: A systematic review and meta-analysis. *BMJ Global Health, 6*(7), Article e006303. https://doi.org/10.1136/bmjgh-2021-006303

Human Rights Watch. (2024). Bangladesh: Events of 2024. In *World Report 2025*. https://www.hrw.org/world-report/2025/country-chapters/bangladesh

Islam, A., & Biswas, T. (2015). Mental health and the health system in Bangladesh: Situation analysis of a neglected domain. *Am J Psychiatry Neurosci, 3*(4), 57–62. https://doi.org/10.11648/j.ajpn.20150304.11

Jahan, R., Amin, R., & Arafat, S. M. Y. (2024). Practical challenges for mental health services among Rohingya refugee in Bangladesh. *Asian Journal of Psychiatry, 97*, Article 104069. https://doi.org/10.1016/j.ajp.2024.104069

Kashmir Conflict Since Partition. (2021). *The Daily Star*. https://www.thedailystar.net/world/south-asia/news/kashmir-conflict-partition-1784887

Lemon, A., & Pinet, M. (2018). Measuring unintended effects in peacebuilding: What the field of international cooperation can learn from innovative approaches shaped by complex contexts. *Evaluation and Program Planning, 68*, 253–261. https://doi.org/10.1016/j.evalprogplan.2017.09.007

Malik, M. S., Afzal, M., Farid, A., Khan, F. U., Mirza, B., & Waheed, M. T. (2019). Disease status of Afghan refugees and migrants in Pakistan. *Frontiers in Public Health, 7*, 185. https://doi.org/10.3389/fpubh.2019.00185

Miao, X.-R., Chen, Q.-B., Wei, K., Tao, K.-M., & Lu, Z.-J. (2018). Posttraumatic stress disorder: From diagnosis to prevention. *Military Medical Research, 5*(1), 32. https://doi.org/10.1186/s40779-018-0179-0

Milton, A. H., Rahman, M., Hussain, S., Jindal, C., Choudhury, S., Akter, S., Ferdousi, S., Mouly, T. A., Hall, J., & Efird, J. T. (2017). Trapped in statelessness: Rohingya refugees in Bangladesh. *International Journal of Environmental Research and Public Health, 14*(8), 942. https://doi.org/10.3390/ijerph14080942

Paul, T. V. (2010). South Asia's weak states: Understanding the regional insecurity predicament. *Stanford University Press*. https://doi.org/10.1515/9780804778534

Riaz, A., Nasreen, Z., & Zaman, F. (2019). Political violence in South Asia. *Routledge, Taylor & Francis Group*. https://doi.org/10.4324/9781351118224

Salih, M., Galappatti, A., Samarasinghe, G., Ganesan, M., & Meemaduma, R. (2025). Integration of MHPSS in post-war transitional justice: A case study of Sri Lanka's 2016 public consultations on and implementation of reconciliation mechanisms. *SSM—Mental Health, 7*, Article 100396. https://doi.org/10.1016/j.ssmmh.2025.100396

Shoib, S., & Arafat, S. M. Y. (2020). Mental health in Kashmir: Conflict to COVID-19. *Public Health, 187*, 65–66. https://doi.org/10.1016/j.puhe.2020.07.034

Shoib, S., Armiya'u, A. Y., Roza, T. H., Saeed, F., Swed, S., Arif, N., Park, C., & Chandradasa, M. (2022). Telepsychiatry for conflict-affected settings: Feasibility, ethics, barriers and prospects. *Asian Journal of Psychiatry, 75*, 103203. https://doi.org/10.1016/j.ajp.2022.103203203

Shoib, S., Chandradasa, M., Saleem, S. M., Ullah, I., & Saeed, F. (2021a). Psychiatry in Kashmir: A call for action. *The Lancet Psychiatry, 8*(12), 1031–1032. https://doi.org/10.1016/S2215-0366(21)00401-6

Shoib, S., Javed, S., Alamrawy, R. G., Nigar, A., Das, S., Saeed, F., Handuleh, J. I. M., Shellah, D., Dazhamyar, A. R., & Chandradasa, M. (2022a). Challenges in mental health and psychosocial care in conflict-affected low-and middle-income countries. *Asian Journal of Psychiatry, 67*, Article 102894. https://doi.org/10.1016/j.ajp.2021.102894

Shoib, S., Rathnayake, L., Badawy, M. M., Swed, S., Saeed, F., & Chandradasa, M. (2022b). International collaboration to address the inevitable mental health burden in Sri Lanka in the context of the economic crisis. *Asian Journal of Psychiatry, 77*, Article 103277. https://doi.org/10.1016/j.ajp.2022.103277

Shoib, S., Islam, S. M. S., Arafat, S. Y., & Hakak, S. A. (2021b). Depression and suicidal ideation among the geriatric population of Kashmir, India. *International Journal of Social Psychiatry, 67*(6), 651–655. https://doi.org/10.1177/0020764020968592

Somasundaram, D. (2010). Collective trauma in the Vanni: A qualitative inquiry into the mental health of the internally displaced due to the civil war in Sri Lanka. *International Journal of Mental Health Systems, 4*, 1–31. https://doi.org/10.1186/1752-4458-4-22

Srof, B. J., Lagerwey, M., & Liechty, J. (2023). Nurses' lived experience of peacebuilding. *Nursing Inquiry, 30*(4), Article e12591. https://doi.org/10.1111/nin.12591

Tarabay, J., & Golm, D. (2024). The transmission of intergenerational trauma and protective factors in survivors of the Lebanese civil war and their adult offspring. *International Journal of Intercultural Relations, 99*, Article 101952. https://doi.org/10.1016/j.ijintrel.2024.101952

Thara, R., & Padmavati, R. (2013). Community mental health care in South Asia. *World Psychiatry, 12*(2), 176. https://doi.org/10.1002/wps.20042

Totten, S., & Parsons, W. S. (2013). Centuries of genocide. *Essays and Eyewitness Accounts, New York-London.* https://doi.org/10.4324/9780203867815

Trivedi, J. K., Goel, D., Kallivayalil, R. A., Isaac, M., Shrestha, D. M., & Gambheera, H. C. (2007). Regional cooperation in South Asia in the field of mental health. *World Psychiatry, 6*(1), 57.

The manufacturer's authorised representative in the EU is Springer
Nature Customer Service Centre GmbH, Europaplatz 3, 69115 Heidelberg,
Germany. If you have any concerns regarding our products, please
contact ProductSafety@springernature.com

Printed and bound by CPI Group (UK) Ltd, Croydon, CR0 4YY
01/10/2026
02225921-0010